Clinical
Companion
FOR

Medical-
Surgical
Nursing

CRITICAL THINKING
FOR COLLABORATIVE CARE

Clinical Companion

FOR

IGNATAVICIUS ■ WORKMAN

Medical-Surgical Nursing

CRITICAL THINKING
FOR COLLABORATIVE CARE

Kathy A. Hausman, PhD, RN, C

Assistant Professor of Nursing
University of Maryland
Baltimore, Maryland

ELSEVIER
SAUNDERS

ELSEVIER
SAUNDERS

11830 Westline Industrial Drive
St. Louis, Missouri 63146

CLINICAL COMPANION FOR MEDICAL-SURGICAL NURSING:
CRITICAL THINKING FOR COLLABORATIVE CARE

NOTICE

Neither the Publisher nor the author assumes any responsibility for any loss
or injury and/or damage to persons or property arising out of or related to
any use of the material contained in this book. It is the responsibility of the
treating practitioner, relying on independent expertise and knowledge of
the patient, to determine the best treatment and method of application for
the patient.

Fifth Edition

ISBN-13: 978-0-7216-0551-7
ISBN-10: 0-7216-0551-6

Acquisitions Editor: Lee Henderson
Developmental Editor: Maureen Iannuzzi
Publishing Services Manager: Deborah L. Vogel
Project Manager: Katherine Hinkebein
Book Designer: Teresa McBryan

Working together to grow
libraries in developing countries

www.elsevier.com | www.bookaid.org | www.sabre.org

ELSEVIER   BOOK AID International   Sabre Foundation

Printed in the United States of America

Last digit is the print number: 9   8   7   6   5   4   3

Preface

The fifth edition of *Clinical Companion for Medical-Surgical Nursing: Critical Thinking for Collaborative Care* is a quick reference to the vital information you need for dealing with conditions commonly seen in the clinical setting. It is designed to be used as a stand-alone reference for nurses in a variety of adult health nursing areas, or as a companion to Ignatavicius and Workman's *Medical-Surgical Nursing: Critical Thinking for Collaborative Care*, Fifth Edition.

The book is divided into two parts. Part I covers special concerns of the clinical nurse, such as nursing care of the client in pain, nursing care of the client with a substance abuse problem, and perioperative nursing care. Part II, by far the larger part of the book, provides need-to-know information about the diseases and disorders that nurses in clinical practice encounter most often. Approximately 225 disorders are included, organized alphabetically for ease of use in all clinical settings. An A-to-Z thumb tab facilitates locating these disorders. Also included are highlighted Cultural, Older Adult, Women's Health, and Genetic Considerations for clients with unique needs.

The fifth edition includes nine appendixes. Appendix 1 is a quick-reference guide to head-to-toe physical assessment of the adult. Appendix 2 lists general laboratory values; Appendix 3 presents common environmental emergencies and care for each; Appendix 4 is a quick reference to biological and chemical weapons that may be seen in a terrorist attack; Appendix 5 is a list of common considerations for discharge planning (details are included in the specific disease sections); Appendix 6 summarizes electrocardiograph complexes, segments, and intervals. Appendix 7 highlights care for the client on a mechanical ventilator; Appendix 8 features Internet and other sources of additional information. Finally, Appendix 9 presents a quick-reference guide for communicating with Spanish-speaking clients.

Whether you use the *Clinical Companion* as a stand-alone reference or in conjunction with *Medical-Surgical Nursing: Critical Thinking for Collaborative Care*, we hope that it will become a trusted companion to your clinical practice.

Acknowledgments

Thank you to the remarkable professional team at Saunders. Marie Thomas provided me with the needed material to make this revision go smoothly. Maureen R. Iannuzzi, Senior Developmental Editor, Nursing Books, ensured meticulous attention to every detail as well as the smooth production of this book. Most important, I have to thank Katherine Hinkebein, Project Manager, for her patience and diligence. Without her gentle reminders, I would not have met deadlines for the production of this book. A special thanks to Lee Henderson, Editor, Nursing, who has guided the team since the first publication of the *Clinical Companion*.

Contents

APPENDIXES

PART ONE

SPECIAL NURSING CONCERNS

Nursing Care of the Client in Pain

OVERVIEW

- Pain is whatever the client says it is and exists whenever the client says it does.
- Pain is an unpleasant sensory and emotional experience associated with actual or potential tissue damage.
- Types of pain
  1. *Acute pain* results from acute injury, disease, or surgery
  2. *Chronic pain* persists or reoccurs for indefinite periods, usually more than 3 months.
     a. Chronic noncancer pain is associated with tissue injury that has healed or is not associated with cancer, such as chronic back pain or arthritis. Neuropathic pain results from some type of nerve injury.
     b. Chronic cancer pain is associated with cancer or another progressive disease such as autoimmune deficiency disease.
- *Complex regional pain syndrome (CRPS)* is a complex disorder that includes debilitating pain, atrophy, autonomic dysfunction (excessive sweating, vascular changes), and motor impairment (motor paresis).
  1. CRPS most often results from traumatic injury and commonly occurs in the feet and hands.
  2. The syndrome tends to pass through three stages:
     a. Stage 1: locally severe, burning pain, edema, vasospasm, and muscle spasm
     b. Stage 2: more severe, diffuse pain and edema, muscle atrophy, and spotty osteoporosis
     c. Stage 3: marked muscle atrophy, intractable (unrelenting) pain, severely limited mobility of the affected area, contractures, and marked diffuse osteoporosis
- Age, gender, sociocultural background, and genetics influence the client's ability to process and react to pain. These factors may put clients at risk for undertreatment.
- One's *pain threshold* or sensation of pain is the amount or degree of noxious stimulus that leads a person to interpret a sensation as painful.

- *Tolerance* is a state of adaptation in which exposure to a drug induces changes that result in a decrease in one or more of the drug's effects over time.
- *Physical dependence* is the adaptation manifested by a drug class–specific withdrawal syndrome. It can be caused by abrupt cessation, rapid dose reduction, and decreasing blood level of the drug or administration of an antagonist.
- Physical dependence occurs in everyone who takes opioids over a period of time.
- It is important to prevent physical withdrawal by slowly tapering drug dosage levels.
- *Withdrawal symptoms* include nausea, vomiting, abdominal cramping, muscle twitching, perfuse perspiration, and delirium.
- *Addiction* is a primary, chronic neurobiologic disease with genetic, psychosocial and environmental factors influencing its development and manifestations. It is manifested by impaired control over drug use, continued use despite harm, and craving.
- *Pseudoaddiction* is an iatrogenic syndrome created by the undertreatment of pain. Client behaviors include anger and escalating demands for more or different medications. Behaviors resolve when pain is adequately treated.

Cultural Considerations

- Pain behaviors are learned and influenced by beliefs.
- Cultural background influences adherence to treatments.
- Inadequate and difficult assessment, language barriers, attitudes toward pain and opioids, and access to health care may all contribute to undertreatment of pain.

Considerations for Older Adults

- Older adults are often undermedicated for pain.
- Older adults hold various beliefs about pain, including that it is something that must be lived with, that expressing pain is unacceptable or a sign of weakness, that nurses are too busy to listen to complaints of pain, that complaints of pain will result in their being labeled a "bad" client, that they might get addicted to pain medication if they take it, and that pain signifies a serious illness or impending death.

- Cognitively impaired adults are often undermedicated for pain. Assume pain is present in clients with diseases and conditions commonly associated with pain. Assess nonverbal indicators of pain.

COLLABORATIVE MANAGEMENT

Assessment

- Record the client's pain experience.
    1. Sequence of events
        a. Length of time the client has experienced pain
        b. Precipitating factors
        c. Aggravating factors
        d. Localization of pain
        e. Character and quality of pain
        f. Duration of pain
    2. Adjustments in the life of the client or family
    3. The client's beliefs about the cause of the pain and what should be done about it
- Assess for
    1. Changes in vital signs
        a. Tachycardia
        b. Blood pressure changes
    2. Diaphoresis
    3. Restlessness, apprehension
    4. Splinting or holding painful body parts while moving
    5. Location of pain
        a. Localized (confined to site of origin)
        b. Projected (along a specific nerve or nerves)
        c. Radiating (diffuse around the site of origin, not well localized)
        d. Referred (perceived in an area distant from the site of painful stimuli)
    6. Character and quality of pain
    7. Intensity of pain
    8. Pattern of pain
    9. Psychosocial factors
    10. Pain indicators in cognitively impaired or critically ill client
        a. Facial expressions
        b. Verbalizations, such as moans and groans

c. Behavioral changes
d. Body language
e. Restlessness

Interventions

DRUG THERAPY

- Refer to current drug book for information regarding adverse side effects and monitoring.
- Non-opioid analgesics
  1. Non-opioid analgesics are first-line therapy for mild to moderate pain.
  2. Aspirin can cause bleeding.
  3. Acetaminophen can cause hepatotoxicity and nephrotoxicity. Restrict the total daily intake to
     a. General population: 4000 mg per day
     b. Chronic use: 3600 mg per day
     c. Older adults: less than 2400 mg per day
  4. Teach clients to be aware of the amount of acetaminophen in their medications.
- Nonsteroidal anti-inflammatory drugs (NSAIDs)
  1. NSAIDs are effective for inflammatory type pain.
  2. NSAIDs may cause gastrointestinal (GI) disturbance.
  3. NSAIDs can prevent platelet aggregation, which results in a tendency toward bleeding or bruising.
  4. Drug-drug interactions may occur particularly with anticoagulants, oral hypoglycemics, and antihypertensives.
  5. NSAIDs may cause renal toxicity. Monitor blood urea nitrogen and creatinine.
  6. NSAIDs may cause sodium and water retention that may lead to heart failure more often in an older client.
  7. The names of over-the-counter drugs may not appear to contain NSAIDs, such as Aleve and WalProfen. Clients may unknowingly be taking several drugs that contain NSAIDs.
- Selective COX-2 inhibitors
  1. COX-2 inhibitors are a newer class of NSAIDs.
  2. COX-2 inhibitors decrease the risk of GI bleeding.
  3. Renal side effects are the same as for older NSAIDs.
- Opioid analgesics
  1. Consult an equianalgesic comparison chart when switching routes of administration of opioids.

2. Side effects include constipation, nausea and vomiting, urinary retention, pruritis, sedation, and respiratory depression.
3. Naloxone (Narcan) may be prescribed to reverse effects of respiratory depression.

- Agonists/antagonists
  1. Administering these medications after a client has been receiving opioids may cause withdrawal symptoms.
  2. Major side effects include drowsiness, nausea, hallucinations, and euphoria.
- Adjuvant analgesics relieve pain either alone or in combination with analgesics by potentiating or enhancing the effectiveness of the analgesic.
- Some antiepileptic drugs (e.g., gabapentin and topiramate) are effective in treating postherpetic neuralgia and other neuropathic pain.
  1. May cause hyponatremia, especially in older adults
- Older tricyclic antidepressants may be beneficial in treating chronic neuropathic pain.
- Oral anesthetics are useful for clients with electric shock–like pain and continuous pain.
- Other agents effective in relieving mild to moderate pain include dextromethorphan and ketamine.
- Topical medications
  1. Liocaine patch for postherpetic neuralgia
  2. EMLA and Ela-Max creams applied 45 minutes before needle sticks
  3. Local, short-acting gels and creams
- The effectiveness of drug therapy should be assessed and evaluated.
- Pain management for the client with a substance abuse problem consists of
  1. Following the principles of opioid use
  2. Use of non-opioid therapies, including medications, cutaneous stimulation techniques, heat for muscle spasm, and cognitive behavioral techniques
  3. Consultation with other health team members (substance abuse counselor, pharmacist, social worker)
- Patient-controlled analgesia (PCA) allows the client to control the dosage of analgesia received.

- PCA is achieved through the use of a PCA infusion pump, which delivers the desired amount of medication through a conventional intravenous (IV) route or through an implantable IV catheter inserted in subcutaneous tissue.
- Drug security with PCA is ensured through a locked syringe pump system or drug reservoir system programmed to deliver a certain amount of drug within a specified interval.
- Teach the client how to use the PCA pump and to report side effects such as dizziness, nausea and vomiting, and the inability to void.
- Monitor the client's vital signs and check sedation level.
- Follow the facility policy regarding documentation.
- *Epidural analgesia* is the instillation of a pain-blocking agent, usually an opioid analgesic alone or in combination with a local anesthetic, into the epidural space. The temporary catheter is not sutured to the skin and is easily dislodged.
- Complications associated with epidural analgesia include catheter displacement, pruritus, nausea, vomiting, infection, respiratory depression, lower motor weakness, and urinary retention.
- *Intrathecal (subarachnoid) analgesia,* sometimes used for the long-term management of intractable pain, is the instillation of a pain-blocking agent into the subarachnoid space.
- A permanent epidural catheter or other implantable device may be used to treat chronic pain.
- Cutaneous (skin) stimulation
  1. Benefits of techniques are highly unpredictable and vary from application to application.
  2. Pain relief is generally sustained only as long as stimulation continues.
  3. Multiple trials may be necessary to establish desired effects.
  4. Stimulation itself may aggravate pre-existing pain or produce new pain.
- Transcutaneous electrical nerve stimulation (TENS)
  1. TENS involves the use of a battery-operated device capable of delivering small electrical current to the skin and underlying tissues.
  2. Electrodes connected to a small box are placed over the painful site. The voltage or current is regulated by adjusting a dial to the point at which the client perceives

a prickly "pins and needles" sensation. The current is adjusted on the basis of client's pain relief and level of comfort.

3. For older adults, TENS may be safer and just as effective as medication.
4. Teach the client to rotate the site of electrode placement to prevent skin irritation.

- Application of heat, cold, and pressure
- Therapeutic touch
- Massage
- Vibration
- Physical therapy
- Cognitive/behavioral measures
  1. Distraction
  2. Imagery
  3. Relaxation
  4. Hypnosis
  5. Music therapy
  6. Aromatherapy
  7. Prayer and meditation
- Other complementary and alternative therapies
  1. Acupuncture
  2. Glucosamine
- *Nerve blocks* can be used for both diagnostic and treatment purposes, and are usually indicated for pain confined to a specific area or nerve root distribution.
  1. Nerve blocks involve localizing a nerve root and injecting it with either a local anesthetic for temporary relief or diagnostic evaluation, or with a chemical agent (phenol or alcohol) to achieve permanent neurolysis or nerve destruction.
  2. Complications may include transient loss of motor function.
  3. Short-term pain relief may occur because of nerve cell regeneration or the development of alternative pathways capable of transmitting pain.
  4. Permanent ablation of nerve roots can be performed using thermal techniques such as radiofrequency ablation (uses heat) or cryoanalgesia (uses cold).
- Spinal cord stimulation involves the use of electrodes implanted under the skin and into the area of the nerve or

nerves responsible for pain, and then connected to an implantable stimulator.

- Surgical management
  1. *Rhizotomy:* the destruction of sensory nerve roots where they enter the spinal cord
  2. *Closed rhizotomy:* insertion of a percutaneous catheter to destroy the sensory nerve roots with a neurolytic chemical, coagulation, or cryodestruction (freezing)
  3. *Open rhizotomy:* requires a laminectomy; the nerve roots are isolated and destroyed
  4. *Cordotomy:* transection of the pain pathways at the midline portion of the spinal cord before nerve impulses ascend to the spinothalamic tract
  5. *Teaching:* involves explaining to the client how to adapt to any neurologic deficits that may be present.

Community-Based Care

- Coordinate effective analgesic regimens or pain-relieving strategies before discharge if the client is still in pain.
- Ensure that the client has prescriptions for pain medication as needed.
- Identify the need for a referral to a pain management specialist or program.

Discharge Planning

- Preparation for home care is carried out with the client, family, and interdisciplinary team.
- Together the team determines whether modifications to the home are necessary for maintaining a reasonably pain-free regimen after discharge.
- Refer the client to specialists, such as home health nursing, physical therapy, a psychiatric clinical specialist, or a social worker to help him or her develop coping strategies, set up a home infusion therapy program, or receive hospice care, for example.
- Health teaching
  1. Involve the client and family in continuing health care behaviors that will relieve pain and improve psychological well-being and overall functional status.
  2. Teach the administration of drug therapy and use of other pain-reduction modalities and how to prevent or treat

constipation commonly associated with opioid analgesics and other pain medication.

3. Explain to the family how to assist the client in adhering to and continuing the proposed medical and nursing plans.
4. Suggest ways that the client can continue to participate in household, social, sexual, and work-oriented activities after discharge.
5. Help the client and family identify coping strategies that have worked in the past.

Nursing Care of the Dying Client

OVERVIEW

- The goals of care for a client near the end of life are to
  1. Control symptoms
  2. Identify client needs
  3. Promote meaningful interaction between client and significant others
  4. Facilitate a peaceful death
- As death nears, clients may manifest fear, anxiety, and physical symptoms of distress that require treatment and control.
- Hospice care seeks to use an interdisciplinary approach to facilitate quality of life and death for clients with terminal disease, using an interdisciplinary approach.

COLLABORATIVE MANAGEMENT

- Obtain client information.
  1. Diagnosis
  2. Past medical history
  3. Recent state of health
- Assess for
  1. Signs and symptoms of impending death
     a. Pain (use visual or verbal analogue scale if possible)
        (1) Location, character
        (2) Level of intensity in the past

   (3) Reaction to medications
   (4) Effect on activities
   (5) Effect on sleep
   (6) Frequency and amount of medications needed to treat and control
  b. Dyspnea
  c. Agitation
  d. Nausea and vomiting
  e. Fatigue, weakness, increased sleeping
  f. Constipation
  g. Anorexia, decreased desire for food and drink
  h. Level of consciousness, delirium
  i. Ability to verbally communicate
  j. Coolness of extremities
  k. Breathing pattern change
 2. Family's perception of client's symptoms
 3. Vital signs
 4. Psychosocial
  a. Cultural considerations
  b. Values and religious beliefs of client and family
  c. Fear, anxiety
  d. Knowledge deficits regarding the process of dying

▌▌▌ Cultural Considerations

- The dying process for many Americans is oriented to the "high-tech" hospital setting; family demands for testing and treatment are common even when clients themselves prefer a palliative approach.
- African American: A definitive statement cannot be made about the dying and mourning process because of the diversity that exists among different communities.
- Asian: Herbal medicine plays an important role. Southeast Asians may feel that discussion of dying brings bad luck, and hospitals and treatments are alien. Some family members may avoid visiting a terminally ill client for fear of contracting the disease.
- Latino/Hispanic: There are many subcultures within this diverse population. Death is viewed as a direct result of life. There is an acceptance of death. Family and family life are important, especially surrounding deaths and funerals.

- Native American: Each tribe has its own belief system. Bereavement follow-up may not be appropriate—some tribes have a taboo against speaking of the dead.
- Judaism: There is a strong belief in the sacredness of life. Funeral and mourning traditions vary. Funerals have two themes: honor the dead and comfort the mourners. The body must not be left unattended until burial, which should take place as soon as possible. Autopsies and cremation are opposed.
- A variety of values, religious beliefs, practices of healing, and family structures may impact dying both in positive and in challenging and negative ways.

Interventions

- For anorexia, dysphagia
  1. Refrain from providing food and drink to the client with impaired swallowing or no desire to eat because of the risk of aspiration.
  2. Reinforce with the family that cessation of food and liquids is thought to be a natural process and that hydration can lead to more discomfort from increased GI secretions, nausea, vomiting, edema, and ascites.
  3. Provide frequent mouth care; apply emollient to the lips.
  4. Identify alternative routes for medication such as sublingual, rectal, subcutaneous, or intravenous.
  5. Identify the need to adjust dosage based on route of administration.
- To manage pain
  1. Assess causes of pain, including tumor pain resulting from the infiltration of malignant cells into organs, nerves, and bones, and disturbance pain resulting from headaches, osteoarthritis, muscle spasms, and stiff joints caused by immobility.
  2. Administer pain medication and bolus dosages as needed.
  3. Depending on the brand of long-acting opioid, oral capsules may be given rectally (same dose and same capsule) when the client is no longer able to swallow.
  4. Liquid morphine can be given sublingually, rectally, or via the buccal mucosa.

- To manage dyspnea
    1. Manifestations include copious secretions, cough, chest pain, fatigue, and air hunger.
    2. Treat the primary cause and relieve psychological distress and autonomic response that accompany dyspnea.
    3. Morphine is used to treat dyspnea and labored respirations; clients already receiving morphine for pain may require a 50% increase to relieve dyspnea.
    4. Diuretics are given for fluid volume overload, heart failure, and pulmonary edema.
    5. Anticholinergics or a diuretic are used to reduce the production of secretions.
    6. Bronchodilators or corticosteroids are given for bronchospasm.
    7. Antibiotics are used to treat dyspnea from a respiratory infection.
    8. Give oxygen as needed; monitor effectiveness and continue if symptoms are relieved.
    9. Sedatives are commonly used to prevent or control dyspnea and anxiety.
    10. Use nonpharmacologic interventions, including
        a. Altering the environment to facilitate the circulation of cool air
        b. Applying wet cloths on the client's face
        c. Positioning the client to facilitate chest expansion
        d. Encouraging imagery and deep breathing
        e. Intervening to conserve the client energy
        f. Facilitating the client's rest
    11. Administer antiemetic agents to manage nausea and vomiting.
- To manage anxiety/agitation
    1. Assess and treat pain, urinary retention, constipation, and other causes.
    2. Consider consultation with the client's spiritual advisor or bereavement counselor.
    3. Ensure adequate sedation around the clock to prevent further restlessness, anxiety, and delirium.
- To manage refractory symptoms of distress
    1. High doses of analgesia may result in sedation; the client may need to be sedated to control symptoms of distress.
    2. Use protocols for doses of medications to alleviate suffering.

- To manage psychosocial issues
    1. Incorporate the client's specific beliefs and customs regarding death when planning and providing care.
    2. Offer physical and emotional support.
    3. Be realistic; avoid reassurance such as "Things will be fine," "Don't be upset," or "Don't cry."
    4. Encourage the client, family, and significant others to reminisce.
    5. Promote spirituality.
    6. Foster hope.
    7. Avoid explanations of the loss in philosophic or religious terms.
    8. Provide referrals to bereavement counselors or hospice agencies.
    9. Teach about the physical signs of death using nontechnical terms.
        a. Coolness of extremities
        b. Increased sleeping
        c. Decreased desire for fluid and food
        d. Incontinence
        e. Congestion and gurgling
        f. Breathing pattern change
        g. Disorientation
        h. Restlessness
        i. Withdrawal
        j. Saying goodbye
- Ensure palliative care.
- Provide care of the client after death.
    1. Ensure that the death certificate is completed.
    2. Prepare the body for viewing by the family according to institutional or home policy.
    3. Remove all tubes and lines, or cut them according to institutional protocol; do not remove these items if the death will be reviewed by the medical examiner.
    4. Close the client's eyes.
    5. Place dentures (if available) in the mouth.
    6. Place the client flat in bed; remove all pillows except one supporting the head.
    7. Place a pad around the perineum to absorb fecal material and fluid.

8. Support the family to say their last words and perform their farewell gestures freely and naturally around the bed.
9. Notify the hospital chaplain or religious leader at the family's request.
10. Follow institutional procedure for preparing the client for transfer to the morgue or funeral home.

Preoperative Nursing Care

OVERVIEW

- The preoperative period begins when the client is scheduled for surgery and ends at the time of transfer to the surgical suite.
- The primary roles of the nurse are educator, advocate, and promoter of health.
- *Inpatient* refers to a client who is admitted to a hospital the day before or the same day of surgery and who requires hospitalization after surgery.
- *Outpatient or ambulatory* refers to a client who goes to the surgical area (surgical center, ambulatory care center) the day of surgery and returns home on the same day.
- The primary reasons for surgery are
  1. Diagnostic
  2. Curative
  3. Restorative
  4. Palliative
  5. Cosmetic
- The urgency of the surgery may be
  1. Elective
  2. Urgent
  3. Emergency
- The extent of surgery can be
  1. Simple
  2. Modified
  3. Radical

Considerations for Older Adults

- The normal aging process decreases immune system functioning and delays wound healing.
- Older adults have a decreased ability to withstand the stresses of surgery and anesthesia.
- Older adults have an increased risk of a change in mental status.
- Older adults often have cardiovascular, respiratory, renal, musculoskeletal, and nutritional deficits that increase the risk of surgery.
- Older adults have a greater incidence of chronic illness, malnutrition, and allergies than younger adults.
- Older adults have an increased risk of cardiopulmonary complications.

COLLABORATIVE MANAGEMENT

Assessment

- Record client information.
    1. Age
    2. Allergies to medication and food
    3. Current medications (prescription, over-the-counter, herbal therapies, folk remedies)
    4. History of medical and surgical problems
        a. Myocardial infarction within the past 6 months
        b. Heart failure or coronary artery disease
        c. Dysrhythmias
        d. Pneumonia
        e. Pulmonary disease such as asthma, emphysema, or chronic bronchitis
    5. Prior surgical procedures and experiences
    6. Prior experience with anesthesia
    7. Tobacco, alcohol, and illicit substance use
    8. Family medical history and problems with anesthetics that may indicate possible intraoperative needs and reactions to anesthesia, such as malignant hyperthermia
    9. Blood transfusion status
        a. Autologous
        b. Directed blood donation
        c. Bloodless surgery

10. Knowledge and understanding about events during the perioperative period
11. Support system availability

- Perform a preoperative assessment to determine baseline data, hidden medical problems, potential complications related to the administration of anesthesia, and potential complications of surgery, assessing the client's
  1. Vital signs
  2. Cardiovascular system
     a. Palpate peripheral pulses; observe for indications of arteriosclerosis.
     b. Auscultate the heart for rate, regularity, and abnormal heart sounds.
     c. Record blood pressure to determine presence of hypertension or increased diastolic pressure.
     d. Report symptoms such as chest pain, shortness of breath, or dyspnea to the physician.
  3. Respiratory system
     a. Observe
        (1) Posture and fingers (for clubbing)
        (2) Rate, rhythm, depth of respirations
        (3) Lung expansion
     b. Auscultate the lungs to determine the presence of abnormal breath sounds.
  4. Renal system
     a. Ask about
        (1) Frequency of urination
        (2) Dysuria
        (3) Nocturia
        (4) Difficulty starting urine flow
        (5) Oliguria
        (6) Appearance and odor of urine
     b. Question the client about usual fluid intake and continence.
     c. Note that scopolamine, morphine, meperidine, and barbiturates may cause confusion, disorientation, apprehension, and restlessness when administered to clients with decreased renal function.

5. Neurologic system
   a. Level of consciousness
   b. Orientation
   c. Ability to follow commands and communicate
   d. Motor or sensory changes
   e. Risk of falling
6. Musculoskeletal system (the following may affect positioning)
   a. Arthritis
   b. Joint replacement
   c. Skeletal deformities
   d. Length of neck and shape of thoracic cavity, which may interfere with respiratory and cardiac function
7. Nutritional status
   a. Malnutrition and obesity can cause poor wound healing and increase surgical risk.
   b. Assess for the following indicators of fluid and electrolyte imbalance and malnutrition
      (1) Brittle nails
      (2) Wasting muscles
      (3) Dry, flaky skin
      (4) Dull, sparse, dry hair
      (5) Decreased skin turgor
      (6) Postural hypotension
      (7) Decreased serum albumin
      (8) Abnormal electrolytes
8. Psychosocial status
   a. Anxiety and fear
   b. Coping mechanisms
9. Laboratory findings
   a. Complete blood count
   b. Electrolytes
   c. Urinalysis
   d. Type and crossmatch
   e. Coagulation studies
10. Other diagnostic studies
    a. Chest x-ray examination
    b. Electrocardiogram

Planning and Implementation

◀**NDx:** Deficient Knowledge

- *Informed consent* for the surgical procedure is obtained by the physician before sedation is given and surgery performed; the nurse may witness the client's signature.
- *Consent* implies that the client has been provided with information necessary to understand the
  1. Nature of and reasons for surgery
  2. Who will be performing the surgery and whether others will be present during the procedure (e.g., students)
  3. Available options and risks associated with each option
  4. Risks of surgical procedure and potential outcomes
  5. Risks associated with the administration of anesthesia
- A competent adult has the right to refuse treatment for any reason, even when refusal might lead to death.
- Interventions include
  1. Notifying the physician of any indications that the client did not understand the information given concerning the procedure or is not adequately informed
  2. Clarifying facts presented by the physician
  3. Dispelling myths about surgery
  4. Ensuring that special permits that may be needed are obtained by the physician
- The client is allowed *nothing by mouth* (NPO) for 6 to 8 hours before surgery. It is customary to place the client on NPO status after midnight.
- Routine preoperative care includes
  1. Emphasizing the consequences of not adhering to NPO restrictions
     a. Increased risk of aspiration during surgery
     b. Possible cancellation of surgery
  2. Consulting the physician concerning the administration of medications such as corticosteroids and those used for hypertension, diabetes mellitus, cardiac disease, glaucoma, and epilepsy
  3. Stopping over-the-counter medications such as aspirin and NSAIDs for several days before and after surgery
- *Bowel preparation* is usually done for clients having major abdominal, pelvic, perineal, or perianal surgery or diagnostic procedures such as a colonoscopy.

- Repeated enemas can cause
  1. Electrolyte (especially potassium) imbalance
  2. Fluid deficit
  3. Postural hypotension
  4. Vagal stimulation
  5. Anorectal discomfort in the client with hemorrhoids
  6. Fatigue
- *Skin preparation* varies depending on the procedure and facility/physician preference.
- Shaving is generally done immediately before the start of the surgical procedure or not at all.
- Prepare the client for the possibility of having tubes, drains, and IV lines postoperatively, including
  1. Foley catheter
  2. Nasogastric tube
  3. Drains that promote the evacuation of fluid from the surgical wound
  3. IV line, which is generally used for all clients
- To reduce apprehension and to increase postoperative cooperation and participation, teach the client and family postoperative exercises before surgery.
  1. Ensure client mastery by observing correct performance on return demonstration.
  2. Encourage the client to regularly practice
     a. Diaphragmatic breathing
     b. Incentive spirometry
     c. Coughing and deep breathing
     d. Splinting the wound
     e. Turning and leg exercises
     f. Early ambulation
     g. Range-of-motion exercises
- Explain the use and importance of antiembolism stockings and sequential compression devices.
- Explain the importance of early ambulation.
- Inform family members about the client's care and allow them to participate if they desire to do so.

NDx: Anxiety

- Assess the client's anxiety level and knowledge base.
  1. Provide information about the surgical procedure and allow time for questions.

2. Provide the client with rest and sleep.
3. Use distractions such as television, radio, or books.
4. Assess the readiness and desire of the family to take an active part in the client's care.

- Review the chart for
  1. Operative permit and other special permits
     a. Confirm that the scheduled procedure, including the identification of left versus right when necessary, is what is listed on the consent form.
  2. Results of all laboratory, radiographic, and diagnostic tests
  3. Allergies, with documentation of any allergies on the front of the chart
  4. Abnormal results that are documented and reported to the physician
  5. Height and weight
  6. Current vital signs
  7. Special needs flagged (e.g., client refusal to allow blood transfusion)
- Client preparation includes
  1. Dressing client in hospital gown
  2. Dressing the client in antiembolism stockings, if ordered
  3. Securing the client's valuables (If rings cannot be removed, cover them with tape and make a note on the preoperative checklist.)
  4. Attaching identification and allergy bands
  5. Removing dentures (including partial plates), hair pins and clips of any type, wigs and toupees, prosthetic devices, and all jewelry such as earrings and watches
  6. Checking facility policy regarding removal of hearing aids and fingernail polish
  7. Instructing the client to void
- If preoperative medication is given, the client should remain in bed with the side rails up. Often, the preoperative medication is given after the client is transferred to the operating room.

Intraoperative Nursing Care

OVERVIEW

- Intraoperative care begins when the client enters the surgical suite.
- A *surgeon* is responsible for the surgical procedure and surgical judgments about the client.
- An *anesthesiologist* is a physician who specializes in the administration of anesthesia.
- A *certified registered nurse anesthetist* is a registered nurse who administers anesthetics under the supervision of an anesthesiologist, a surgeon, a dentist, or a podiatrist.
- A *holding room nurse* manages the client's care while the client is in this area waiting for the operating suite to be ready. The nurse assesses the client's physical and emotional status, provides emotional support, answers questions, and ensures that the necessary permits and other paperwork are completed.
- A *circulating nurse* is a registered nurse who ensures that the necessary supplies and equipment are available, safe, and functional before surgery; helps to position the client on the operating room table; comforts and reassures the client; ensures that sterile technique and the sterile field are maintained by the surgical team; documents that drains or catheters are in place; and documents the length of surgery and the count of sponges, sharps, and instruments.
- A *surgical assistant,* who might be another surgeon, resident, nurse, physician assistant, or surgical technologist, holds retractors, suctions the wound, cuts tissue, and sutures and dresses the wound.
- A *scrub nurse* or *technologist* sets up the surgical field; assists with positioning and draping the client; hands surgical instruments or sterile supplies to the surgeon and assistants; and maintains an accurate count of sponges, sharps, and instruments.
- A *specialty nurse* is educated in a particular type of surgery and is responsible for nursing care specific to clients needing that type of surgery. The nurse assesses, maintains, and

recommends equipment, instruments, and supplies used in the specialty.

- A *laser specialty* nurse is specially trained in the use of laser technology and ensures all safety procedures are followed.
- The types of anesthesia are
  1. *General anesthesia* is a reversible loss of consciousness by inhibiting neuronal impulses in several areas of the central nervous system, causing analgesia, amnesia, and loss of muscle tone and reflexes.
  2. *Balanced anesthesia* is a combination of IV medications and inhalation agents used to provide hypnosis, amnesia, analgesia, muscle relaxation, and reduced reflexes with minimal disturbance to the client's physiologic function.
  3. *Local or regional anesthesia* temporarily interrupts the transmission of sensory nerve impulses to and from a specific area or region; motor function may or may not be involved, and the client does not lose consciousness.
     a. *Topical anesthesia* involves the use of an anesthetic agent applied directly to the surface of the area to be anesthetized, usually in the form of an ointment or spray.
     b. *Local infiltration* is the injection of an anesthetic agent directly into the tissue surrounding an incision, wound, or lesion.
     c. *Field block* is produced by a series of injections around the operative field.
     d. A *nerve block* involves the injection of a local anesthetic into or around a nerve or around a group of nerves supplying the involved areas.
     e. *Spinal* or *intrathecal block* is administered by injecting an anesthetic into the cerebral spinal fluid in the subarachnoid space.
     f. An *epidural block* is the injection of an anesthetic agent into the epidural space so that the protective coverings of the spinal cord (dura mater and arachnoid mater) are not entered.
- *Conscious sedation* refers to the IV administration of sedative, hypnotic, and opioid medication to reduce the level of consciousness but allow the client to maintain a patent airway and respond to verbal commands.

- Complications of general anesthesia may include
  1. Malignant hyperthermia, an acute, life-threatening complication manifested by hyperthermia, tachycardia or other dysrhythmias, muscle rigidity, hypotension, tachypnea, skin mottling, cyanosis, and cola-colored urine (Malignant hyperthermia is treated with dantrolene sodium, a skeletal muscle relaxant.)
  2. Overdose, if the client's pharmacokinetics are such that they do not respond or react as expected
  3. Difficult intubation, resulting in broken or injured teeth or caps, swollen lips, or trauma to vocal cords
- Complications of local or regional anesthesia are usually attributed to overdosage, incorrect administration technique, systemic absorption, or client sensitization to the anesthetic (anaphylaxis).

COLLABORATIVE MANAGEMENT

Assessment

- The circulating room or holding room nurse
  1. Verifies the client's identity with two types of identifiers (name, birth date, medical record number, identification bracelet, asking the patient to state his or her name, birth date)
  2. Validates that the surgical consent form has been signed and witnessed
     a. The client is asked, "What kind of operation are you having today?"
     b. When the procedure involves a specific site, the nurse validates the side on which a procedure is to be performed (e.g., right arm or left arm).
     c. The surgeon initials the correct surgical site.
  3. Validates that all aspects of the preoperative checklist are complete and information is on the chart
     a. Allergies are noted—most facilities require a separate identification band with allergies listed.
     b. Previous anesthesia and any reactions are documented.
     c. The history of blood transfusions and reactions, if any, are noted.
     d. Reports on laboratory, radiographic, and diagnostic tests are reviewed for completeness.

    e. The client's history and physical examination are reported.

    f. Medications routinely taken by the client are noted.

4. Ensures that the client is attired correctly and that items such as jewelry, hearing aids, contact lenses, prostheses, and dentures are removed.

5. Validates whether an autologous blood transfusion is being used.

6. Validates the status of advance directives and do not resuscitate (DNR) orders.

7. Reviews the medical record, particularly the history and physical.

Planning and Implementation

◆**NDx:** Risk for Perioperative Positioning Injury

- The surgical team observes for and treats complications of general anesthesia.
- Ensure proper positioning by assessing for
  1. Proper padding of operating bed or table with foam, silicone gel pads, or both; placement of grounding pads
  2. Physiologic alignment
  3. Minimal interference with circulation and breathing
  4. Protection of skeletal and neuromuscular structures
  5. Optimal exposure of the operative site and IV line
  6. Access for the anesthesiologist
  7. Preservation of the client's dignity
  8. Client comfort and safety
- Observe for complications of special positioning, such as wrist or foot drop, loss of sensation, and inflammation.

◆**NDx:** Impaired Skin Integrity and Impaired Tissue Integrity

- The surgeon applies a plastic drape after the skin has been prepped and is dry.
- Skin closures include
  1. Sutures
     a. Absorbable
     b. Nonabsorbable
  2. Clamps
  3. Staples
  4. Steri-Strips

- After the wound is sutured, the plastic drape is carefully removed and the surgeon applies a sterile dressing.
- Special attention is paid to older adults and clients with fragile skin to prevent skin tearing when the adhesive drape is removed.

NDx: Potential for Hypoventilation

- The nurse, surgeon, or anesthesia provider
  1. Continuously monitors the client's breathing, circulation, and cardiac rhythm
  2. Records the client's blood pressure and heart rate every 5 minutes
  3. Ensures the continuous presence of an anesthesia provider during the case

Postoperative Nursing Care

OVERVIEW

- Postoperative care starts at the completion of surgery and transfer of the client to the postanesthesia care unit (PACU), the same day surgery unit (ambulatory care unit), or the intensive care unit.
- The postoperative period continues after the client's condition is stabilized until after the client is discharged from the ambulatory surgery facility or hospital.
- Time spent in the PACU varies with the client's age and physical health, type of procedure, anesthesia used, and postoperative complications.

COLLABORATIVE MANAGEMENT

Assessment

- The postanesthesia nurse initiates assessment and the inpatient unit nurse continues assessment until the client is discharged. Assessment includes
  1. Postanesthesia score (PACU nurse)
     a. Vital signs

    b. Level of consciousness

    c. Examination of the surgical area for bleeding

2. Respiratory function
   a. Patent airway
   b. Adequate respiratory exchange
   c. Breath sounds bilaterally
   d. Symmetric movement of the chest wall
   e. Indications of diaphragmatic breathing and sternal retraction

3. Cardiovascular function
   a. Vital signs; cardiac monitoring
   b. Peripheral vascular assessment
   c. Presence of Homans' sign
   d. Edema, redness, and pain in the lower extremities (indications of thrombophlebitis)

4. Fluid and electrolyte balance
   a. Intake and output
   b. Monitor IV fluids
   c. Complete blood count
   d. Electrolytes
   e. Hydration status

5. Neurologic system
   a. Level of consciousness
   b. Orientation
   c. Ability to follow commands
   d. Motor movement
   e. Sensation and pain
   f. Eye opening

6. Genitourinary system
   a. Output and color of urine
   b. Inspection, palpation, and percussion of the client's abdomen for bladder distention

7. GI system
   a. Auscultation for bowel sounds
   b. Palpation of the abdomen
   c. Patency of the nasogastric tube or any abdominal tubes and drains
   d. Nausea and vomiting

8. Integumentary system, integrity of the wound site

9. Dressings and drains
   a. Color, amount, and consistency of drainage

b. Integrity of Penrose drains (a single-lumen, soft latex tube inserted into or close to the surgical site)
   c. Patency and integrity of Hemovac, VacuDrain, or Jackson-Pratt drains to ensure maintenance of suction
   d. Patency of all other drains or tubes
10. Pain
11. Psychosocial: anxiety, restlessness, and fear
12. Complications
   a. Acute urinary retention
   b. Allergic reaction
   c. Atelectasis, pneumonia
   d. Congestive heart failure
   e. Deep vein thrombosis
   f. Disseminated intravascular coagulation
   g. Dysrhythmias
   h. Electrolyte imbalance
   i. GI bleed
   j. Hypotension/hypertension
   k. Hypothermia/hyperthermia
   l. Hypovolemic shock
   m. Laryngeal edema
   n. Pulmonary embolism
   o. Renal failure
   p. Wound evisceration

Planning and Implementation

- Interventions include
  1. Monitoring vital signs every 4 hours or more frequently if clinically indicated (significant changes in blood pressure may indicate myocardial depression, hemorrhage, oversedation, or pain)
  2. Performing a complete systems assessment every shift
  3. Measuring and recording intake and output
  4. Observing for and reporting postoperative complications as noted in number 12 above

NDx: Impaired Gas Exchange

- Interventions in the PACU include
  1. Monitoring for stridor or snoring, which are signs of upper airway obstruction from tracheal or laryngeal

spasm, mucus in the airway, or occlusion of the airway from relaxation of the tongue

2. To prevent possible aspiration, positioning the client on the side or with the head turned
3. Unless contraindicated, keeping the head of the bed flat until the client regains a gag reflex and to prevent hypotension
4. When appropriate, raising the head of the bed to promote respiratory function
5. Encouraging the client to cough (splint the wound as needed) and deep breathe, using incentive spirometer if needed

■ Interventions for the inpatient include

1. Assisting the client out of bed to ambulate as soon as possible
2. Ensuring that the client performs breathing and leg exercises

NDx: Impaired Skin Integrity

■ The expected outcome is that the client's skin will remain intact. To facilitate this outcome

1. Observe the wound for separation.
   a. Check for *dehiscence*, the partial or complete separation of the upper layers of the wound.
      (1) Apply a sterile nonadherent or saline dressing to the wound.
      (2) Notify the surgeon immediately.
   b. Check for *evisceration*, the total separation of the layers and extrusion of internal organs or viscera through an open wound.
      (1) Cover the wound with a sterile towel or nonadherent dressing moistened with normal saline.
      (2) Notify the surgeon immediately.
      (3) Do not attempt to reinsert the protruding organ or viscera.
   c. Monitor vital signs and assess for signs of shock.
   d. Support and reassure the client.
   e. Prepare the client for surgery to repair the wound.
2. Perform dressing changes as ordered (with the first change usually performed by the physician).

a. Reinforce the dressing if it becomes wet from drainage.
b. Document the color, type, amount, and odor of drainage and note time of observation on the client's chart.
c. Notify the surgeon of excessive drainage; document the time of the call and the physician's response.
d. Recognize that wet dressings are a source of infection; obtain an order from the surgeon for dressing changes using aseptic technique.
e. Follow facility procedure for dressing changes and wound care.

3. Observe the wound for infection; antibiotics may be administered prophylactically.
4. Inspect surgical drains.
   a. The Penrose drain drains directly onto the dressing and skin around the incision. Change the dressing carefully to avoid pulling the drain out. Record amount and color of drainage.
   b. Jackson-Pratt and Hemovac drains are two self-contained drainage systems that drain wounds directly through a tube via gravity and vacuum. Empty the reservoir and record the amount and color of drainage every 8 hours.
5. Examine the client's skin for areas of redness or lost integrity that may occur from positioning during surgery, prolonged contact with damp surgical linens, or contact with unpadded surfaces.

◀ **NDx:** Acute Pain

■ Opioids and non-opioids are routinely given immediately postoperatively.
■ Other interventions include
   1. Assessing the type, location, and intensity of the pain before giving the medication
   2. Assessing and documenting the effectiveness of the medication
   3. Monitoring PCA, as ordered, via an IV or internal pump, with the rate or dosage of infusion of an opioid analgesic adjusted by the client on the basis of his or her pain level and physical response to the drug

4. Tapering pain medication as recovery progresses and administering non-opioid medication such as acetaminophen (Tylenol, Atasol ✣) and nonsteroidal anti-inflammatory drugs such as ibuprofen (Motrin, Novoprofen ✣, Amersol ✣, Advil), as ordered
5. Positioning the client based on surgical procedure and medical condition
6. Turning the client every 2 hours or more often as needed
7. Providing back rubs, relaxation techniques, and distractions to control pain
8. Cushioning and elevating painful areas; avoiding pressure and tension

◆**NDx:** Potential for Hypoxia

- The highest incidence of hypoxemia after surgery occurs on the second postoperative day.
- Monitor respiratory status carefully and implement interventions as discussed under Impaired Gas Exchange.
- Provide oxygen as prescribed with careful attention to the client's past medical history.

Community-Based Care

- Discharge planning includes assessing information about the home environment as described in Appendix 5.
- The teaching plan for the client and significant others includes
  1. Care of the surgical wound (provide written instructions as needed)
     a. Prevention of infection
     b. Care and assessment of the surgical wound
     c. The importance of handwashing
     d. Disposal procedure for soiled dressing
     e. Return demonstration of wound care
     f. Signs and symptoms of infection and complications and what to do if infection occurs
  2. Diet therapy and how to obtain a dietary consultation if necessary. Advise a diet that is high in protein, calories, and vitamin C to promote wound healing unless the client is on a restricted or special diet. Collaborate with the dietitian to determine whether the client needs dietary supplements.

3. Information on drug therapy, instructing the client to notify the physician if pain is not relieved or suddenly increases
4. Restrictions for activity and exercise. Teach the client to increase activity level slowly, rest often, and avoid straining the wound or surrounding area.
5. Proper body mechanics
6. Written discharge instructions
   a. Permissible activities
   b. Activity restrictions
   c. When driving may be resumed
7. References to home health care and community resources

Rehabilitation

OVERVIEW

- A *chronic illness* or condition is one that has existed for at least 3 months.
- A *disabling condition* is any physical or mental health problem that can cause a disability.
- *Rehabilitation* is the process of learning to live with chronic and disabling conditions.
  1. Clients participate in rehabilitation programs to prevent disability, maintain functional ability, and restore as much function as possible.
- *Impairment* is an abnormality of a body structure or structures or an alteration in the function of a body system resulting from any cause. It may be temporary or permanent.
- *Disability* is the consequence of impairment, usually described in terms of a client's altered functional ability.
- A *handicap* is the disadvantage that a person feels as a result of impairments and disabilities. It is based on interactions the client experiences in society.
- Settings for rehabilitation include
  1. Freestanding rehabilitation hospitals
  2. Rehabilitation units within acute care hospitals or within skilled nursing or long-term care facilities
  3. Ambulatory care rehabilitation centers

4. Subacute units and transitional living centers, which are a step between a rehabilitation center and an independent living center (ILC), with the goal of preparing the client to live at home or in the ILC
5. Group homes in which the client shares an apartment or home with other disabled clients and has supervision and support available

- In addition to the client, family, and significant others, the rehabilitation team members typically include
    1. Case manager
    2. Cognitive therapist
    3. Nurse specializing in rehabilitation
    4. Nursing or therapy assistants
    5. Occupational therapist
    6. Orthotist
    7. Physicians such as a physiatrist who specializes in rehabilitation
    8. Physical therapist
    9. Psychologist
    10. Recreational or activity therapist
    11. Respiratory therapist
    12. Speech language pathologist
    13. Social worker or case manager
    14. Vocational counselor

COLLABORATIVE MANAGEMENT

Assessment

- Record the client's health history with a rehabilitation focus.
    1. History of present condition
        a. Current medications
        b. Current treatment program
    2. General background data
        a. Financial status
        b. Occupation
        c. Educational level
        d. Cultural background
    3. Home situation
        a. Architectural features; layout of house or apartment
        b. Proximity of shopping centers, transportation

  c. Availability of support for help in the home such as cooking and cleaning

 4. Daily schedule and activities of daily living (ADLs)

  a. Hygiene practices

  b. Eating

  c. Elimination

  d. Sexual activity

  e. Sleep

  f. Dietary patterns

  g. Food likes and dislikes

  h. Bowel and bladder dysfunction

  i. Exercise

  j. Recreational activities

■ Assess body systems.

 1. Cardiovascular system

  a. Manifestations of decreased cardiac output (chest pain, fatigue)

  b. Manifestations of activity intolerance and unwillingness to return to *any* activity because of fear of cardiac failure

 2. Respiratory system

  a. Level of activity the client can perform without becoming short of breath

  b. Fear of inability to breathe

 3. GI system

  a. Oral intake and eating pattern

  b. Indications of anorexia, dysphagia, nausea, vomiting, and discomfort related to or interfering with oral intake

  c. Height, weight, hemoglobin and hematocrit levels, and serum albumin and blood glucose concentrations

  d. Elimination patterns and habits

  e. Ability to manage bowel functions independently.

 4. Renal and urinary systems

  a. Baseline urinary patterns

   (1) Number of times the client usually voids and at what time of day

   (2) Determine whether client routinely awakens during night to empty bladder

   (3) Problems with incontinence or retention

  b. Usual fluid intake patterns and volume, including types of fluids ingested and times of fluid consumption

     c. Problems with urinary retention or incontinence

     d. Results of laboratory tests

  5. Neurologic system

     a. Functional aspects of cognition, motor ability, and sensation

     b. Pre-existing problems, general physical condition, and communication abilities

     c. Presence of paresis or paralysis

     d. Sensory-perceptual alterations: response to hot or cold temperatures and to light touch; ability to receive and understand what is heard and seen; ability to express appropriate motor and verbal responses

  6. Musculoskeletal system

     a. Routine musculoskeletal and functional assessment

     b. Impact of deficits on the client's home, work, or school environment

     c. Endurance level

     d. Active and passive range of motion (ROM)

     e. Muscle strength

  7. Integumentary system

     a. Actual and potential interruptions in skin integrity

     b. Risk of skin breakdown (use facility assessment tool to predict)

     c. Client's understanding of the cause and treatment of skin breakdown

■ Perform assessments.

  1. Functional assessment, with various tools used to assess a client's abilities

     a. ADLs

     b. Self-care

     c. Sphincter control

     d. Mobility and locomotion

     e. Communication

     f. Cognition

  2. Psychological assessment

     a. Changes in body image and self-esteem

     b. Defense mechanisms

     c. Manifestations of anxiety

     d. Availability of support systems such as family and significant others

3. Vocational assessment, including information on the client's work environment to determine whether environment is conducive to the client's return
   a. Provide information to a client in the United States about the Americans with Disabilities Act.
   b. Assess cognitive and physical demands of the client's job.

Planning and Implementation

◆NDx: Impaired Physical Mobility

- Interventions include
  1. Using and teaching correct transfer techniques as identified by the physical or occupational therapist
     a. Bed to wheelchair or chair
        (1) Place the chair at an angle to the bed on the client's strong side.
        (2) Lock the wheelchair brakes or secure the chair position.
        (3) Assist the client to stand and to move his or her strong hand to the armrest.
        (4) Keep the client's body weight forward while you and the client pivot.
        (5) When the client's legs touch the chair edge, assist the client in sitting.
     b. Wheelchair or chair to bed
        (1) Place the chair with the client's strong side next to the bed.
        (2) Lock or secure the wheelchair brakes.
        (3) Assist the client to stand and move the client's strong hand to the armrest.
        (4) Keep the client's body weight forward while you and the client pivot.
        (5) Assist the client in sitting and then reclining when the client's legs touch the bed edge.
     c. Use of a sliding board
        (1) Place the chair or wheelchair as close to the bed as possible.
        (2) Remove the armrest from the chair (if removable) or wheelchair.
        (3) Powder the sliding board.

    (4) Place the sliding board under the client's buttocks.

    (5) Instruct the client to reach toward his or her side.

    (6) Assist the client in sliding gently to the bed or chair.

2. Assisting the client in gait training
   a. Walker assisted
      (1) Apply a gait belt around the client's waist.
      (2) Assist the client to a standing position.
      (3) Assist the client in placing both hands on the walker.
      (4) Ensure that the client is well balanced.
      (5) Assist the client repeatedly to perform the following sequence:
         (a) Lift the walker.
         (b) Move the walker 2 feet forward and set it down on all legs.
         (c) While resting on the walker, take small steps.
         (d) Check balance.
   b. Cane assisted
      (1) Apply a gait belt around the client's waist.
      (2) Assist the client to a standing position.
      (3) Assist the client in placing his or her strong hand on the cane.
      (4) Ensure that the client is well balanced.
      (5) Assist the client repeatedly to perform the following sequence:
         (a) Move the cane forward.
         (b) Move the weaker leg one step forward.
         (c) Move the stronger leg one step forward.
         (d) Check balance.
3. Assessing for and intervening to prevent complications of immobility
   a. Contractures
      (1) Perform active-assist or passive ROM exercises at least once daily.
   b. Footdrop
      (1) Provide foot support while client is in bed.
      (2) Have client wear high-top tennis shoes.
   c. Osteoporosis
      (1) Provide ROM exercises.
      (2) Have the client ambulate if possible.

    d. Constipation or decreased GI motility

        (1) Assist the client in increasing his or her activity level.

        (2) Encourage the client to increase fluid intake unless contraindicated.

    e. Decreased cardiac output

        (1) Monitor vital signs and pulse.

        (2) Assess for changes in levels of consciousness.

    f. Increased venous stasis, thrombus formation, embolism

        (1) Apply antiembolism stockings or support hose.

        (2) Avoid leg massage.

        (3) Perform ROM exercises.

        (4) Monitor vital signs.

    g. Disorientation

        (1) Help the client maintain a normal sleep-wake schedule.

        (2) Orient the client as needed.

        (3) Control sensory stimulation.

    h. Postural hypotension

        (1) Avoid sudden position changes.

    i. Renal calculi

        (1) Decrease dietary calcium.

        (2) Increase client's fluid intake.

        (3) Maintain acidic urine.

        (4) Apply intermittent catheterization if necessary; avoid indwelling catheter.

    j. Pneumonia

        (1) Encourage the client to turn, cough, and deep breathe at least once every 2 hours.

        (2) Teach respiratory exercises.

    k. Pressure ulcers

        (1) Reposition the client frequently (at least once every 2 hours).

        (2) Apply pressure-relief devices as appropriate.

        (3) Provide skin care.

        (4) Monitor skin integrity.

3. Performing ROM exercises

    a. Exercise all joints.

    b. Complete full range of movement of each joint (include the fingers, hands, and toes) five or more times.

    c. Perform exercises at least three times daily.

    d. Do not move the joint beyond the point at which the client expresses pain or you perceive stiffness or difficulty.

◀NDx: Self-Care Deficit

- Nursing interventions include
  1. Collaborating with physical and occupational therapy to
     a. Encourage the client to perform as much self-care as possible
     b. Identify ways self-care activities can be modified so the client can perform them independently
     c. Reinforce the correct use of adaptive devices
     d. Develop strategies for energy conservation to reduce effort and energy expenditure
  2. Reinforcing the correct use of assistive devices

◀NDx: Risk for Impaired Skin Integrity

- Nursing interventions include
  1. Assessing the client for risk level
  2. Turning and repositioning
     a. Reposition the client once every 2 hours or more based on skin assessment.
     b. Teach the client to perform "wheelchair push-ups" by using his or her arms to lift buttocks off the seat for 10 seconds or longer at least once every hour.
  3. Encouraging the client to eat a balanced diet
     a. Monitor the client's weight and serum prealbumin level.
     b. Collaborate with the dietitian to assess the client's food selection to ensure it contains adequate protein and carbohydrates.
  4. Providing frequent skin care
     a. Remove the client's shoes and assess for pressure areas.
     b. Check the client's lower legs where the leg of the chair or wheelchair could rub against the skin.
     c. Assess skin using facility assessment tool.
     d. Provide skin care with turning, repositioning, and bathing.
     e. Use topical barrier cream if the client is incontinent.
     f. Do not rub reddened areas.

5. Obtaining mechanical devices as appropriate
   a. Waterbed
   b. Foam or gel mattress
   c. Air mattress, low air loss overlap
   d. Alternating-pressure mattress
   e. Air-fluidized bed

NDx: Impaired Urinary Elimination

- *Reflex* or *spastic bladder* (upper motor neuron) causes incontinence characterized by sudden gushing voids. The bladder does not empty completely.
- *Flaccid bladder* (lower motor neuron) results in overflow (dribbling) and urinary retention.
- *Uninhibited bladder* results in incontinence and incomplete emptying of the bladder. The client has little sensorimotor control and cannot wait until he or she is on the commode before voiding.
- Design a bladder-training program.
  1. Initiate a bladder-training program as appropriate.
     a. Intermittently catheterize client and determine residual urine.
     b. Schedule consistent toileting routine.
     c. Teach facilitating or triggering techniques to stimulate voiding such as using the Valsalva and Credé maneuvers, stroking the medial aspect of the thigh, pinching the area above the groin, pulling pubic hair, or digitally stimulating the anus.
  2. Provide drug therapy.
     a. Cholinergics to promote bladder emptying and decrease urinary retention from a flaccid bladder
     b. Antispasmodics to prevent incontinence
     c. Skeletal muscle relaxants to decrease spasticity, which promotes self-care
  3. Provide and teach importance of fluid intake.
     a. Encourage fluid intake of 2000 to 2500 mL per day unless contraindicated.
     b. Encourage intake of fluids that promote an acidic urine, such as tomato juice, prune juice, cranberry juice, and bouillon.
     c. Discourage excessive intake of milk, citrus juices, and carbonated beverages, which promote alkaline urine.

    d. Discourage overweight clients from drinking high-calorie fluids.

  4. Intervene to prevent complications such as urinary tract infections and urinary calculi or stasis.

◆**NDx:** Risk for Constipation

- Design a bowel program.
  1. Plan and implement the program based on the cause.
     a. *Upper motor neuron* disease may result in a reflex (spastic) bowel pattern with defecation occurring suddenly and without warning.
     b. *Lower motor neuron* disease may result in a flaccid bowel pattern with defecation occurring infrequently and in small amounts.
        (1) Teach the client facilitating and triggering mechanisms such as pulling pubic hair, digitally stimulating the anus, and gently pinching the anus.
        (2) Provide a high-fiber diet.
        (3) Administer suppositories, as prescribed.
        (4) Maintain a consistent toileting schedule.
        (5) Perform manual disimpaction if other techniques fail, unless the client has cardiac disease.
     c. Uninhibited bowel pattern may result in frequent defecation, urgency, and complaints of constipation.
        (1) Maintain a consistent toileting schedule.
        (2) Provide a high-fiber diet.
        (3) Administer stool softeners, as prescribed.
  2. Modify the bowel program if complications such as constipation, diarrhea, or flatulence occur.

◆**NDx:** Ineffective Coping

- Assist the client to learn to cope and participate in a rehabilitation program.
  1. Encourage the client to discuss his or her feelings and ask questions to elicit specific information that can help in assessing his or her acceptance of and ability to cope with the disability.
  2. Assess the coping strategies and support systems the client used in the past and assist during rehabilitation.

3. Help the client use spiritual and religious beliefs to cope, as appropriate; some clients may benefit from alternative therapies such as acupuncture, imagery, and music.

Community-Based Care

- Discharge planning includes
  1. Predischarge home assessment
     a. Assess the current home environment to determine potential needs after discharge such as modifications to the entryway of the house or apartment and accessibility of the bedroom, bathroom, and kitchen.
     b. Determine whether there is sufficient space in each room depending on the client's need to use a wheel chair, walker, or cane.
  2. Leave-of-absence visit (generally lasts a few hours)
     a. Nurse meets with patient and family to set goals for visit and identify specific tasks to be attempted while at home.
     b. The client is interviewed after the trial visit to determine success and to assess additional training or education needs before final discharge.
  3. Referral
     a. Some clients may not be able to go home and are referred to a nursing home, skilled nursing facility, or assisted-living facility.
  4. Health teaching
     a. Determine the client's learning potential and cognitive capacity and verify his or her understanding of skill needed to be performed at home.
     b. Assess reading level of the client and family and provide written material explaining steps of procedures, if appropriate, taking into account their reading ability and language skills.
     c. Encourage the client to verbalize feelings and emotions surrounding changes in lifestyle and body image. Talk about ways to prevent worries from becoming reality after discharge.
  5. Health care resources
     a. Collaborate with the health care team to determine need for physical or occupational therapy, home care nursing, or vocational counseling.

Nursing Care of the Client with a Substance Abuse Problem

- Substance abuse is the overindulgence of a chemical substance and the resulting dependence that interferes with life's activities.
- It is a documented nursing diagnosis when the following criteria are present: The client
  1. Loses control of use of the drug
  2. Takes the drug even though the drug has caused adverse conditions in the body
  3. Demonstrates cognitive, behavioral, and physiologic disturbances with the abuse of drugs or inhalants
- Dependence is characterized as a condition that causes a habitual, compulsive, and uncontrollable urge to use a substance; and without the substance, the body experiences severe physiologic, psychological, and emotional disturbances.
- It is important to understand the client's culture to avoid making assumptions about substance abuse based on body language.
- Do not overlook substance abuse in the older adult.
  1. Identify patterns of drug use that are harmful to the client.
  2. Misuse of prescription drugs can occur.
  3. Toxicity is a common situation due to problems with metabolizing.
- Risk factors for substance abuse include
  1. Family history
  2. Stress
  3. Biologic response to stress
- Genetic predisposition has not been established.

Stimulants

- Stimulants are drugs that excite the cerebral cortex of the brain, producing a variety of behavioral responses.
  1. Commonly abused stimulants include

a. Amphetamines ("black beauties," "cross," "hearts")
b. Methamphetamines ("chalk," "speed," "crank," "glass," "ice")
c. Cocaine ("coke," "crack," "flake," "rocks," "snow")

2. Signs and symptoms of overdose include
   a. Respiratory distress
   b. Ataxia
   c. Fever
   d. Convulsions
   e. Coma
   f. Myocardial infarction
   g. Stroke
   h. Death

3. Interventions for overdose include
   a. Maintain a safe environment for the client both physically and psychologically.
   b. Monitor airway, breathing, and circulation.
   c. Provide respiratory support.
   d. Apply cooling blanket.
   e. Administer anticonvulsants.
   f. Give antipsychotics.
   g. Give ammonium chloride to acidify urine for excretion of amphetamines.

4. Signs and symptoms of withdrawal include
   a. Fatigue
   b. Depression
   c. Agitation
   d. Apathy
   e. Anxiety
   f. Insomnia
   g. Disorientation
   h. Craving

5. Interventions for withdrawal include
   a. Antianxiety medication
   b. Antidepressants
   c. Dopamine agonists to reduce tremors

Hallucinogens

- *Hallucinogens* are chemical substances that possess mind-altering or mental perception–altering properties.

LSD

- Lysergic acid ("LSD," "acid") abuse is manifested by
    1. Dilated pupils
    2. Tachycardia
    3. Palpitations
    4. Diaphoresis
    5. Tremors
    6. Poor coordination
    7. Elevated temperature; increased pulse and respiration
    8. Paranoid ideas, anxiety, and depression
    9. With overdose, brain damage, psychosis, or death
- Interventions for LSD crisis include
    1. One-to-one observation
    2. Calming environment, comfortable temperature, few disturbances
    3. Antianxiety medications
    4. Other medications to control symptoms

PHENCYCLIDINE

- Phencyclidine ("PCP," "angel dust") abuse is manifested by
    1. Feeling of detachment, unawareness of surroundings
    2. Flushing, increased perspiration
    3. Aggression, incoherence
    4. Shallow respirations
    5. Generalized numbness of the extremities
    6. Vomiting
    7. Loss of balance
    8. Visual disturbances
    9. Seizures, coma, death
    10. Lasting effects: memory loss, speech difficulties, and interference with thinking processes

KETAMINE

- Ketamine, a disassociate anesthetic, is referred to as a "techno" drug because of its attractiveness to the "Rave" culture. Symptoms of overdose include
    1. Tunnel vision
    2. Shortness of breath
    3. Loss of balance
    4. Numbness of the body
    5. Clinical depression

6. No sense of time
7. Seizures
8. Coma
- Interventions for ketamine abuse include
  1. Calm, stimulus-free environment
  2. Supportive therapies
  3. Respiratory support if needed

METHYLENEDIOXYMETHAMPHETAMINE

- 3,4 Methylenedioxymethamphetamine ("MDMA," "Ecstasy," "date rape drug") is an oral amphetamine that is altered to become a hallucinogen. Signs and symptoms of abuse include
  1. Development of trust in others, which eases inhibitions between people
  2. Increased confidence
  3. Euphoria
  4. Physical energy
  5. Relaxation of voluntary muscles
  6. Amnesiac effect for period in which drug is in body
  7. Confusion
  8. Depression
  9. Sleep disturbances
  10. Drug craving
  11. Severe anxiety
  12. Paranoia
  13. Nervousness
  14. Muscle tension
  15. Involuntary teeth clenching
  16. Nausea, chills, sweating
  17. Brain damage
  18. Malignant hyperthermia
- Interventions for MDA abuse
  1. Safety and relief of symptoms
  2. Medications to reduce or eliminate adverse effects of the drug

MARIJUANA

- Physical and psychological effects of marijuana use include
  1. Euphoria, happiness
  2. Relaxation

3. Increased heart rate
4. Impaired short-term memory
5. Paranoia
6. Restlessness
7. Anxiety or panic attacks
8. Increased appetite
9. Altered perceptions
- Withdrawal effects from marijuana include insomnia, decreased appetite, nausea, irritability, and anxiety and are treated symptomatically.

Depressants

- Benzodiazepine users can develop high tolerance causing increasing amounts to be needed to achieve desired feelings.

ROHYPNOL

- *Rohypnol* ("rophies," "ruffies," "R2s," "Rib," "roach") is used to engage in destructive or violent activities without feelings of guilt.
  1. Effects of drug include
     a. Relief from tension
     b. Anticonvulsant action
     c. Sedation
     d. Amnesia
     e. Muscle relaxation
     f. Slowing of motor performance
     g. Loss of inhibition
     h. Dizziness
     i. Tranquility
     j. Slurred speech
  2. Signs and symptoms of withdrawal from Rohypnol include
     a. Headache
     b. Muscle pain
     c. Extreme anxiety
     d. Tension and restlessness
     e. Confusion and irritability
     f. Depersonalization
     g. Hypersensitivity to light, noise, and physical contact
     h. Delirium
     i. Respiratory depression
     j. Cardiovascular collapse

3. Interventions are directed toward treating signs and symptoms.

GAMMA HYDROXYBUTYRATE

- Gamma hydroxybutyrate ("GHB," "liquid ecstasy") reduces social inhibitions and increases libido.
  1. Signs and symptoms of abuse include
     a. Euphoria
     b. Anxiety
     c. Increased sexual pleasure
     d. Impaired judgment
     e. Loss of coordination
     f. Loss of inhibition
  2. Signs and symptoms of overdose include
     a. Respiratory depression
     b. Memory loss
     c. Bradycardia
     d. Muscular fatigue
     e. Coma
  3. Interventions to treat overdose include
     a. Careful assessment and measures based on signs and symptoms
     b. Psychological support and nonjudgmental communications
     c. Client may be fearful and respond in various behaviors.

BARBITURATES

- Barbiturates depress the central nervous system causing sedation, drowsiness, and decreased motor activity. Dependence can occur in a short time and lead to withdrawal systems if discontinued abruptly.
  1. Withdrawal symptoms include
     a. Nausea, vomiting, abdominal cramping
     b. Seizures
     c. Varied behavioral responses
  2. Symptoms of overdose include
     a. Respiratory depression
     b. Coma
     c. Pinpoint pupils
  3. Interventions are based on signs and symptoms.

ALCOHOL

- *Alcoholism* (alcohol dependence syndrome) is a disease in which the person has a strong need or compulsion to consume alcohol, is unable to quit once drinking begins, experiences physical dependence, and has a need to increase the amount of alcohol to get "high."
- *Alcohol abuse* exists when a person does not have a strong craving for alcohol, loss of control, or physical dependence, but does have problems related to alcohol use.
- Blood alcohol levels
  1. 80–200 mg/dL: mild to moderate intoxication manifested by mood and behavior changes, impaired judgment, poor motor coordination, and hypertension
  2. 250–400 mg/dL: marked intoxication manifested by the above plus staggering ataxia and emotional lability, which may progress to confusion, stupor, or coma
  3. Greater than 500 mg/dL: severe intoxication manifested by respiratory depression, which may lead to death
- Alcohol withdrawal
  1. Mild: manifested by restlessness, anxiety, sleeping difficulties, agitation, tremors, tachycardia, low-grade fever, diaphoresis, and elevated blood pressure
  2. Major: in addition to mild signs and symptoms, manifested by visual or auditory hallucinations, delirium tremens (DTs), tachycardia, increased diastolic blood pressure, pronounced diaphoresis, and vomiting
  3. Life-threatening DTs: disorientation, global confusion, and inability to recognize familiar objects or people. This is a medical emergency.
- Interventions for alcohol withdrawal
  1. Focus on preventing client from harming self or others.
  2. Reorient client to reality, creating a low-stimulation environment.
  3. Give medications, as ordered, such as diazepam, anticonvulsants, pain relievers, IV fluids, and vitamins. Diet is determined in collaboration with the dietitian.
  4. Provide emotional support.

Opiates

- Manifestations of opiate intoxication
  1. Constricted pupils
  2. Decreased blood pressure
  3. Decreased respirations
  4. Drowsiness
  5. Slurred speech
  6. Initial euphoria followed by dysphoria (depression)
  7. Cognitive impairments resulting in judgment and memory losses
- Manifestations of opiate withdrawal
  1. Yawning
  2. Insomnia
  3. Irritability
  4. Rhinorrhea
  5. Diaphoresis
  6. Abdominal cramps
  7. Nausea and vomiting
  8. Muscle aches
  9. Chills, cold flashes with goose bumps (referred to as "cold turkey")
- Manifestations of opiate overdose
  1. Dilated pupils
  2. Respiratory depression
  3. Coma
  4. Shock
  5. Convulsions
  6. Respiratory arrest
  7. Death
- Interventions for opiate overdose
  1. Medications such as anticonvulsants, opioid antagonists, and antianxiety agents
  2. Vital signs and neurologic checks
  3. Supportive measures

INHALANT ABUSE

- Inhalant abuse ("glue," "kick," "bang," "huffing," "poppers," "whippets," "sniff," "Texas Shoe-shine")
  1. Commonly abused inhalants include
     a. Solvents such as paint thinners, gasoline, glues, felt tip markers

b. Gases such as butane lighters, propane tanks, hair spray, or other sprays

   c. Nitrates such as cyclohexyl nitrite, amyl nitrite, and butyl nitrite

2. Signs of inhalant use include

   a. Slurred speech

   b. Drunk, dizzy, or dazed appearance

   c. Chemical smell on the person

   d. Paint stains on body or face

   e. Red eyes

   f. Rhinorrhea

3. Treatment is based on presenting symptoms and supportive care.

Discharge Planning for Substance Abuse

- Referral to drug treatment program
- Referral to social services
- Referral to community agencies

Nursing Care to Promote Sexual Health

OVERVIEW

- Sexual health includes one's freedom from physical and psychological impairment, the awareness of open and positive attitudes toward sexual functioning, and accurate knowledge of sexuality.
- *Homosexuality* is erotic attraction to persons of the same sex.
- *Bisexuality* refers to a preference for intimate relationships with members of either sex.
- A person who is *transsexual* is completely dissatisfied with his or her gender assignment and is convinced that he or she is trapped within the wrong body; sex reassignment surgery may be performed.
- A *transvestite* wears clothes associated with the opposite sex for the sake of sexual arousal, but there is no conflict about

his or her gender; cross-dressing occurs more frequently in men than in women.

- *Pedophilia* is a sexual preference for children and is considered to be a psychiatric disorder.

||| Cultural Considerations

- ◆ Cultural or religious background may influence a person's willingness to discuss sexual health.

COLLABORATIVE MANAGEMENT

Assessment

- Record client information.
  1. Injury or disease of the genitourinary system
  2. Contraceptive use
  3. Development of secondary sex characteristics
  4. Unwanted or traumatic sexual events such as rape
  5. Changes of sexual functioning related to drug or alcohol use
  6. Changes in sexual functioning since the current illness, injury, or surgery
  7. Current physical condition causing the change in body image
  8. Changes in usual activities and roles
  9. Changes in beliefs and practices about sexual functioning that have occurred as a result of illness
- Assess for
  1. Changes in external genitalia and breasts (e.g., thickening of or discharge from genitalia or breasts)
  2. Dyspareunia (painful intercourse)
  3. Inhibited sexual desire: loss of interest in sexual activity or decline in libido
  4. Vaginismus: powerful contraction of the muscles of the outer third of the vaginal barrel, preventing insertion of a tampon or other object
  5. Orgasmic dysfunction: the inability to achieve orgasm (primary dysfunction) or to achieve orgasm with intercourse or at an appropriate time during intercourse (secondary dysfunction)

6. Erectile dysfunction: the inability to attain or maintain an erection of the penis of sufficient firmness to permit penetration
7. Ejaculatory dysfunction, premature: ejaculation after penetration but sooner than either partner desires
8. Retrograde ejaculation, or dry orgasm: semen discharged into the urinary bladder
9. Sexual aversion: irrational fear or phobic reaction to the thought of sexual activity or to the actual activity
10. Psychological and social factors related to past and present functioning

Planning and Implementation

◆**NDx:** Sexual Dysfunction: Dyspareunia

- In females, dyspareunia may be related to
  1. An intact hymen: refer the client to a gynecologist or nurse practitioner.
  2. Scarring from an episiotomy or pathologic conditions of the reproductive organs: refer the client to a gynecologist or nurse practitioner.
  3. Infections of the vagina or vulva
     a. Explain methods to decrease risk of infection.
     b. Administer drug therapy such as antibiotics.
     c. Teach the client to avoid sexual intercourse until the infection is resolved.
     d. Encourage the client to rest and to increase fluid intake.
  4. Insufficient vaginal lubrication: instruct the client to use a water-soluble lubricant before sexual activity or intercourse.
  5. Irritation from chemical products such as contraceptives or douches
     a. Instruct the client to avoid excessive use of these products or to stop their use completely.
     b. Encourage the use of products without scents.
  6. Psychogenic factors: refer the client to a competent therapist.
- In males, dyspareunia may be related to
  1. Inflammation or infection of the organs within the genitourinary system.
     a. Administer prescribed antibiotics.
     b. Encourage the client to drink fluids and to rest.

    c. Teach the client to avoid sexual intercourse until the acute condition is resolved.

  2. Exposure to vaginal contraceptive cream, jelly, or foam, or irritation from an intrauterine device: provide information and alternatives to the client and his sexual partner.

  3. Psychosocial factors: refer the client to a competent therapist.

◆NDx: Sexual Dysfunction: Vaginismus and Orgasmic Dysfunction

- Interventions for the client with sexual dysfunction include
  1. Identifying and relieving underlying psychogenic factors, such as rape trauma syndrome, conflicts surrounding homosexual experimentation, or strong religious teachings
    a. Encourage the client to express feelings of anxiety and conflict, if present.
    b. Refer the client to a competent therapist.
  2. Helping to identify and relieve underlying physical factors such as sexual activity too soon after childbirth, abnormality of the hymen, or atrophy of the vagina
    a. Refer the client to a gynecologist or nurse practitioner.
    b. Encourage the client to explore alternatives to vaginal intercourse during the healing process.
    c. Explain the relationship between physical factors and involuntary muscular response.
- Help the client with orgasmic dysfunction by
  1. Referring the client to a gynecologist or nurse practitioner
  2. Instructing the client in the performance of Kegel exercises
  3. Giving the client permission to talk about the problem
  4. Providing information about the relationship between stressors and the physical response of orgasm
  5. Referring the client to a therapist who specializes in treating sexual disorders

◆NDx: Sexual Dysfunction: Erectile Dysfunction, Premature Ejaculation, Dysfunctional or Retrograde Ejaculation

- Erectile dysfunction may be related to
  1. Spinal cord injury
  2. Diabetes mellitus

3. Alcoholism
4. Neurologic disease
5. Infections of the genitourinary system
6. Drug use or abuse
7. Psychogenic factors
- Interventions include
  1. Referring the client to a urologist or competent therapist, as appropriate
  2. Instructing the client and his partner in "sensate focus" technique
- For the client with premature ejaculation
  1. Educate the client and his partner about the relationship between emotions and the sexual response cycle.
  2. Teach systematic relaxation exercises.
- When the client's problem is retrograde ejaculation
  1. Refer the client to a urologist.
  2. Assist the client with coping skills and provide education and counseling.

Community-Based Care

- Teach the importance of follow-up visits with the physicians and other therapists.

PART TWO

DISEASES
and
DISORDERS

Abscess, Anorectal

OVERVIEW

- Anorectal abscesses result from obstruction of the ducts of glands in the anorectal region by feces, foreign bodies, or trauma.
- Stasis of the obstructing contents results in infection that spreads into adjacent tissue.

COLLABORATIVE MANAGEMENT

- Rectal pain is the first clinical manifestation.
- Local swelling, erythema, and tenderness on palpation appear a few days after the onset of pain.
- The diagnosis is made by physical examination and history.
- Simple perianal and ischiorectal abscesses can be excised and drained with local anesthesia.
- Clients with more extensive abscesses require incision under regional or general anesthesia.
- Interventions include
    1. Giving systemic antibiotics only to clients who are immunocompromised or who have diabetes, valvular disease or prostheses, or extensive cellulitis
    2. Assisting the client to maintain comfort and optimal perineal hygiene by providing warm sitz baths, analgesics, bulk-forming agents, and stool softeners, as ordered
    3. Emphasizing the importance of ongoing perineal hygiene and the maintenance of a regular bowel pattern with a high-fiber diet

Abscess, Brain

OVERVIEW

- A brain abscess is a purulent infection of the brain in which pus forms in the extradural, subdural, or intracerebral area.
- The number of clients with a brain abscess secondary to immunosuppression, organ transplantation, and acquired immunodeficiency syndrome (AIDS) has rapidly increased over the past two decades.
- The causative organisms are most often bacteria, such as *Streptococcus* and *Staphylococcus*.
- Most brain abscesses occur in the frontal and temporal lobes.

COLLABORATIVE MANAGEMENT

- A brain abscess is typically manifested by symptoms of a mass and of mildly increased intracranial pressure, including
  1. Headache
  2. Fever
  3. Focal neurologic deficits
  4. Lethargy and confusion
  5. Visual field deficits
  6. Nystagmus and dysconjugate gaze
  7. Generalized weakness, hemiparesis
  8. Ataxic gait
  9. Seizures
  10. Varying degrees of aphasia if frontal or temporal lobe abscess
  11. Elevated white blood cell (WBC) count
  12. Elevated erythrocyte sedimentation rate
- Drug therapy includes
  1. Antibiotics
  2. Metronidazole (Flagyl, Novonidazol) if an anaerobic organism is the causative agent
  3. Antiepileptic drugs, as ordered, to prevent or treat seizures
  4. Analgesics, as ordered, to treat the client's headache
- Surgical drainage of an encapsulated abscess or a craniotomy may be performed.

Abscess, Hepatic

- Hepatic (liver) abscesses occur when the liver is invaded by bacteria or protozoa.
- Liver tissue is destroyed, producing a necrotic cavity filled with infected agents, liquefied liver cells and tissue, and leukocytes.
- Liver abscess occurs infrequently and is associated with a high mortality rate.
- Pyrogenic abscesses are caused by bacteria such as *Escherichia coli, Klebsiella, Enterobacter, Salmonella, Staphylococcus,* and *Enterococcus.*
- Abscesses can result following acute cholangitis, liver trauma, peritonitis, or sepsis, or an abscess can extend to the liver after pneumonia or bacterial endocarditis.
- Amebic hepatic abscesses occur following amebic dysentery as a single abscess in the right upper quadrant of the liver.

COLLABORATIVE MANAGEMENT

- Assessment findings include
  1. Right upper quadrant abdominal pain
  2. Tender, palpable liver
  3. Anorexia
  4. Weight loss
  5. Nausea and vomiting
  6. Fever and chills
  7. Shoulder pain
  8. Dyspnea
  9. Pleural pain if the diaphragm is involved
- Hepatic abscesses are usually diagnosed by contrast-enhanced computed tomography (CT) scan or ultrasound.
- Abscesses may be drained under CT or ultrasound guidance. Drainage is sent for laboratory analysis so optimal antibiotic treatment can be selected.

Abscess, Lung

- A lung abscess is a localized area of lung destruction caused by liquefaction necrosis, which is usually related to pyogenic bacteria.

COLLABORATIVE MANAGEMENT

- Assessment findings include
  1. History of influenza
  2. Pneumonia
  3. Febrile illness
  4. Cough and foul-smelling sputum production
  5. Decreased breath sounds
  6. Bronchial breath sounds, crackles
  8. Fatigue, cachectic
  7. Abnormal chest x-ray examination results
- Nursing diagnoses and interventions are similar to those for pneumonia.
- Medical treatment is directed toward drainage of the abscess and antibiotics.

Abscess, Pancreatic

- A pancreatic abscess consists of infected, necrotic pancreatic tissue.
- Pancreatic abscess usually occurs after severe acute pancreatitis, exacerbations of chronic pancreatitis, and biliary tract surgery.
- The problem may occur as a single abscess or multiloculated abscesses resulting from extensive inflammatory necrosis of the pancreas readily invaded by infectious organisms such as *Escherichia coli, Klebsiella, Bacteroides, Staphylococcus,* and *Proteus.*
- Temperature spikes may be as high as 104° F (40° C).

- The mortality rate is 100% if the abscess is not surgically drained; multiple drainage procedures are often required.
- Antibiotic therapy alone does not resolve the abscess.
- Pleural effusions often accompany the abscess.

Abscess, Peritonsillar

- Peritonsillar abscess is a complication of acute tonsillitis.
- Acute infection spreads from the tonsil to the surrounding peritonsillar tissue, forming an abscess.
- The common cause is group A beta-hemolytic *Streptococcus*.
- One sided swelling and deviation of the uvula from pus collection cause difficult swallowing, drooling, severe throat pain radiating to the ear, dysphagia, voice change, trismus, and difficulty breathing.
- Treatment includes
  1. Warm saline gargles or irrigations
  2. Ice collar
  3. Analgesics
  4. Antibiotics
  5. Incision and drainage of the abscess
  6. Tonsillectomy after healing

Abscess, Renal

- A renal abscess is a collection of fluid and cells resulting from an inflammatory response to bacteria in the renal parenchyma, renal fascia, or flank.
- An abscess is suspected when fever and symptoms are unresponsive to antibiotic therapy.
- Symptoms include
  1. Fever
  2. Flank pain

3. General malaise
   4. Local edema
- Treatment includes
   1. Broad-spectrum antibiotics
   2. Drainage by surgical incision or needle aspiration

Achalasia

OVERVIEW

- Achalasia is an esophageal motility disorder in which the lower esophageal sphincter (LES) fails to relax properly with swallowing and the normal peristalsis of the esophagus is replaced with abnormal contractions.
- Clinical manifestations include progressively worsening dysphagia as evidenced by chronic and vague complaints of difficulty swallowing and of food sticking in the throat.

COLLABORATIVE MANAGEMENT

Assessment

- Record client information.
   1. Symptoms, including dysphagia, chest pain, regurgitation, and halitosis (foul mouth odor)
   2. Factors that aggravate the symptoms, such as position or diet
   3. Home treatments that relieve the symptoms, including over-the-counter drugs
   4. History of previous esophageal trauma or surgery
   5. Respiratory history and current respiratory-associated symptoms
   6. Nutritional history, including diet habits, food intolerance, nutritional status, and weight loss
   7. Results of the barium swallow, which usually show a narrow "bird's-beak" junction at the esophageal hiatus and esophageal dilation above the junction

NONSURGICAL MANAGEMENT

- A combination of dietary measures, medication, esophageal dilation, and surgery may be used.
  1. Teach the client to avoid foods or habits that aggravate symptoms.
  2. Encourage the client to experiment with diet changes, including semisoft foods, warm foods, and liquids that may be better tolerated.
  3. Teach the client to eat four to six small meals per day instead of three large meals.
  4. Advise the client to experiment with various changes in position while eating because these changes can reduce pressure sensation during meals.
  5. Drug therapy is given for symptom relief and is not recommended as an alternative to more definitive therapy.
     a. Calcium channel blockers or nitrates to reduce LES
     b. Botulism toxin (Botox) injected directly into the LES muscle to denervate cholinergic nerves in the distal esophagus by suppression of acetylcholine release
  6. Instruct the client to sleep with the head of the bed elevated on blocks or reclining in a semi-sitting position.

SURGICAL MANAGEMENT

- Surgery may be necessary and is aimed at facilitating food passage by dilating the unrelaxed esophageal sphincter or destroying the sphincter by esophagomyotomy.
- *Esophageal dilation* for achalasia is performed under local anesthesia with a pneumatized dilator (a pressurized bag filled with water). After the procedure
  1. Monitor the client for complications of bleeding and signs of perforation such as chest and shoulder pain, elevated temperature, subcutaneous emphysema, or hemoptysis.
  2. Instruct the client to take nothing by mouth for 1 hour and to consume only liquids for 24 hours after the procedure.
- An *esophagomyotomy* is performed to obliterate the sphincter and requires a thoracotomy approach to expose the

esophagus. Muscle fibers are cut to open the esophagus to provide less obstruction for food passage.

■ Nursing care for the client undergoing esophagomyotomy is similar to that described for thoracotomy under Cancer, Lung.

Acidosis, Metabolic

OVERVIEW

■ Metabolic acidosis is characterized by a low pH, low bicarbonate level, normal partial pressure of arterial carbon dioxide ($PaCO_2$), normal oxygen tension, elevated serum potassium level, elevated serum chloride level, acid access, and high anion gap.
■ Common causes include
  1. Overproduction of hydrogen ions
     a. Diabetic ketoacidosis
     b. Starvation
     c. Heavy exercise
     d. Fever
     e. Hypoxia, ischemia
     f. Ethanol, methanol, or ethylene glycol intoxication
     g. Salicylate intoxication
  2. Underelimination of hydrogen ions (renal failure)
  3. Underproduction of bicarbonate ions (liver failure, pancreatitis, dehydration)
  4. Overelimination of bicarbonate ions
     a. Diarrhea
     b. Buffering of organic acids

COLLABORATIVE MANAGEMENT

■ Record client information.
  1. Age
  2. Use of prescribed and over-the-counter medications, especially those containing aspirin or alcohol
  3. Current and past medical history
     a. Respiratory problems
     b. Renal failure

    c. Diabetes mellitus

    d. Pancreatitis

    e. Fever

4. Diet history, especially fasting or strict dieting the week before seeking health care

5. Behavior or personality changes

- Assessment findings include

  1. Central nervous system changes: lethargy, confusion, stupor, coma

  2. Neuromuscular changes

     a. Hyporeflexia

     b. Skeletal muscle weakness

     c. Flaccid paralysis

  3. Cardiac changes

     a. Delayed electrical conduction

        (1) Bradycardia

        (2) Tall T waves

        (3) Widened QRS complex

        (4) Prolonged PR interval

     b. Hypotension

     c. Thready peripheral pulses

  4. Respiratory changes: Kussmaul respiration (respirations that are deep, rapid, and not under voluntary control)

  5. Integumentary changes: warm, flushed, dry skin

- Metabolic acidosis is managed by

  1. Treating the underlying cause of the acid imbalance

  2. Monitoring arterial blood gas levels

  3. Administering intravenous (IV) fluids and maintaining IV access

  4. Monitoring intake and output

Acidosis, Respiratory

OVERVIEW

- An alteration in some area of respiratory function results in reducing the exchange of oxygen and carbon dioxide, which results in retention of carbon dioxide.

- Respiratory acidosis is characterized by a low pH level, elevated carbon dioxide partial pressure (PCO_2) and variable bicarbonate level, and decreased oxygen tension (PO_2).
- Elevated serum potassium levels result.
- Common causes include
  1. Respiratory depression
     a. Chemical depression
        (1) Anesthetics
        (2) Drugs
        (3) Poisons
     b. Physical depression
        (1) Trauma
        (2) Cerebral edema
        (3) Overhydration
        (4) Stroke, aneurysm
  2. Inadequate chest expansion
     a. Skeletal deformities and trauma, such as broken ribs or spinal cord injury
     b. Respiratory muscle weakness, such as muscular dystrophy
     c. Nonrespiratory conditions
        (1) Obesity
        (2) Abdominal or thoracic masses
        (3) Ascites
        (4) Hemothorax or pneumothorax
  3. Airway obstruction that may be due to regional lymph node involvement, asthma, emphysema, tight clothing
  4. Reduced alveolar-capillary diffusion
     a. Atelectasis
     b. Acute respiratory distress syndrome
     c. Chest trauma
     d. Emphysema
     e. Pneumonia
     f. Pulmonary edema
     g. Pulmonary emboli
     h. Tuberculosis

Considerations for Older Adults

- The older adult is more susceptible than the younger adult to acid-base imbalance secondary to cardiac, renal, or pulmonary problems.
- Medications that interfere with acid-base balance and fluid and electrolyte balance include diuretics, aspirin, and alcohol.

COLLABORATIVE MANAGEMENT

Assessment

- Record client information.
  1. Age
  2. Prescribed and over-the-counter medications, especially those containing aspirin or alcohol
  3. Current and past medical history
     a. Respiratory problems
     b. Renal failure
     c. Diabetes mellitus
     d. Pancreatitis
     e. Fever
  4. Diet history
  5. Behavior or personality changes
- Assessment findings include
  1. Central nervous system changes
     a. Lethargy, confusion, stupor
     b. Depression
  2. Neuromuscular changes
     a. Hyporeflexia
     b. Skeletal muscle weakness
     c. Flaccid paralysis
  3. Cardiac changes
     a. Delayed electrical conduction
        (1) Bradycardia
        (2) Tall T waves
        (3) Widened QRS complex
        (4) Prolonged PR interval
     b. Hypotension
     c. Thready peripheral pulses

4. Respiratory changes
   a. Diminished respiratory efforts
   b. Shallow and rapid respirations
5. Integumentary changes: pale to cyanotic skin

- Treat respiratory acidosis.
  1. Perform a respiratory assessment every 2 hours or more often as indicated by the client's clinical condition, including
     a. Rate and depth of respirations
     b. Auscultation of breath sounds
     c. Ease with which the client moves air in and out of the lungs
     d. Presence of retractions
  2. Administer drugs to increase the diameter of the upper and lower airway and thin pulmonary secretions and improve gas exchange, such as albuterol (Novo-Salmol, Proventil) or salbutamol (Ventolin).
  3. Administer drugs that increase bronchodilation by reducing inflammation of bronchial luminal tissues such as beclomethasone (Vanceril) or dexamethasone (Dexasone).
  4. Administer medication to thin bronchial secretions such as acetylcysteine (Mucomyst, Mucosil).
  5. Administer nebulized oxygen cautiously, particularly if the client has chronic airway limitation and carbon dioxide narcosis.
  6. Place the client in the Fowler or semi-Fowler's position.
  7. Monitor for respiratory compromise.
     a. Examine nail beds and mucous membranes for color.
     b. Assess breath sounds.

Acute Respiratory Distress Syndrome

OVERVIEW

- Acute respiratory distress syndrome (ARDS) is a form of acute respiratory failure characterized by refractory hypoxemia, decreased pulmonary compliance, dyspnea, noncardiac-associated bilateral pulmonary edema, and the presence of pulmonary infiltrates.

- The major site of injury in the lung is the alveolar capillary membrane.
- Interstitial edema causes compression and obliteration of terminal airways, thereby reducing lung volume and lung compliance.
- Causes include serious nervous system injury, trauma, shock, sepsis, near-drowning, hemolytic disorders, drug ingestion, inhalation of toxic gases, pulmonary infections, pancreatitis, burns, fat and amniotic fluid emboli, pulmonary infections, pulmonary aspiration, multiple blood transfusions, and cardiopulmonary bypass.
- Some factors produce ARDS by direct injury to the lung such as aspiration of gastric contents, which leads to mechanical obstruction or produces an acid burn to the airway when the pH level of the gastric contents is less than 2.5.
- Clients have a rapidly deteriorating respiratory status with increased work of breathing and deteriorating blood gas levels; hypoxemia persists despite high concentrations of oxygen.
- A major goal in the prevention of ARDS is early recognition of the client who is at high risk for the syndrome.

COLLABORATIVE MANAGEMENT

Assessment

- Assessment findings include
    1. Respirations (rate and quality); usually increased work of breathing as indicated by hyperpnea, grunting respirations, and suprasternal or intercostal retractions
    2. Cyanosis
    3. Pallor
    4. Diaphoresis
    5. Mental status changes
    6. Lung sounds, which are typically normal because edema is in the interstitial spaces, not the airways
    7. Hypotension
    8. Tachycardia
    9. Dysrhythmias

10. Lowered arterial PO_2
11. Haziness or "white out" appearance on chest x-ray film
12. Normal to low pulmonary capillary wedge pressure (diagnostic tool to differentiate ARDS from cardiogenic pulmonary edema in which pressure is high)

Interventions

- The course of ARDS and its management are divided into four phases.

  Phase 1: This phase includes early changes with the client exhibiting dyspnea and tachypnea. Support the client and provide oxygen.

  Phase 2: Patchy infiltrates form from increasing pulmonary edema. Interventions include endotracheal intubation and mechanical ventilation with positive end-expiratory pressure (PEEP) and continuous positive airway pressure, and prevention of complications. Assess lung sounds to monitor for the development of tension pneumothorax, a side effect of PEEP. Sedation and paralysis may be necessary for adequate ventilation and for reducing oxygen requirements.

  Phase 3: This phase occurs over 2 to 10 days and the client exhibits progressive refractory hypoxemia. Interventions focus on maintaining adequate oxygen transport, preventing complications, and supporting the failing lung until it has had time to heal.

  Phase 4: Pulmonary fibrosis pneumonia with progression occurs after 10 days. Interventions focus on preventing sepsis, pneumonia, and multiple organ dysfunction syndrome, as well as weaning the client from the ventilator. Antibiotics are given to treat infections identified by culture, and diuretics may be given to decrease lung edema.

- Intravenous fluid volume is titrated to maintain adequate cardiac output and tissue perfusion.
- Nutritional status is monitored and enteral or parenteral nutrition may be initiated.

AIDS

OVERVIEW

- Acquired immunodeficiency syndrome (AIDS) is the late stage of a continuum of symptoms that results from infection with the human immunodeficiency virus (HIV), a retrovirus.
- HIV is transmitted in three ways:
  1. Sexual: genital anal or oral sexual contact with exposure of mucous membranes to infected semen or vaginal secretions
  2. Parenteral: sharing needles or equipment contaminated with infected blood or receiving contaminated blood products
  3. Perinatal: through the placenta from contact with maternal blood and body fluids during birth, or from breast milk from an infected mother to child
- Needle stick or "sharps" injuries are the primary means of HIV infection for health care workers. Infection also occurs through exposure of nonintact skin and mucous membranes to blood and body fluids.
- Not everyone who has an HIV infection has AIDS.
- A diagnosis of AIDS requires that the client be HIV-positive and have *either*
  1. A CD4+ cell count of less than 200 cells/mm^3

     or
  2. An opportunistic infection
- A person with HIV infection can transmit the virus to others at all stages of the disease.
- HIV infection results in immune system dysfunctions.
  1. Lymphocytopenia (decreased number of lymphocytes)
  2. Increased production of incomplete and nonfunctional antibodies
  3. Abnormally functioning macrophages
- As a result of these immune system dysfunctions, the client is susceptible to bacterial, fungal, and viral infections (opportunistic infections) and some cancers.
- Opportunistic infections are those caused by organisms that are present as part of the normal environment and are kept in check by normal immune function.

- The time from the beginning HIV infection to development of AIDS ranges from several months to years. The range depends on
  1. How HIV was acquired
  2. Personal factors such as frequency of re-exposure to HIV, presence of other sexually transmitted diseases, nutritional factors, pregnancy, and stress
  3. Interventions

 ## Genetic Considerations

- Long-term nonprogressors (LTNP) are clients with HIV infection for more than 10 years, who are asymptomatic and have CD4+ cell counts within a normal range. This population has a mutation of CCR5 receptors, forming a CCR5Δ32 receptor, which resists the entrance of HIV.
- Epidemiologic and demographic data have shown that most people with AIDS in the United States are men who have had sex with other men or persons of either sex who have used injection drugs.
- Women and minorities are the fastest-growing group with HIV infection and AIDS.

 ## Women's Health Considerations

- Women with HIV infection appear to have a poorer outcome with shorter survival time than men with HIV infection.
- Gynecologic symptoms, particularly persistent or recurrent vaginal candida infections, may be the first sign of HIV infection.
- Most women with HIV infection are of childbearing age; the effects on pregnancy are not known.

 ## Considerations for Older Adults

- Assess older adults for risk factors including sexual history and drug use history.
- Decline in immune factor may increase the risk for HIV infection.

Assessment

- Assessment findings include
  1. Immunologic manifestations
     a. Low white blood cell (WBC) count
     b. Hypergammaglobulinemia
     c. Opportunistic infections
     d. Lymphadenopathy
     e. Fatigue
  2. Integumentary manifestations
     a. Dry skin
     b. Poor wound healing
     c. Skin lesions
     d. Night sweats
  3. Respiratory manifestations
     a. Shortness of breath
     b. Cough
  4. Gastrointestinal manifestations
     a. Diarrhea
     b. Weight loss
     c. Nausea and vomiting
  5. Central nervous system manifestations
     a. Confusion
     b. AIDS dementia complex
     c. Fever
     d. Headache
     e. Visual changes
     f. Memory loss
     g. Personality changes
     h. Pain
     i. Peripheral neuropathies
     j. Gait changes, ataxia
     k. Seizures
  6. Abnormal laboratory findings
     a. Decreased T4 cells
     b. Positive ELISA (enzyme-linked immunosorbent assay) and Western blot analysis
     c. Positive quantitative ribonucleic acid (RNA) analysis
     d. Leukopenia

7. Opportunistic infections
    a. Protozoal infections
        (1) *Pneumocystis carinii* pneumonia (PCP)
        (2) Toxoplasmosis
        (3) Cryptosporidiosis
    b. Fungal infections
        (1) *Candida*
        (2) *Cryptococcosis*
        (3) *Histoplasmosis*
    c. Bacterial infections
        (1) *Mycobacterium avium*-intracellulare complex infection
        (2) Tuberculosis
    d. Viral infections
        (1) Cytomegalovirus infection
        (2) Herpes simplex virus infection
        (3) Varicella zoster virus infection
    d. Malignancies
        (1) Kaposi's sarcoma
        (2) Hodgkin's lymphoma
        (3) Non-Hodgkin's lymphoma
        (4) Invasive cervical carcinoma
    e. Endocrine complications
        (1) Gonadal dysfunction
        (2) Body shape changes
        (3) Adrenal insufficiency
        (4) Diabetes mellitus
8. Availability of a support system, such as family and significant others
    a. Learn who in this support system is aware of the client's diagnosis.
    b. Identify whether there is a health care proxy or a durable power of attorney has been signed, if appropriate.
9. Employment, activities of daily living (ADLs)
10. Social activities and hobbies
11. Self-esteem and body image changes
12. Suicidal ideation, depression
13. Involvement with community resources or support groups

Planning and Implementation

NDx: Risk for Infection

- Clients with HIV are at high risk for *opportunistic* infections.
- Administer medication as prescribed for specific infection and monitor for adverse effects.
- Monitor for systemic and localized signs of infection.
- Monitor WBC count (differential, T4/T8 ratios, and viral load test).
- Follow neutropenic precautions as indicated.
- Screen all visitors for communicable disease.
- Inspect skin and mucous membranes for redness, warmth, drainage, and presence of fissures or abscesses.
- Obtain cultures as needed.
- Promote sufficient nutritional intake.
- Monitor for changes in energy level, malaise, and fatigue.
- Encourage activity at appropriate level for client's current health status.
- Instruct client to take medication as prescribed.
- Research is being conducted to determine the effectiveness, if any, of therapies such as bone marrow transplantation and lymphocyte transfusion.
- Teach client and family how to avoid infections.
- Perform interventions for the client who is immuno-suppressed.
    1. Place the client in a private room when possible.
    2. Keep frequently used equipment in the room for use by the client only (blood pressure cuff, stethoscope, thermometer).
    3. Change intravenous tubing daily.
    4. Change wound dressings daily.
    5. Use strict aseptic technique for all invasive procedures.
    6. Avoid the use of indwelling urinary catheters.
    7. Keep fresh flowers and potted plants out of the client's room.
    8. Do not use supplies from common areas for immuno-suppressed clients; for example, keep a supply of paper cups in the client's room, and do not share this supply with any other client; other articles include gloves and dressing materials.

9. Monitor body temperature: minor temperature elevation may suggest early infection.
- Drug therapy for HIV/AIDS continues to change as the result of intense research.
- Antiretroviral therapy only inhibits viral replication and does not kill the virus.
  1. Multiple drugs are used together called "cocktails"; this approach is termed highly active antiretroviral therapy (HAART).
  2. Nucleoside analogue reverse transcriptase inhibitors (NRTIs) suppress production of reverse transcriptase and inhibit DNA synthesis and genetic reproduction.
  3. Non-nucleoside reverse transcriptase inhibitors (NNRTIs) inhibit synthesis of the enzyme reverse transcriptase.
  4. Protease inhibitors block the HIV protease enzyme, preventing viral replication and release of viral particles.
  5. Fusion inhibitors work by blocking the fusion of HIV with a host cell. Without fusion, infection of new cells does not occur.
- Drawbacks to HIV/AIDS drug therapy includes expense of drugs, side effects, food and timing requirements, and number of daily drugs needed.

◆**NDx:** Impaired Gas Exchange

- Nursing interventions include
  1. Assessing respiratory status frequently
  2. Monitoring arterial blood gases
  3. Providing oxygen and room humidification
  4. Performing chest physiotherapy
  5. Encouraging fluid intake as tolerated
  6. Elevating the head of the bed to facilitate breathing
  7. Helping the client pace activities to minimize shortness of breath
  8. Administering antipyretics to reduce fever
  9. Assisting with ADLs as needed
  10. Administering trimethoprim-sulfamethoxazole (Apo-Sulfatrim, Bactrim, Cotrim), pentamidine (Pentam, Pentacarinat), dapsone (Avlosulfon), and atovaquone (Mepron), as ordered, for PCP.

◆**NDx:** Acute Pain

- Pain relief measures include
  1. Providing a pressure-relieving mattress pad
  2. Providing warm baths or other forms of hydrotherapy
  3. Giving a massage
  4. Applying heat or cold to the painful area
  5. Taking care when moving and repositioning the client; use lift sheets to reposition the client.
- The type of drug used to relieve pain is dependent on the cause of the pain.
- Complementary and alternative therapies such as guided imagery, distraction, progressive relaxation techniques, and biofeedback may be used to control pain.

◆**NDx:** Imbalanced Nutrition: Less than Body Requirements

- Interdisciplinary treatment for this nursing diagnosis includes
  1. Determining the exact cause of the nutritional problems
  2. Obtaining a calorie count and recording the client's intake and output
  3. Weighing the client daily
  4. Providing small frequent meals or snacks that are high calorie, high protein, low microbial, and nutritionally sound
  5. Assessing the client's food preferences and dietary, cultural, and religious practices and helping the client select foods to meet these needs
  6. Giving enteral or parenteral feedings if needed
  7. Providing meticulous mouth care and assisting the client to rinse the mouth with sodium bicarbonate and normal saline; providing the client with a soft toothbrush, and intervening to treat mouth pain
  8. Administering supplemental vitamins as needed
  9. Administering ketoconazole (Nizoral), fluconazole (Diflucan), or amphotericin B, as ordered. Monitor for side effects that may further alter nutritional status.

◆**NDx:** Diarrhea

- Nursing interventions include
  1. Administering diphenoxylate hydrochloride (Lomotil, Diarsed ✦), as prescribed, to control diarrhea

2. Collaborating with the dietitian to provide a diet low in roughage and with less fatty, spicy, and sweet food. Alcohol, dairy products, and caffeine should be avoided.
3. Providing the client with a bedside commode or bedpan as needed

◆NDx: Impaired Skin Integrity

- Kaposi's sarcoma is the most common skin lesion.
  1. Lesions may be localized or widespread; monitor for progression.
  2. Treatment is with local radiation therapy, intralesional chemotherapy, or cryotherapy.
  3. Treat with chemotherapy with interferon-alpha or interferon-alpha plus zidovudine.
  4. Large lesions may cause pain and restrict movement and ambulation.
- Avoid pressure on lesions (use egg crate, air, or water mattress).
- Use careful hygienic measures.
- Provide meticulous skin care.
- Document pain score and provide appropriated medications.
- Minimize changes in appearance by the use of makeup, long-sleeved shirts, and hats.
- Note that herpes simplex virus abscess is also a commonly seen skin lesion in clients with HIV infection.
- If an abscess occurs, clean it with normal saline or a diluted solution of povidone-iodine and leave it open to the air or use a heat lamp to help it dry.
- Administer drug therapy, as ordered, with acyclovir (Zovirax), which is potentially toxic to the kidneys; thus the client must maintain adequate hydration.
- Give analgesics, assist with positioning, and provide other comfort measures.
- Implement wound and skin precautions.

◆NDx: Disturbed Thought Processes

- Nursing interventions include
  1. Establishing baseline neurologic and mental status
  2. Evaluating subtle changes in memory, ability to concentrate, affect, and behavior

3. Observing for and reporting changes in behavior that may be related to the loss and psychological stress experienced by the client

4. Assisting with ADLs, as needed
5. Reorienting the client to the environment; using calendars, clocks, and radios; and putting the bed near the window if possible
6. Pacing the client's activities, giving simple directions, and using short and uncomplicated sentences
7. Teaching the family and significant others techniques to use to help orient the client, such as bringing in familiar items from home
8. Making the environment safe and comfortable
9. Administering psychotropic, antidepressant, and anxiolytic medications as prescribed

◆**NDx:** Risk for Situational Low Self-Esteem

- Self-esteem is affected by changes in appearance, relationships with others, day-to-day activities, job performance, and possibly by guilt about lifestyle.
- Nursing interventions include
  1. Providing a climate of acceptance
  2. Allowing for privacy, but not avoiding or isolating the client
  3. Offering a safe environment
  4. Encouraging self-care, independence, control, and decision making
  5. Helping to formulate attainable short-term goals
  6. Using complementary therapies such as imagery to increase the client's sense of control and enhance self-esteem

◆**NDx:** Social Isolation

- Nursing interventions include
  1. Explaining the rationale for Standard Precautions to the client and visitors
  2. Visiting the client frequently and providing for diversional activities
  3. Encouraging the client to verbalize feelings about self, coping skills, and sense of ability to control the situation

4. Educating the client, family, and significant others about prevention of HIV transmission

Community-Based Care

- Collaborate with the health care team members, client, and family to plan what will be needed and how they will manage at home with self-care and ADLs.
  1. Identify the actual and potential need for care, such as help with ADLs, around-the-clock nursing care, medications, and nutritional support.
  2. Assess available resources, including family members and significant others.
  3. Refer the client to a support group, financial counselor, or legal services.
  4. Determine the need for assistance with health insurance, housing, and making funeral arrangements when appropriate.
- Teach the client and family
  1. The mode of transmission of HIV infection and preventive behaviors
  2. Guidelines for safe sex; the need to notify sexual contacts
  3. Not to share razors, toothbrushes, or other potentially blood-contaminated articles
  4. Signs and symptoms of infections
  5. The importance of not changing pet litter boxes
  6. Self-care strategies such as good hygiene, balance of rest and exercise, and skin and oral care
  7. How to safely administer medications
  8. The importance of follow-up visits with the physician or other health care provider
- Teach good dietary habits, including
  1. Proper nutrition
  2. The importance of avoiding raw fish, fowl, or meat
  3. Thorough washing of fruits and vegetables
  4. Proper food handling and refrigeration practices
- Psychosocial preparation includes
  1. Helping identify ways to avoid problems with social stigma and rejection
  2. Helping to identify coping strategies for difficult situations
  3. Encouraging the client to continue as many usual activities as possible

4. Making referrals to community agencies, mental health professionals, and support groups as needed

Alkalosis, Metabolic

OVERVIEW

- Metabolic alkalosis is characterized by a high pH level, elevated bicarbonate level (above 28 mEq/L), normal oxygen tension, rising carbon dioxide partial pressure, decreased serum potassium level, and decreased serum calcium level.
- Common causes include
    1. Increase of base components
        a. Excessive use of antacids, bicarbonates
        b. Milk-alkali syndrome
        c. Blood transfusion
        d. Total parenteral nutrition (TPN)
    2. Decrease of acid components
        a. Prolonged vomiting
        b. Nasogastric suctioning
        c. Cushing's syndrome
        d. Hyperaldosteronism
        e. Use of thiazide diuretics

COLLABORATIVE MANAGEMENT

- Assessment findings include
    1. Central nervous system changes
        a. Light-headedness
        b. Changes in the ability to concentrate
        c. Anxiety, irritability, agitation
        d. Tetany, seizures
        e. Positive Chvostek's sign
        f. Positive Trousseau's sign
        g. Paresthesia
    2. Neuromuscular changes
        a. Hyperreflexia
        b. Muscle cramping and twitching
        c. Skeletal muscle weakness

3. Cardiac changes
    a. Increased heart rate
    b. Normal or low blood pressure
    c. Increased digitalis toxicity
4. Respiratory changes: decreased respiratory effort associated with skeletal muscle weakness
- Manage metabolic alkalosis by treating the underlying cause of the alkalosis and restoring normal fluid, electrolyte, and acid-base balance.

Alkalosis, Respiratory

OVERVIEW

- Respiratory alkalosis results from the excessive loss of carbon dioxide through hyperventilation and direct stimulation of the respiratory centers.
- Common causes include
    1. Hyperventilation
    2. Anxiety and fear
    3. Improperly set ventilators
    4. Drugs
        a. Salicylates
        b. Catecholamines
        c. Progesterone
    5. Hypoxemia
    6. Asphyxiation
    7. High altitudes
    8. Shock
    9. Pneumonia
    10. Asthma
    11. Pulmonary emboli

COLLABORATIVE MANAGEMENT

- Assessment findings include
    1. Central nervous system changes
        a. Memory changes
        b. Changes in the ability to concentrate

    c. Anxiety, irritability
    d. Tetany, seizures
    e. Positive Chvosteck's sign
    f. Positive Trousseau's sign
    g. Paresthesia
  2. Neuromuscular changes
    a. Hyperreflexia
    b. Muscle cramping and twitching
    c. Skeletal muscle weakness
  3. Cardiac changes
    a. Increased heart rate
    b. Normal or low blood pressure
    c. Increased digitalis toxicity
  4. Respiratory changes (increased rate and depth of ventilation)

- Manage respiratory alkalosis by treating the underlying cause of the alkalosis, usually with drug therapy.

Allergy, Latex

- Latex allergy is a type I hypersensitivity reaction in which the specific allergen is a protein found in processed natural latex rubber products.
- Allergic reaction varies from anaphylaxis to contact dermatitis to a reaction that may occur days later.
- All clients should be questioned regarding use of and known reactions to natural latex products.
- Use of latex-free products is essential.
  1. Persons in contact with the patient should wash their hands before entering the client's room and wear a cover (isolation) gown.
  2. Latex products must be restricted from coming into contact with the patient.
  3. Health care personnel must remove personal equipment that may contain latex before entering the client's room.
- Emergency equipment should include latex-free products.

Alzheimer's Disease

OVERVIEW

- Alzheimer's disease (AD), also known as dementia, Alzheimer's type (DAT), is a chronic, progressive, degenerative disease that accounts for 60% of the dementias occurring in persons older than 65 years of age.
- AD is also seen in people in their 40s and 50s, which is referred to as early dementia, or *presenile dementia, Alzheimer's type.*
- The disease is characterized by memory loss and progressive cognitive impairment caused by neurofibrillary tangles and senile plaques in the brain.
- The exact cause of AD is unknown; genetic predisposition, chemical changes, environmental agents, and immunologic causes are theories and risk factors.
- Current research is focusing on the role of a balanced diet, eating dark-colored fruits and vegetables, use of soy products, and sufficient amounts of folate, vitamins B_{12}, C, and E in preventing AD.
- The use of ibuprofen and other nonsteroidal anti-inflammatory drugs has been demonstrated to reduce the risk of developing AD if taken years before symptoms develop. However, the long-term use of these agents may result in significant complications.

COLLABORATIVE MANAGEMENT

Assessment

- Record client information.
  1. Age
  2. Current employment status and work history
  3. Ability to fulfill household responsibilities: grocery shopping, laundry, meal planning
  4. Driving ability
  5. Ability to handle routine financial transactions
  6. Language and communication skills
  7. Behavior

8. Changes in ability to smell or change in the sense of smell

9. Family history of AD
10. Past medical history, with particular attention to head trauma, viral illness, or exposure to metal or toxic waste

- Assess for
    1. Indicators of the stages of the disease
        a. Early (stage I) AD is characterized by forgetfulness, misplacing household items, mild memory loss, short attention span, decreased performance, loss of judgment, subtle changes in personality and behavior, and the inability to travel alone to new destinations. There are no associated social or employment problems.
        b. Middle (stage II) AD is characterized by severe impairments in all cognitive functions; gross intellectual impairments; complete disorientation to time, place, and event; physical impairment; loss of ability to care for self; visual-spatial deficits; speech-language problems; and incontinence.
        c. Late (stage III) AD is characterized by lost motor and verbal skills and by severe physical and cognitive deterioration and total dependence for activities of daily living (ADLs).
    2. Cognitive changes, such as deficits in attention, concentration, judgment, perception, learning, and memory
    3. Alterations in communication abilities
    4. Indications of tremors, myoclonus, and seizure activity
    5. Reaction to changes in routine and environment
    6. Impaired social interaction, disinterest in hobbies, loss of interest in current affairs
    7. Behavioral changes such as aggressiveness, sexual acting out, rapid mood swings, and increased confusion at night or when fatigued
    8. Wandering
    9. Hoarding of other's or own belongings
    10. Paranoia, delusions, hallucinations
    11. Depression
    12. Dependency in self-care
- Genetic testing, specifically for apolipoprotein E (apo-E), may be helpful as an ancillary test (not a predictive test) for the differential diagnosis of AD.

- A variety of laboratory or radiographic tests are performed to rule out other treatable causes of dementia or delirium.

Planning and Implementation

◆NDx: Chronic Confusion

- Collaborate with the health care team to prevent over-stimulation and provide a structured and orderly environment.
  1. Assess the room for pictures on the wall that could be misinterpreted as people, animals, or events that could harm the client.
  2. Ensure that the room has adequate, nonglare lighting and no potentially frightening shadows.
  3. Place the client in a quiet area of the unit, away from obvious exits and within easy view of the staff, preferably in a private room.
  4. Arrange the client's schedule to provide as much un-interrupted sleep at night as possible. Fatigue increases confusion and behavioral problems such as agitation and aggression.
  5. Establish a daily routine, explaining changes in routine before they occur and again immediately before they take place.
  6. Place familiar objects, clocks, and single-date calendars in easy view of the client. Encourage the family to provide pictures of family members and close friends that are labeled with the person's name on the picture.
  7. Keep the environment free of distractions; provide an unobstructed environment.
  8. Regularly reorient the client to the environment (during early stages).
  9. Use validation therapy for later stages of the disease to prevent agitation.
  10. Collaborate with the physical and occupational therapist to assist the client to maintain independence in ADLs as long as possible through the use of assistive devices (grab bars in the bathroom) and exercise programs.
  11. Develop an individualized bowel and bladder program for the client.
  12. Attract the client's attention before conversing.
  13. Speak slowly and distinctly in short, clear sentences.

14. Allow sufficient time for the client to respond.

15. In the home environment, place complete outfits on a single hanger for the client to choose from; encourage the family to include the client in meal planning, grocery shopping, and other household routines as able.

16. Provide drug therapy.
    a. Cholinesterase inhibitors are approved for symptomatic treatment of AD.
    b. Selective serotonin reuptake inhibitors are used to treat depression; tricyclic antidepressants should not be used because of their anticholinergic effect.
    c. Psychotropic drugs, also called antipsychotic and neuroleptic drugs, should be reserved for a client with emotional and behavioral health problems that may accompany dementia, such as hallucinations and delusions.
    d. Many drugs are currently under investigation for use in clients with AD.

17. Use art, massage, dance, and music therapy in the long-term care setting to minimize agitation.

◆NDx: Risk for Injury

■ The following nursing interventions are used to decrease the risk for injury.
1. Ensure that the client always wears an identification bracelet or badge.
2. Ensure that alarms or other distractions for outside doors are working properly at all times.
3. Check on the client frequently.
4. Take the client for walks several times per day and encourage the client to participate in activities to decrease his or her restlessness.
5. Talk calmly and softly, redirecting the client as needed and using diversion.
6. Keep the client busy with structured activities such as puzzles, board games, and music and art activities.
7. Remove and secure all dangerous items such as medications, needles, and syringes.
8. Implement seizure precautions if there is a history of seizures.

9. Keep an updated photo of the client that can be used if the client wanders away.
10. Inform the client's family about the Safe Return program, a national government-funded program of the Alzheimer Association that assists in the identification and safe, timely return of individuals with AD and related dementias who wander off and become lost.

◀**NDx:** Compromised Family Coping/Caregiver Role Strain

- The following nursing interventions are used to increase family coping and decrease caregiver role strain.
  1. Advise the family to seek legal counsel regarding the client's competency and the need to obtain guardianship or durable power of attorney.
  2. Refer the family to a local support group affiliated with the Alzheimer's Disease Association.
  3. Assess the family and other caregivers for signs of stress, such as anger, social withdrawal, anxiety, depression and lack of concentration, sleepiness, irritability, and health problems; refer them to their health care provider.
  4. Encourage the family to maintain its own social network and to obtain respite care periodically.
  5. Assist the family to identify and develop strategies to cope with the long-term consequences of the disease.

◀**NDx:** Disturbed Sleep Pattern

- To establish the usual day-night pattern
  1. Establish a pre-bedtime ritual.
     a. Personal hygiene
     b. Quiet environment
     c. Backrub or small snack
  2. Keep the client active during the day with a balance between active and passive activities; if possible, discourage the client from taking a nap.
  3. Give a mild antianxiety agent or hypnotic if conventional measures fail to induce sleep.

Community-Based Care

- When possible, the client should be assigned to a case manager who can assess the client's need for health care resources and facilitate appropriate placement throughout the continuum of care.

- The client is usually cared for in the home until late in the disease process. Therefore, teach the client and family
  1. How to assist the client with ADLs
  2. How to use adaptive equipment
  3. With dietary consultation, how to select and prepare food that the client is able to chew and swallow
  4. How to prevent the client from wandering
  5. What to do if the client has a seizure
  6. How to prevent the client from injury
  7. Drug information (if drugs are prescribed)
  8. How to implement the prescribed exercise program
  9. How to obtain respite services
  10. Strategies that caregivers can use to reduce their stress, including
     a. Maintaining realistic expectations for the person with AD
     b. Taking one day at a time
     c. Trying to find positive aspects of each incident or situation
     d. Using humor with the person who has AD
     e. Setting aside time each day for rest or recreation, away from caregiving duties if possible
     f. Seeking respite care periodically
     g. Exploring alternative care settings early in the disease process for possible use later
     h. Establishing advance directives with the person who has AD early in the disease process
     i. Taking care of themselves by watching their diet, exercising, and getting plenty of rest
     j. Being realistic about what they can do, and getting and accepting help from family, friends, and community resources
- Refer the client's family and significant others to the local chapter of the Alzheimer's Disease Association.

Amenorrhea

- *Amenorrhea* is the absence of menstrual periods.
- *Primary amenorrhea*, menstruation that has failed to occur by age 16, is associated with congenital factors or ovarian, pituitary, or hypothalamic disease.
- *Secondary amenorrhea*, menstruation that has started but has stopped and has not recurred for 3 months, is associated with functional conditions such as pregnancy, menopause, and lactation.

COLLABORATIVE MANAGEMENT

Assessment

- Assess for
  1. Menstrual and obstetric history
  2. Sexual activity and symptoms of pregnancy
  3. Current eating habits and history of dieting
  4. Strenuous exercises
  5. Hormonal deficiencies
  6. Medications (prescribed, over-the-counter, and illegal)
  7. Emotional stress
  8. Galactorrhea
  9. Hirsutism (unusual hair growth in women)
- Direct management at correcting the underlying cause.
  1. Hormone replacement
  2. Corrective surgery
  3. Stimulation of ovulation
  4. Periodic progesterone withdrawal
  5. Counseling and emotional support

Amputation

- Amputation is the removal of a part of the body.
- The psychological ramifications of the procedure are often more devastating than the physical impairment that results.
- *Traumatic amputation* occurs when a body part is severed unexpectedly, such as by a saw; attempts to replant it may be made.
- *Prehospital care* of a severed digit or other body part includes
  1. Wrapping the body part in a cool, dry cloth, moistened with saline, if possible
  2. Placing the body part in a sealed plastic bag and placing the bag in ice water
- Methods of *surgical amputation* include
  1. *Open,* or guillotine, amputation, used for clients who have or are likely to develop an infection; the wound remains open, with drains to allow drainage to escape from the site until the infection clears
  2. *Closed,* or flap, amputation, in which skin flaps are pulled over the bone end and are sutured in place as part of the amputation procedure
- Loss of all or any of the small toes presents minor disability.
- Loss of the great toe is significant because it affects balance, gait, and "push-off" ability during walking.
- Midfoot amputations (e.g., Lisfranc and Chopart procedures) and the Syme procedure (most of the foot is removed, but the ankle remains intact) are performed for peripheral vascular disease.
- Other *lower extremity amputations* are below-knee amputation (BKA), above-knee amputation (AKA), hip disarticulation (removal of the hip joint), and hemicorporectomy (hemipelvectomy and translumbar amputation).
- *Upper extremity amputations* are generally more incapacitating because the arms and hands are needed for activities of daily living (ADLs).
- Complications of elective or traumatic amputations include hemorrhage, infection, phantom limb pain, problems associated with immobility, neuroma, and flexion contractures.

COLLABORATIVE MANAGEMENT

Assessment

- Assess for
  1. Skin color, temperature, sensation, and pulses in both the affected and unaffected extremities
  2. Capillary refill
  3. Concurrent medical problems
  4. Psychological preparation for an amputation
  5. Disturbed self-concept, self-esteem, and body image
  6. The client's willingness and motivation to withstand prolonged rehabilitation after the amputation
  7. How the client has dealt with previous life crises
  8. The family's reaction to the surgery
  9. Ankle-brachial index (obtained by dividing ankle systolic pressure by brachial systolic pressure [should be greater than or equal to 1.00])
  10. Results of blood flow studies such as ultrasound, plethysmography, and laser Doppler flowmetry

Considerations for Older Adults

- Primary indication for surgical amputation is ischemia from peripheral vascular disease; rate of lower extremity amputation is greatest among clients with diabetes.
- Hip disarticulation and higher amputations are not performed on older adults because the prostheses are cumbersome and increased energy is required for ambulation.
- Complications of immobility may be more common in older than in younger clients.

Interventions

- Tissue perfusion assessment
  1. Monitor for signs indicating that there is sufficient tissue perfusion but no hemorrhage: skin at the end of the residual limb should be pink in a light-skinned person and not discolored (lighter or darker than other skin pigmentation) in a dark-skinned client.
  2. Assess the closest proximal pulse for strength and compare it with the pulse in the other extremity, noting that

comparison of limbs is not an accurate way of measuring blood flow if the client has bilateral vascular disease.

 3. The area should be warm but not hot.

- Pain management related to stump pain is not unlike that for any client in pain.
- Phantom pain management
  1. The client complains of pain in the removed body part.
  2. The pain is described as burning, crushing, or cramping or as a numbness or tingling; the client feels that the missing part is in a distorted position.
  3. Pain is triggered by touching the stump and by increased stress, anxiety, or depression.
  4. Opioids may not be effective for phantom limb pain but are effective for stump pain.
  5. Beta-blocking agents are used for constant, dull burning pain; anticonvulsants may be used for knifelike pain, and antispasmodics may be used for muscle spasms or cramping.
  6. Other treatment measures include ultrasound, massage, exercises, biofeedback, distraction therapy, hypnosis, and psychotherapy.
  7. It is not therapeutic to remind the client that the limb cannot be hurting because it is missing.
- Infection prevention
  1. The surgeon typically removes the pressure dressings for the wound to drain for 48 to 72 hours after surgery.
  2. Inspect the wound for signs of inflammation, such as redness and swelling.
  3. Record the characteristics of drainage.
  4. Follow hospital procedure for wrapping the stump; a stump shrinker or heavy stockinette may be used in place of an elastic bandage.
  5. Monitor the skin flap for adequate tissue perfusion.
  6. Change the soft dressing every day until sutures are removed.
- Ambulation promotion
  1. Follow the exercise program initiated by the physical therapist and assist the client to perform range-of-motion (ROM) and muscle strengthening exercises.

2. Teach the client to use adaptive devices (e.g., crutches, walker) before surgery, if appropriate.
3. Arrange for the client to see a prosthetist before surgery to begin planning for postoperative needs; some clients are fitted with temporary prostheses at the time of surgery.
4. Initiate special measures for lower extremity amputations.
   a. Ensure that the bed is equipped with a firm mattress and a trapeze and overhead frame.
   b. Assist the client into a prone position every 3 to 4 hours for 20 to 30 minutes to prevent hip contractures.
   c. Instruct the client to push the residual limb down toward the bed while supporting it on a pillow (for BKAs).
   d. Elevate the limb on a pillow for 24 hours after surgery (this is controversial; follow hospital policy).
   e. Inspect the limb daily to ensure that it lies flat on the bed surface.
5. Take measures to prevent complications of immobility, such as atelectasis, pneumonia, confusion, or thromboembolism.

- Prosthesis care and application
   1. Several devices help shape and shrink the residual limb in preparation for receiving a prosthesis; rigid removal devices are preferred.
   2. Most surgeons prefer elastic bandages to a shrinker sock; reapply (using a figure-8 wrapping) every 4 to 6 hours or more often as the bandage becomes loose.

- Body image promotion
   1. Assess the client's verbal and nonverbal references to the affected area.
   2. Ask the client to verbalize his or her feelings about changes in body image and self-esteem; the client may verbalize acceptance but refuse to look at the area during a dressing change.
   3. Provide realistic information about potential changes in lifestyle, job, and recreational activities; however, many clients are able to return to previous activities through use of prosthetic devices.
   4. Refer to a vocational counselor for evaluation as appropriate.

5. Help the client set realistic goals and objectives.
6. Stress the client's personal strengths.
7. Reassure the client and his or her sexual partner that an intimate relationship is possible, assist the client to adjust to changes, and refer the client to a sexual counselor as needed.

Community-Based Care

- The client is discharged directly to home or a rehabilitation facility depending on the extent of the amputation.
- If the client is discharged to home, collaborate with the case manager and physical therapist to determine need for referrals and adaptive equipment.
- Teach the client
  1. Care for the residual limb and prosthesis
  2. Care for the socket and inserts, the importance of wearing correct liners, and how to assess shoewear.
- Schedule the client for follow-up care with the health care provider.
- Refer the client to home health nursing and vocational counseling.

Amyotrophic Lateral Sclerosis

- Amyotrophic lateral sclerosis (ALS), also known as Lou Gehrig's disease, is a progressive degenerative disease involving the motor system.
- Mental status changes do not occur.
- The disease is characterized by fatigue while talking, tongue atrophy, dysphagia, weakness of the hands and arms, nasal quality to speech, fasciculations of the face, and dysarthria.
- As the disease progresses, muscle atrophy and eventually flaccid quadriplegia develop and respiratory muscles become involved, leading to pneumonia and death.
- There is no known cure.
- Treatment is symptomatic and directed toward the following: preventing complications of immobility, promoting comfort, providing ongoing support and counseling to the client

and family, and informing the client about the need for advance directives such as a living will and durable power of attorney.
- The drug riluzole (Rilutek) is associated with increased survival time.

Anaphylaxis

- Anaphylaxis is the rapid, systemic, simultaneous occurrence of a type I hypersensitivity reaction.
- It affects many organs within seconds to minutes after allergen exposure; episodes can vary in severity.

COLLABORATIVE MANAGEMENT

Assessment

- Assessment findings include
  1. Apprehension, uneasiness
  2. Weakness
  3. Anxiety (the client may complain of a feeling of impending doom)
  4. Generalized pruritus and urticaria (hives)
  5. Erythema
  6. Diffuse swelling of the eyes, lips, or tongue
  7. Cutaneous wheals or hives that are intensely pruritic and sometimes merge to form large, red blotches
  8. Bronchoconstriction, as well as mucosal edema and excess secretion of mucus
  9. Respiratory assessment that reveals congestion, rhinorrhea, dyspnea, wheezing, crackles, and reduced breath sounds
  10. Laryngeal edema (hoarseness, stridor)
  11. Respiratory failure causes hypoxemia
  12. Hypotension

13. Rapid, weak, and possibly irregular pulse
14. Diaphoresis
15. Confusion
16. Dysrhythmias
17. Shock
18. Respiratory and cardiac arrest

Interventions

- Provide emergency respiratory management.
    1. Establish an airway *immediately* and have a tracheostomy set available (emergency care).
    2. Administer supplemental oxygen through a nasal cannula or face mask.
    3. Elevate the head of bed unless contraindicated secondary to hypotension.
- Medications that may be administered include
    1. Epinephrine (1:1000), 0.3 to 0.5 mL as soon as the client displays symptoms of systemic anaphylaxis; may repeat every 15 to 20 minutes if needed
    2. Diphenhydramine (Benadryl, Allerdryl ✦), 25 to 100 mg, to treat angioedema and urticaria
    3. Aminophylline, 6 mg/kg intravenously (IV) for severe bronchospasm, then initiate maintenance therapy at 0.3 to 0.5 mg/kg/hr
    4. Inhaled beta-adrenergic agonist such as metaproterenol (Alupent) or albuterol (Proventil) every 2 to 4 hours
    5. Corticosteroids for persistent symptoms
- Monitor arterial blood gases.
- Suction as needed.
- Perform frequent respiratory assessments.
- Monitor the client's cardiac rhythm (dysrhythmias can occur secondary to anaphylaxis or treatment).
- Carefully observe the client for fluid overload from rapid administration of medications and IV fluids.
- Instruct the client to wear a medical alert bracelet.
- Consult with the physician about the need for the client to carry an emergency anaphylaxis kit.

Anemia, Aplastic

- Aplastic anemia is a deficiency of circulating red blood cells because of failure of the bone marrow to produce these cells. It is usually accompanied by leukopenia (reduction in white blood cells) and thrombocytopenia (decreased platelets).
- Deficiency of all three types of cells is called *pancytopenia.*
- The cause is often unknown but may be associated with exposure to toxic agents, ionizing radiation, or infection.

COLLABORATIVE MANAGEMENT

- Blood transfusions are the mainstay of treatment.
- Drugs to treat underlying disease may be given in addition to general immunosuppressive agents.
- Splenectomy and bone marrow transplantation may be necessary for client survival.

Anemia, Folic Acid Deficiency

- Folic acid deficiency is often produced by vitamin B_{12} deficiency; primary folic acid deficiency may also occur.
- Causes of folic acid deficiency include poor nutrition (especially in clients with alcoholism); malabsorption syndromes, such as Crohn's disease; and drugs such as methotrexate, some anticonvulsants, and oral contraceptives, which block folic acid conversion to its active form.

COLLABORATIVE MANAGEMENT

- Clinical manifestations of folic acid deficiency are similar to those for vitamin B_{12} deficiency without the accompanying nervous system manifestations.
- Prevention is aimed at identifying high-risk clients, such as alcoholics, others susceptible to malnutrition, and those

with increased folic acid requirements, by routinely assessing dietary habits in the health history.

- Treatment includes
    1. Teaching the client to consume foods high in folic acid, such as green leafy vegetables, liver, yeast, citrus fruits, dried beans, and nuts
    2. Encouraging the client to take a folic acid supplement

Anemia, Iron Deficiency

- In iron deficiency anemia, depletion of iron stores occurs first, followed by a reduction in hemoglobin. As a result, the red blood cells (RBCs) are small (microcytic).
- Iron deficiency anemia can result from blood loss, poor intestinal absorption, and dietary inadequacy.

COLLABORATIVE MANAGEMENT

- Abnormal bleeding is identified and treated.
- The client is instructed to increase his or her oral intake of iron from common food sources such as liver and other organ meats, red meat, kidney beans, whole wheat breads and cereals, green leafy vegetables, carrots, egg yolks, and raisins and other dried fruit.
- In the case of iron deficiency, iron is administered orally or parenterally. Explain that iron preparations often change the color of stool to black.

Anemia, Sickle Cell

- Sickle cell anemia is a genetic disorder with an autosomal recessive pattern of inheritance.
- It occurs when at least 40% of the total hemoglobin contains an abnormality of the beta chains known as hemoglobin S

(HbS), which are sensitive to changes in the oxygen content of the red blood cell (RBC).

- Insufficient oxygen causes the RBCs containing HbS to become sickle shaped. As a result, they clump together and form clusters that obstruct capillary blood flow. Capillary obstruction leads to further tissue hypoxia and more sickling, causing blood vessel obstructions and infarctions in the locally obstructed tissue.

||| Cultural Considerations

- Sickle cell anemia occurs most commonly in African Americans. It also occurs commonly in African, Mediterranean, Asian, Caribbean, Middle Eastern, and Central American populations.

COLLABORATIVE MANAGEMENT
Assessment

- Question the client about previous crises, including precipitating events, severity, and usual treatments.
- Review all activities and events during the previous 24 hours with the client to obtain information about fatigue, activity tolerance, and participation in activities of daily living (ADLs).
- The physical assessment reveals
  1. Pain (the most common symptom during sickle cell crisis)
  2. Extremities distal to blood vessel occlusion that are cool to the touch with slow capillary refill
  3. Pale or cyanotic skin; gray lips and tongue; blue-tinged soles, conjunctiva, and nail beds
  4. Jaundice
  5. Stasis ulcers or pressure ulcers on the lower extremities
  6. Damaged abdominal organs (usually the first to be damaged as a result of multiple episodes of hypoxia and ischemia)
  7. Damaged joints that may undergo necrotic degeneration; limited range of motion in all joints

8. Seizure activity or clinical manifestations of a stroke secondary to central nervous system infarct or hypoxia
9. Behavioral changes from hypoxia
10. Symptoms of heart failure from anemia (shortness of breath, dyspnea on exertion, weakness), heart murmurs, tachycardia

- Laboratory findings indicative of sickle cell disease include a large percentage of HbS present on electrophoresis, low hematocrit, elevated reticulocyte, and elevated white blood cell (WBC) count.
- Bone changes may be seen on x-ray.
- Electrocardiographic changes may be present.
- Soft tissue and organ degenerative changes may be seen on computed tomography, magnetic resonance imaging, and ultrasonography images.

☀ Women's Health Considerations

- Explain the hereditary nature of the disease, especially as related to childbearing.
- Clients who show evidence of damage to vital organs are advised against becoming pregnant.
- The use of oral contraceptives is controversial.

Interventions

- Pain management is based on the client's past pain history, previous drug use, disease complication, and current pain assessment.
- Pain management during a sickle cell crisis includes
  1. Administering morphine or hydromorphone (Dilaudid) intravenously (IV) on a *routine* schedule or via patient-controlled analgesia (PCA) pump until relief is obtained; dose is then tapered
  2. Treating moderate pain with oral doses of opioids or nonsteroidal anti-inflammatory drugs (NSAIDs)
  3. Avoiding intramuscular medications because they may lead to sclerosing of tissue, and absorption may be impaired as a result of poor circulation

- Hydroxyurea (Droxia) may be used for pain management in adults; however, it is associated with an increased incidence of leukemia, bone marrow suppression, and birth defects.
- IV hydration helps reduce the duration of pain episodes.
- Nonpharmacologic pain management includes
  1. Relaxation techniques
  2. Proper positioning
  3. Aromatherapy, warm room
  4. Warm soaks or compresses
- Interventions to prevent infection include
  1. Monitoring complete blood count (CBC) with differential WBC count
  2. Assessing lung sounds every 8 hours
  3. Inspecting the oral mucosa for lesions indicating a fungal or viral infection
  4. Inspecting the urine for odor and cloudiness and asking the client about sensation of urgency, burning, or pain with urination
  5. Using strict aseptic technique for all invasive procedures
  6. Giving prophylactic antibiotic therapy
  7. Encouraging the client to have a yearly influenza vaccination
- Management of sickle cell anemia focuses on prevention and treatment of crises.
  1. Teach the client the early signs and symptoms of hypoxia, hypoxemia, and sickle cell crisis.
  2. Treat crises using pain management, fluid replacement, oxygen therapy, and correction of the condition contributing to hypoxia.
     a. Perform nursing interventions.
     b. Remove constrictive clothing.
     c. Encourage the client to keep extremities extended to promote venous return.
     d. Check circulation in the extremities every hour.
     e. Keep room temperature at 72° F.
     f. RBC transfusion may be helpful to increase HbA levels and dilute HbS levels
- Bone marrow transplantation may be undertaken to permanently correct the problem of abnormal hemoglobin.

Anemia, Vitamin B$_{12}$ Deficiency

- A deficiency of vitamin B$_{12}$ indirectly causes anemia by inhibiting folic acid transportation and limiting DNA synthesis in red blood cell precursor cells. As a result, the immature precursor cells increase in size. This is called megaloblastic (macrocytic) anemia.
- Anemia caused by failure to absorb vitamin B$_{12}$ is called *pernicious* anemia.

COLLABORATIVE MANAGEMENT

- Anemia as a result of vitamin B$_{12}$ deficiency may be mild or severe, usually develops slowly, and produces few symptoms.
- Assessment findings include
  1. Pallor
  2. Jaundice
  3. Glossitis (smooth, red, "beefy" tongue)
  4. Fatigue
  5. Weight loss
  6. Paresthesias in the feet and hands
  7. Disturbances of balance and gait
- Treatment includes
  1. Teaching the client to eat foods high in vitamin B$_{12}$ such as animal proteins, eggs, and dairy products
  2. Providing vitamin supplements
  3. For pernicious anemia, administering vitamin B$_{12}$ parenterally on a regular basis
  4. Encouraging the client to rest as needed

Aneurysms

OVERVIEW

- An aneurysm is a permanent localized dilation of an artery, which enlarges the artery to at least two times its normal diameter.

- An aneurysm forms when the media, or the middle layer of the artery, is weakened, producing a stretching effect in the intima (the inner layer) and adventitia (the outer layer of the artery).
- The effect of blood pressure on the artery wall produces further weakness in the media and enlarges the aneurysm.
- The most common cause is arteriosclerosis; atheromatous plaque forms and weakens the intimal surface.
- Hypertension and cigarette smoking are contributing factors.
- The three types of aneurysms are
  1. *Saccular,* an outpouching from a distinct portion of the artery wall
  2. *Fusiform,* the diffuse dilation involving the total circumference of the artery
  3. *Dissecting,* a cavity formed when blood separates the layers of the artery wall; more commonly referred to as aortic dissection
- The most common aneurysm site is the aorta.
- Abdominal aneurysms arise below the level of renal arteries but above the iliac bifurcation.
- Thoracic aneurysms develop between the origin of the left subclavian artery and the diaphragm.
- The thoracic aorta is the most common site for dissecting aneurysms.
- Femoral and popliteal aneurysms are relatively uncommon.
- Aneurysms can thrombose, embolize, or rupture (rupture being the most frequent and life-threatening complication).

COLLABORATIVE MANAGEMENT

Assessment

- Most clients with abdominal or thoracic aneurysm are asymptomatic.
- Assess for clinical manifestations of abdominal aortic aneurysms.
  1. Prominent pulsation in the upper abdomen (do not palpate)
  2. Abdominal bruit
  3. Abdominal, flank, or back pain (Pain is usually steady with a gnawing quality, is unaffected by movement, and may last for hours or days.)

4. Severe sudden pain (which may radiate), abdominal distention, and hypovolemic shock (*if* rupture occurs)

- Assess for aortic dissection
  1. Pain that is described as tearing, ripping, and stabbing
  2. Pain that is located in the anterior chest, back, neck, throat, jaw, or teeth
  3. Diaphoresis
  4. Nausea, vomiting
  5. Faintness, apprehension
  6. Elevated blood pressure
  7. Decreased or absent peripheral pulses
  8. Neurologic deficits such as change in level of consciousness, paraparesis, stroke
- Assess for clinical manifestations of thoracic aneurysms.
  1. Hoarseness
  2. Shortness of breath
  3. Difficulty swallowing
  4. Visible mass above the suprasternal notch (occasional)
  5. Sudden and excruciating back or chest pain (*if* rupture occurs)
- Assess also for the following:
  1. Presence of mass on x-ray or computed tomography (CT) scan
  2. Results of ultrasonography

Interventions

NONSURGICAL MANAGEMENT

- Antihypertensive drugs are prescribed to maintain normal blood pressure and to decrease stress on the aneurysm.
- Teach the client the importance of keeping scheduled CT scan appointments to monitor growth of the aneurysm.
- Review with the client the clinical manifestations of aneurysms that need to be promptly reported.

SURGICAL MANAGEMENT

- Surgical removal of the aneurysm and replacement of the excised portion with graft placement may be performed as an elective or emergency procedure. Ruptures always require emergency surgery.

- Provide preoperative care.
  1. Administer large volumes of intravenous fluids if the aneurysm has ruptured to maintain tissue perfusion and blood pressure.
  2. Assess all peripheral pulses to serve as a baseline for comparison after surgery; mark where the pulse is heard.
  3. Provide routine preoperative care.
- Postoperative care varies with the type of aneurysm repair.
- Care of the client with an abdominal aneurysm repair is similar to that provided for clients with other abdominal surgeries. The client is admitted to the critical care unit and is often maintained on a mechanical ventilator overnight.
- In addition to routine postoperative care,
  1. Assess vital signs every hour.
  2. Assess circulation by checking pulses distal to the graft site.
  3. Report signs of occlusion immediately to the physician, such as pulse changes, severe pain, cool to cold extremities below the graft, white or blue extremities or flanks, abdominal distention, and decreased urinary output.
- Abdominal aortic aneurysm repair requires assessment of renal function because the aorta is clamped during the repair, potentially compromising the blood flow to the kidneys.
- Other interventions include
  1. Assessing hourly urinary output and urine color
  2. Monitoring daily blood urea nitrogen and creatinine levels
  3. Limiting elevation of the head of the bed to 45 degrees to avoid flexion of the graft
  4. Assessing the client's respiratory rate and depth and breath sounds hourly
  5. Administering opioid analgesics for pain
  6. Maintaining nasogastric tube suction for 3 or 4 days until bowel sounds return
  7. Monitoring for complications such as myocardial infarction, graft occlusion or rupture, hypovolemia or renal failure, respiratory distress, and paralytic ileus
- Care of the client undergoing thoracic aneurysm repair is similar to other thoracic surgeries. (See Cancer, Lung.)
- Additional postoperative care includes
  1. Assessing vital signs and reporting signs of hemorrhage immediately; assessing for bleeding and separation at the

graft site by monitoring chest tube drainage for excess drainage

2. Monitoring for cardiac dysrhythmias, paraplegia, and respiratory distress
3. Teaching the client with abdominal aortic aneurysms to report abdominal fullness or pain or back pain
4. Instructing the client with thoracic aneurysm repair to report back pain, shortness of breath, difficulty swallowing, or hoarseness

- Endovascular stent grafts provide an alternative choice for some clients who are at high risk for major abdominal surgery. The stent graft is inserted through a skin incision into the femoral artery by way of a catheter-based system, and advanced to a level above the aneurysm, away from the renal arteries. The graft is deployed into place with a series of hooks. Monitor closely in the hospital and at home for the development of complications such as bleeding, aneurysm rupture, peripheral embolization, and mis-deployment of the stent graft. All of these complications require surgical intervention.

Community-Based Care

- Emphasize the importance of compliance with the schedule of CT scans to monitor the size of the aneurysm in clients who have not had surgery.
- Emphasize the importance of controlling hypertension.
- Educate the client and family.
  1. Teach the client to restrict activities (if surgery was performed), including
     a. Avoiding lifting heavy objects for 6 to 12 weeks postoperatively
     b. Using discretion in activities that involve pulling, pushing, or straining, such as vacuuming, changing bed linens, moving furniture, mopping or sweeping, raking leaves, mowing grass, and chopping wood
     c. Avoiding hobbies such as tennis, swimming, golf, and horseback riding
     d. Deferring driving a car for several weeks
  2. Provide written and oral wound care instructions, if needed.
  3. Provide pain management instruction.

- Refer to home health nursing and other community agencies as needed.

Anthrax, Cutaneous

- Cutaneous anthrax is an infection caused by the spores of the bacterium *Bacillus anthracis*.
- The skin lesion appears initially as a raised vesicle that may itch and resemble an insect bite. The center of the vesicle becomes hemorrhagic and sinks inward and an area of necrosis and ulceration begins. The tissue around the wound swells and becomes edematous.
- It is distinguished from insect bites or other skin lesions in that it is painless and eschar forms regardless of treatment.
- Treatment includes ciprofloxacin (Cipro) or doxycycline (Doryx, Vibramycin)

Anthrax, Inhalation

- Inhalation anthrax is a bacterial infection caused by the gram-positive, rod-shaped organism *Bacillus anthracis*, which lives as a spore in contaminated soil.
- Infection can occur through the skin, intestinal tract, or lungs.
- It is *not* spread by person-to-person contact.

COLLABORATIVE MANAGEMENT

Assessment

- Illness and manifestation may not begin until as long as 8 weeks after exposure.
- Diagnosis of the prodromal stage (early) is difficult.
- Prodromal stage (early)
  1. Fever
  2. Fatigue

3. Mild chest pain
4. Dry cough
5. *No manifestations of upper respiratory infection* or rhinitis, headache, watery eyes, or sore throat
6. Possible improvement in 2 to 4 days
7. Diagnostic tests
   a. Slightly elevated white blood cell count with increasing numbers of band neutrophils
   b. Positive Gram stain of serum
   c. Mediastinal "widening" seen on chest x-ray

- Fulminant stage (late)
  1. Begins after the client feels a little better
  2. Sudden onset of breathlessness, progressing to severe respiratory distress
  3. Diaphoresis
  4. Stridor on inhalation and exhalation
  5. Hypoxia
  6. High fever
  7. Mediastinitis and pleural effusion
  8. Hypotension
  9. Septic shock, meningitis
  10. Death within 24 to 36 hours after onset of breathlessness, even if antibiotics are started at this stage

Interventions

- Combination therapy is with ciprofloxacin, doxycycline, and amoxicillin.
- These same drugs are used individually in oral form for prophylaxis after exposure to inhalation anthrax.

Appendicitis

OVERVIEW

- Appendicitis is an acute inflammation of the vermiform appendix, the small finger-like pouch attached to the cecum of the colon.
- Inflammation of the appendix can occur when the lumen of the appendix is obstructed.

- Inflammation leads to infection as bacteria invade the wall of the appendix.
- Appendicitis is the most common cause of acute inflammation in the right lower abdominal quadrant.
- Appendicitis may occur at any age, but the peak incidence is between 20 and 30 years of age.

Considerations for Older Adults

- Appendicitis is not common in older adults, but when it occurs, perforation is a common complication.
- The diagnosis of appendicitis is difficult to establish for the older adult because symptoms of pain and tenderness are not as pronounced in older adults as they are in younger persons.

COLLABORATIVE MANAGEMENT

Assessment

- Assessment findings include
    1. Abdominal pain originating in the epigastric or periumbilical area and shifting to the right lower quadrant (McBurney's point); pain may not be localized
    2. Nausea and vomiting
    3. Anorexia after the initial diagnosis of pain
    4. Urge to defecate or pass flatus
    5. Muscle rigidity and rebound tenderness
    6. Normal or slightly elevated temperature
    7. Increased white blood cell (WBC) count
- Abdominal pain that increases with cough or movement and is relieved by flexion of the right hip or knees suggests a perforated appendix with peritonitis.

Interventions

- Keep the client on nothing by mouth (NPO) status and administer fluids intravenously, if ordered, before emergent surgical appendectomy (removal of the appendix).
- Keep the client in a semi-Fowler's position so that abdominal drainage, if any, can be contained in the lower abdomen.
- Appendectomy may be performed as a *traditional* procedure through a small incision or by means of *laparoscopy.*
- If abscess is present, surgical drains are inserted during surgery.

- If peritonitis is present, the client will have a nasogastric tube in place to prevent gastric distention.
- Routine postoperative care for a *traditional* appendectomy includes
  1. Assessing the abdominal drains for excess drainage
  2. Maintaining the client's nasogastric tube or other drainage devices if inserted intraoperatively for peritonitis
  3. Administering intravenous antibiotics
  4. Assisting the client out of bed on the evening of surgery
  5. Administering opioid analgesia
- Care after a *laparoscopic* procedure includes
  1. Monitoring vital signs and puncture sites
  2. Preparing the client for discharge on the day of surgery or the next day

Arterial Disease, Peripheral

OVERVIEW

- Peripheral vascular disease (PVD) includes disorders that alter the natural flow of blood through the arteries and veins of the peripheral circulation.
- Peripheral arterial disease (PAD) is a chronic condition in which partial or total arterial occlusion deprives the lower extremities of oxygen and nutrients.
- Tissue damage generally occurs below the arterial destruction, and the location of the occlusion determines the location of tissue damage.
- Obstructions are characterized as inflow or outflow according to the arteries involved and their relationship to the inguinal ligament.
- Clients with chronic PAD seek treatment for the characteristic leg pain known as intermittent claudication.
- The four stages of PAD are
  Stage I: asymptomatic
    a. No claudication is present.
    b. Bruit or aneurysm may be present.
    c. Pedal pulses are decreased or absent.

Stage II: claudication
  a. Muscle pain, cramping, or burning is exacerbated by exercise and relieved by rest.
  b. Symptoms are reproducible with exercise.

Stage III: rest pain
  a. Pain while resting commonly awakens the client at night.
  b. Pain is described as a numbness, burning, toothache-type of pain.
  c. Pain usually occurs in the distal portion of the extremity (toes, arch, forefoot, or heel) and only rarely the calf or ankle.
  d. Pain is relieved by placing the extremity in a dependent position.

Stage IV: necrosis/gangrene
  a. Ulcers and blackened tissue occur on the toes, forefoot, and heel.
  b. A distinctive gangrenous odor is present.

- To detect cyanosis in a dark-skinned client, assess their skin and nail beds for a dull, lifeless color.
- Acute peripheral vascular disease occurs when there is an acute obstruction by a thrombus or embolus, causing severe, acute pain below the level of the obstruction.
- Risk factors for acute disease include hypertension, hyperlipidemia, diabetes mellitus, cigarette smoking, obesity, and familial predisposition.

COLLABORATIVE MANAGEMENT

Assessment

- Assessment findings include
  1. Leg pain with exercise or rest
  2. Discomfort in the lower back, buttocks, or thighs (inflow disease)
  3. Burning or cramping in the calves, ankles, feet, and toes (outflow disease)
  4. History of acute or chronic pain
  5. Ischemic changes of the extremity
     a. Loss of hair on the lower calf, ankle, and foot
     b. Dry, scaly skin
     c. Thickened toenails

    d. Color changes (elevation pallor or dependent rubor)

    e. Mottled and cool or cold extremity

6. Presence or absence of pulses

7. Ulcer formation

    a. Arterial ulcers develop on the toes, between the toes, or on the upper aspect of the foot; they are painful.

    b. Diabetic ulcers develop on the plantar surface of the foot, over metatarsal heads, on the heel, or on pressure areas; they may not be painful.

    c. Venous stasis ulcers occur at the ankles, with discoloration of the lower extremity at the ulcer; they cause minimal pain.

- Diagnostic assessment includes

    1. Segmental systolic blood pressure measurement

    2. Exercise tolerance test

    3. Plethysmography

Planning and Implementation

NONSURGICAL MANAGEMENT

- Teach the following methods of increasing arterial blood flow in chronic arterial disease.

    1. Exercise, which promotes collateral circulation

    2. Positioning to promote circulation and decrease swelling

        a. Legs should be elevated but not above the level of the heart.

        b. Teach clients to avoid crossing their legs and wearing restrictive clothing.

    3. Providing warmth to the affected extremity

        a. Teach the client to wear socks or insulated bedroom shoes and maintain a warm home environment.

        b. Caution the client not to apply direct heat to the lower limbs, which may cause burns because of decreased sensitivity.

    4. Decreasing exposure to cold and avoiding nicotine, caffeine, and emotional stress

    5. Drug therapy, including hemorheologic and antiplatelet therapy

    6. Control of hypertension

- *Percutaneous transluminal angioplasty* (PTA) dilates arteries that are occluded or stenosed with a balloon catheter.

- *Laser-assisted angioplasty* may be used to open an occluded artery.
- *Mechanical rotational abrasive atherectomy* is used to improve blood flow to ischemic limbs for scraping plaque while minimizing danger to the vessel wall.
- Prepare the client for PTA or laser-assisted angioplasty by giving the client nothing by mouth (NPO) after midnight.
- After PTA, care of the client includes
  1. Observing the puncture site for bleeding
  2. Closely monitoring vital signs
  3. Checking the distal pulses of both limbs
  4. Encouraging the client to maintain bedrest for 6 to 8 hours, as ordered, with the limb straight
  5. Administering anticoagulation therapy, which may continue for 3 to 6 months after the procedure
  6. Encouraging the client to take aspirin on a permanent basis, as ordered

SURGICAL MANAGEMENT

- An emergency surgical *embolectomy* is performed on clients who experience an acute peripheral artery occlusion by an embolus.
- Acute arterial insufficiency often presents with the 6 P's of ischemia:
  1. Pain
  2. Pallor
  3. Pulselessness
  4. Paresthesia
  5. Paralysis
  6. Poikilothermia
- Arterial revascularization surgery is used to increase arterial blood flow in an affected limb and includes *inflow* procedures such as aortoiliac bypass, aortofemoral bypass, and axillofemoral bypass and *outflow* procedures, including femoropopliteal bypass and femorotibial bypass.
- Grafting materials for bypass surgeries include the autogenous saphenous vein and synthetic graft material such as polytetrafluoroethylene.
- Provide postoperative care.
  1. Monitor for the patency of the graft by checking for changes in the extremity.

a. Color
b. Temperature
c. Pulse intensity
d. Pain intensity (Typical pain is described as throbbing pain, which occurs from increased blood flow to the affected limb.)

2. Mark the site of the distal pulses, which are best palpated or auscultated with Doppler ultrasonography.
3. Monitor the client's blood pressure, notifying the physician for increases and decreases beyond desired ranges.
4. Avoid bending the knee and hip of the affected limb.
5. Encourage the client to cough, deep breathe, and use an incentive spirometer.
6. Maintain NPO status for at least 1 postoperative day; record intake and output.
7. Monitor for signs and symptoms of infection at or around the graft and incision sites, such as hardness, tenderness, redness, or warmth.

- Thrombectomy (removal of the clot) is the most common treatment for acute graft occlusion; thrombolytic therapy may be used.
- Compartment syndrome occurs when tissue pressure within a confined body space becomes elevated and restricts blood flow.
  1. Assess the extremity for worsening pain, fullness, swelling, and tenseness.
  2. Notify the physician, remove or loosen the dressing, and place the extremity at the level of the heart when compartment syndrome is suspected.
- Use sterile technique when in contact with the incision and observe for symptoms of infection.

Community-Based Care

- The client benefits from a case manager who can follow the client across the continuum of care.
- Client and family education includes
  1. Reinforcing the need for individualized positioning and an exercise plan
  2. Teaching the client to avoid raising the legs above the level of the heart unless he or she also has venous stasis

3. Providing written and oral foot care instructions, instructing the client to
   a. Keep the feet clean by washing with a mild soap in room temperature water.
   b. Keep the feet dry, especially between the toes and ankles.
   c. Avoid injury or extended pressure to the feet and ankles.
   d. Always wear comfortable, well-fitting shoes.
   e. Keep the toenails clean and cut the nails straight across.
   f. Prevent dry, cracked skin.
   g. Prevent exposure to extreme heat or cold.
   h. Avoid heating pads.
   i. Avoid constricting garments.
4. Providing dressing change and incision care instructions, if necessary
5. Providing instructions concerning discharge medications
6. Encouraging the client to avoid smoking and to limit daily intake of fat to less than 30% of total calories

- Identify the need for a home care nurse or home health aide.
- Home care assessment of the client includes
  1. Assessing tissue perfusion to affected extremity
     a. Distal circulation, sensation, and motion
     b. Presence of pain, pallor, paresthesias, pulselessness, paralysis, coolness
     c. Ankle-brachial index
  2. Assessing adherence to therapeutic regimen
     a. Following foot care instructions
     b. Quitting smoking
     c. Maintaining dietary restrictions
     d. Participating in exercise regimen
     e. Avoiding both exposure to cold and constrictive clothing
  3. Assessing client ability to manage wound care and prevent further injury
  4. Assessing coping ability of client and family members
  5. Assessing home environment for safety hazards

Arteriosclerosis and Atherosclerosis

OVERVIEW

- Arteriosclerosis is a thickening or hardening of the arterial wall of the vascular system.
- Atherosclerosis, a type of arteriosclerosis, involves the formation of a plaque within the arterial wall and is the leading contributor to coronary artery disease (CAD) and cerebrovascular disease.
- The exact pathophysiologic mechanism of atherosclerosis is unknown but is thought to occur from vascular damage.
- Atherosclerosis begins as a fatty streak on the intimal surface of an artery and develops into a fibrous plaque that partially or completely occludes the blood flow of the artery.
- The final stage of atherosclerosis occurs when the fibrous lesion becomes calcified, hemorrhagic, ulcerated, or thrombosed, affecting all layers of the vessel.
- The rate of progression of this process is believed to be influenced by genetic factors, certain diseases, such as diabetes mellitus, and certain behaviors, including smoking, poor diet, and lack of exercise.

COLLABORATIVE MANAGEMENT

Assessment

- Assess as follows.
  1. Take blood pressure in both arms.
  2. Palpate pulses at all major sites and note any differences.
  3. Assess for prolonged capillary refill.
  4. Assess temperature differences in lower extremities.
  5. Assess for pallor around lips and nail beds.
  6. Assess arterial bruits.
  7. Assess for elevated serum cholesterol (elevated low-density lipoprotein [LDL] and low or normal high-density lipoprotein [HDL]), triglyceride, and homocysteine levels.

Interventions

- Nursing interventions include
  1. In collaboration with the dietitian, teaching the client to limit cholesterol intake following the Step One diet of the American Heart Association
     a. Limit dietary fat to 30% of total calories per day.
        (1) Less than 10% of total calories from saturated fat
        (2) Up to 10% of total calories from polyunsaturated fat
        (3) 10% to 15% of total calories from monounsaturated fat
  2. If the Step One diet does not significantly lower the clients cholesterol, collaborating with the dietitian to teach the client the Step Two diet, which limits saturated fat to 7% of total calories and cholesterol to less than 200 mg/day
  3. Reinforcing the need for a routine exercise program
  4. Administering cholesterol-lowering agents as prescribed for clients who do not respond to diet therapy and other nondrug measures
  5. Encouraging the client to stop smoking (cigarette smoking lowers levels of HDL cholesterol), to avoid secondary smoke, and to seek a smoking cessation group such as the American Cancer Society's Fresh Start program if needed
     a. Client's who smoke may consider using a nicotine patch or nicotine gum. Teach the client the adverse effects that could occur if they continue to smoke while using these products.
     b. Other complementary and alternative therapies to stop smoking include acupuncture, hypnosis, and biofeedback.

Arthritis, Rheumatoid

OVERVIEW

- Rheumatoid arthritis (RA) is a chronic, progressive, systemic inflammatory autoimmune disease process that primarily affects synovial joints. It is characterized by natural remissions and exacerbations.
- Onset may be acute and severe or slow and insidious.
- Other areas of the body can be affected; vasculitis can cause malfunction and eventual failure of an organ or system.

Genetic Consideration

- Some humans may have a predisposition for RA, or a gene-environment interaction may come into play.
- Female reproductive hormones may influence the development of RA because the disease affects more women than men.
- Infectious organisms may play a role, particularly the Epstein-Barr virus.

Cultural Considerations

- Incidence rates among Pima Indians are substantially higher than those among non–Native Americans.

COLLABORATIVE MANAGEMENT

Assessment

- Assess for early disease manifestations, including
  1. Joint stiffness, swelling, pain
  2. Fatigue, generalized weakness
  3. Anorexia, weight loss
  4. Persistent low-grade fever
  5. Initial involvement of upper extremity joints
  6. Typical pattern of bilateral, symmetric joint involvement
  7. Migrating symptoms known as *migratory arthritis*
  8. Joint infection, manifested by presence of only one hot, swollen, painful joint (out of proportion to the other joints)

- Assess for late disease manifestations.
  1. Joints become progressively inflamed and quite painful.
  2. Morning stiffness lasts longer than 45 minutes.
  3. Synovitis and effusions result in a softness or a spongy feeling.
  4. Muscles atrophy.
  5. Range of motion decreases.
  6. Most or all of the synovial joints are eventually affected.
  7. Cervical disease may result in subluxation that may be life threatening.
     a. Cervical pain with loss of range of motion should be reported to the physician.
- Assess for joint involvement by palpating the tissues around the joint to elicit pain or tenderness associated with other rheumatoid complications.
- Assess for systemic complications.
  1. Exacerbations, often called "flares"
     a. Increased joint swelling and tenderness
     b. Moderate to severe weight loss
     c. Fever
     d. Extreme fatigue
  2. Subcutaneous nodules, which may become open and infected or interfere with activities of daily living
  3. Inflammation of blood vessels, resulting in vasculitis, particularly of small to medium-sized vessels
     a When arterial involvement occurs, major organs and body systems become ischemic and malfunction.
     b. Ischemic skin lesions (periungual lesions) appear in small groups as small, brownish spots. Monitor the number and location each day.
     c. Larger skin lesions that appear on the lower extremities may lead to ulceration, which heal slowly as a result of decreased circulation.
  4. Peripheral neuropathy, causing foot drop and paresthesias
  5. Respiratory complication, including pleurisy, pneumonitis, diffuse interstitial fibrosis, and pulmonary hypertension
  6. Cardiac complications, including pericarditis and myocarditis
  7. Ocular involvement, such as iritis or scleritis

8. Sjögren's syndrome
9. Felty's syndrome, which is characterized by RA, hepatosplenomegaly (enlarged liver and spleen), and leukopenia
10. Caplan's syndrome, characterized by the presence of rheumatoid nodules in the lungs and pneumoconiosis, which is noted primarily in coal miners and asbestos workers

- Psychosocial assessment
  1. Fear of becoming disabled and dependent
  2. Altered body image
  3. Devaluation of self
  4. Frustration
  5. Depression
- Laboratory data
  1. Positive rheumatoid factor
     a. Positive Rose-Waaler test
     b. Positive latex agglutination test
  2. Elevated erythrocyte sedimentation rate
  3. Elevated C reactive protein (hsCRP)
  4. Positive antinuclear antibody test
  5. Decreased serum complement
  6. Increased serum protein electrophoresis
  7. Elevated serum immunoglobulins
  8. Altered CBC and platelet count
- Other diagnostic tests
  1. Standard x-rays
  2. Computed tomography or magnetic resonance imaging
  3. Arthrocentesis, a procedure to aspirate a sample of the synovial fluid to relieve pressure and analyze the fluid for inflammatory cells and immune complexes, including rheumatoid factor
  4. Bone scan

Interventions

- Drug therapy used to treat RA includes
  1. Nonsteroidal anti-inflammatory drugs (NSAIDs)
     a. NSAIDs are often the drug of choice to relieve pain and inflammation; they are discontinued if pain is not decreased within 6 to 8 weeks.

    b. NSAIDs may be given with misoprostol (Cytotec) to minimize gastrointestinal problems.

2. Salicylates may not be used as often in the United States because of potential complications.
3. Disease-modifying antirheumatic drugs (DMARDs)
       a. DMARDs, such as hydroxychloroquine (Plaquenil), sulfasalazine (Azulfidine), and minocycline (Minocin), are used to slow the progression of mild rheumatoid disease before it progresses.
4. Immunosuppressants
       a. Methotrexate (Rheumatrex) is the mainstay of therapy because it is effective and relatively inexpensive. Strict birth control is recommended for women of childbearing age because birth defects are possible.
       b. Cyclophosphamide (Cytoxan) may be given to control RA vasculitis. It may cause sterility; strict birth control is recommended.
5. Leflumonide (Arava)
       a. It is a slow-acting immune modulator that helps diminish inflammatory arthritis symptoms of joint swelling and stiffness, and improves mobility.
       b. Strict birth control is recommended for women of childbearing age because birth defects are possible.
6. Biologic response modifiers (BRMs)
       a. These medications are extremely expensive and all insurance companies may not pay for their use.
       b. Clients with multiple sclerosis and tuberculosis are not prescribed these medications.
       c. BRMs include etanercept (Enbrel), infliximab (Remicade), adalimumab (Humira), or anakinra (Kineret)
7. Adjunctive therapy
       a. It is not unusual for a client to be taking several DMARDs and a BRM, as well as Arava and an adjunct medication. Each drug works differently to relieve symptoms and slow progression of the disease.
       b. Long-term steroid therapy may be used if the client does not have relief of symptoms with other medications.

8. Gold therapy, used less frequently than other therapies, may be used to modify RA disease and reduce pain and inflammation.

9. Analgesic drugs, including
   a. Acetaminophen (Tylenol, Exdol, Datril)
   b. Propoxyphene (Darvon, Novapropoxyn)
   c. Propoxyphene with acetaminophen (Darvocet-N 100)

10. Plasmapheresis (or plasma exchange) to remove the antibodies causing the disease

11. Other pain-relief measures: rest, positioning, ice and heat, and stress management

- Some clients achieve pain relief with hypnosis, acupuncture, magnet therapy, imagery, or music therapy.
- Encourage good nutrition, including foods that contain omega-3 fatty acids (salmon, tuna); fish oil capsules; and antioxidant vitamins A, C, and E.
- Promote self-care as much as possible; identify assistive devices to allow the client as much independence as possible.
- If pain is not controlled, synovectomy, osteotomy, or total joint replacement may be necessary.
- Identify factors that contribute to fatigue.

1. Anemia
   a. Treat with iron, folic acid, vitamin supplements, or a combination of these.
   b. Assess the client for drug-related blood loss, such as that caused by salicylate therapy, by testing the stool for occult blood.
   c. Assess for drug-related blood loss by checking the stool for gross or occult blood.

2. Muscle atrophy
   a. Implement a daily exercise program.

3. Inadequate rest
   a. Arrange for a quiet environment
   b. Encourage the client to drink a warm beverage before bedtime.
   c. Teach the principles of energy conservation.
      (1) Pacing activities
      (2) Setting priorities
      (3) Allowing rest periods

        (4) Obtaining assistance when possible; delegating activities to the family
- Identify factors to enhance body image.
  1. Determine the client's perception of changes and the impact of the reactions of family and significant others
  2. Communicate acceptance of the client by establishing a trusting relationship.
  3. Encourage the client to wear street clothes and his or her own night clothes or bathrobe.
  4. Assist with grooming, such as shaving and makeup.
  5. The client may use coping strategies that range from denial or fear to anger and depression. The client may appear to be manipulative and demanding; however, he or she is trying to cope with the effects of the illness and should be treated with patience and understanding.

Community-Based Care

- Discharge planning includes
  1. Assisting the client and family to identify structural changes needed in the home before discharge
  2. Health teaching, including
     a. Consulting with the health care provider before trying any over-the-counter or home remedies
     b. Checking with the Arthritis Foundation for the latest information on arthritis myths and quackery
     c. Supplying information about drug therapy
     d. Reviewing energy conservation measures
     e. Reviewing the prescribed exercise program
     f. Teaching joint protection measures
     g. Asking for help to prevent further joint damage and disease progression
  3. Referring the client to local and national support groups such as the Arthritis Foundation
  4. Referring the client to the dietitian, counselor, home health nurse, rehabilitation therapist, financial counselor, and local and state support groups as needed

Asthma

OVERVIEW

- *Bronchial asthma* is an intermittent, *reversible* airflow obstruction affecting only the airways, not the alveoli.
- Airway obstruction can occur in two ways.
  1. Inflammation obstructs the lumen or the insides of airways.
  2. Airway hyperresponsiveness results in airway obstruction by constricting bronchial smooth muscle, causing a narrowing of the airway from the outside.
- Many people with asthma have concurrent airway inflammation and airway hyperresponsiveness.
- Asthma may occur in some clients after taking aspirin or other nonsteroidal anti-inflammatory drugs (NSAIDs).
- Severe airway obstruction can be fatal.

COLLABORATIVE MANAGEMENT

Assessment

- Obtain information during the history-gathering phase.
  1. Pattern of episode of dyspnea, chest tightness, coughing, wheezing, and excessive mucus production
  2. When symptoms occur (e.g., continuously, seasonally, in association with specific activities or exposures, or more often at night)
- Other allergic symptoms such as rhinitis, skin rash, or pruritus may occur with atopic or allergic asthma.
- Clinical manifestations during an attack include
  1. Audible wheeze, which is louder on expiration
  2. Increased respiratory rate
  3. Increased coughing if inflammation is present
  4. Use of accessory muscles to assist in respiratory effort
  5. Muscle retraction at the sternum, suprasternal notch, and between the ribs
  6. Barrel chest in clients with persistent or severe asthma
  7. Increased anterior-posterior (AP) diameter of the chest
  8. Longer respiratory cycle, which requires greater effort

9. Possible cyanotic nail beds and circumoral cyanosis
10. Possibly unable to complete a sentence of more than five words between breaths
11. Pulse oximetry showing poor oxygen saturation
12. Hypoxemia as evidenced by change in level of consciousness and tachycardia
- Other assessment data include
    1. Arterial blood gases (ABGs)
    2. Pulmonary function tests
    3. Chest x-ray
    4. Therapeutic blood levels of selected medications

Interventions

- The goal of therapy is to improve airflow, relieve symptoms, and prevent episodes by including the client as a key partner in the management plan.
- Client education includes
    1. How to assess symptom severity at least twice daily with a peak flowmeter
    2. How to adjust medications to manage inflammation and bronchoconstriction to prevent or relieve symptoms
    3. How to use a symptom and intervention diary to learn his or her triggers of asthma symptoms, early cues for impending attacks, and personal response to medication
    4. How to use a metered dose inhaler (MDI) if appropriate
    5. How to determine when to consult the health care provider
- Drug therapy includes bronchodilators, which increase bronchiolar smooth muscle relaxation. Bronchodilators have no effect on inflammation.
    1. Short-acting beta$_2$ agonists are most useful when an attack begins or as premedication when the client is about to begin an activity that is likely to induce an asthma attack.
    2. Long-acting beta$_2$ agonists are delivered by MDI directly to the bronchioles, are useful in preventing an asthma attack, but have no value during an acute attack.
    3. Cholinergic antagonists allow for increased bronchodilation and decreased pulmonary secretions.

4. Methylxanthines (i.e., theophylline) are given systemically, have narrow therapeutic ranges, and have many side effects.

5. Anti-inflammatory agents decrease the inflammatory responses in the airways; they may be administered systemically or as an inhalant.

6. Corticosteroids decrease inflammatory and immune responses.

7. Nonsteroidal inhaled anti-inflammatory agents are helpful for preventing an asthma episode.

8. Mast cell stabilizers prevent mast cell membranes from opening when an allergen binds to IgE; they are helpful for preventing symptoms of atopic asthma but are not useful during an acute attack.

9. Monoclonal antibodies prevent allergens from triggering the release of mediators from mast cells and basophils.

10. Leukotriene antagonists are used to prevent an asthma episode.

- Regular exercise, including aerobic exercise, is encouraged; the client's exercise routine is adjusted to ensure that it does not trigger an episode–for example, adjusting the environment in which the activity takes place.

- Supplemental oxygen with high flow rates or concentration may be used during an asthma attack.

- Status asthmaticus is a severe, life-threatening acute episode of airway obstruction that intensifies once it begins and often does not respond to common therapy:

1. Clinical manifestations include extremely labored breathing and wheezing, use of accessory muscles, and distended neck veins.

2. The client may develop a pneumothorax and cardiac or respiratory arrest.

3. Status asthmaticus is treated with intravenous fluids, systemic bronchodilators, steroids, epinephrine, and oxygen.

4. The client may require intubation.

5. If status asthmaticus is not reversed, it may lead to cor pulmonale, pneumothorax, and cardiac or respiratory arrest.

Bleeding, Dysfunctional Uterine

- Dysfunctional uterine bleeding (DUB) is bleeding that is excessive or abnormal in amount or frequency without predisposing anatomic or systemic conditions.
- DUB occurs in the absence of ovulation related to ovarian function.
- DUB is associated with polycystic ovary disease, stress, extreme weight changes, and long-term use of drugs, including anticholinergics, morphine, and oral contraceptives.

COLLABORATIVE MANAGEMENT

Assessment

- Assess the client for
  1. Menstrual history
  2. Symptoms of systemic disease, such as renal or hepatic disease
  3. Variations in weight, obesity
  4. Undernutrition
  5. Abnormal hair growth
  6. Abdominal pain or masses
  7. Anatomic abnormalities

Interventions

NONSURGICAL MANAGEMENT

- Provide drug therapy.
  1. Treat women with anovulatory DUB with hormone therapy, which includes medroxyprogesterone or combination oral contraceptives.
  2. Treat women with ovulatory DUB with progestins during the luteal phase, oral contraceptives, prostaglandin inhibitors, or danazol.
  3. Explain the side effects of these drugs and evaluate the woman's knowledge of the effects, dosage, and administration schedule.

SURGICAL MANAGEMENT

- Surgical management includes diagnostic dilation and curettage (D&C), which involves scraping the endometrial tissue to assess for possible causes of bleeding or to remove bleeding tissue; laser endometrial ablation; and hysterectomy.
- Interventions for the perioperative period include
  1. Preparing the client for surgery and providing routine postoperative care, including assessment of vaginal bleeding
  2. Reviewing postoperative care, instructing the client to
     a. Avoid sexual intercourse, tub bathing, and the use of tampons for 2 weeks.
     b. Note that slight bleeding is normal, but if bleeding is as heavy as the normal menstrual period or persists for 2 weeks, client should notify the health care provider.
     c. Use a hot water bottle or heating pad to relieve abdominal cramping.
     d. Take mild analgesics such as acetaminophen for abdominal pain.

Blindness

- Blindness may be total or diminished vision in one or both eyes.
- Types of blindness include
  1. Color blindness: unable to distinguish certain colors; primary colors seen as gray
  2. Legal blindness: best visual acuity with corrective lenses in the better eye of 20/200 or less, or if the widest diameter of the visual field in that eye is no greater than 20 degrees
  3. Loss of peripheral vision
  4. Loss of central vision

COLLABORATIVE MANAGEMENT

- Nursing interventions include
  1. Teaching the client to make use of existing vision
     a. Moving the head slightly up and down can enhance a three-dimensional effect.
     b. When shaking hands or pouring water, the client can line up the object and move toward it.
     c. Choose a position that favors the good eye.
  2. Orienting the client to the immediate environment
     a. Describe the approximate size of the room.
     b. Describe a focal point in the room to serve as a point of reference, such as a chair or the bed, and then describe all other objects in relation to the focal point.
     c. Accompany the client to other important areas in the room (e.g., bathroom).
     d. Never leave the client in the middle of an unfamiliar room.
  3. Assisting the client in establishing the location of personal objects, such as the call light, clock, and water pitcher.
  4. Never changing the location of objects without the client's consent.
  5. Setting up the meal tray using an imaginary clock placement to orient the client to food placement.
  6. When assisting with ambulation, instructing the client to grasp your elbow while keeping your elbow close to your body; alerting the client to hazards such as steps or a narrow doorway
  7. Monitoring the client's use of a cane (held in the client's dominant hand) to help detect obstacles
  8. Knocking before entering the client's room; identifying yourself and the purpose of the visit
  9. Providing for diversional activities
- Newly blind clients may experience a brief period of physical or psychological immobility, hopelessness, anger, or denial.

Breast Disease, Fibrocystic

OVERVIEW

- Fibrocystic breast disease (FBD) consists of fibrotic changes or physiologic nodularity of the breast.
- The *first stage* commonly occurs between the late teens and early 20s and is characterized by premenstrual bilateral fullness and tenderness, especially in the outer upper quadrant; symptoms resolve after menstruation and recur before the next menstrual cycle.
- In the *second stage*, which occurs in women in their late 20s and their 30s, bilateral, multicentric nodular areas appear that feel like small marbles, with fullness and soreness.
- The *third stage* occurs in clients between 35 and 55 years of age, when microscopic or macroscopic cysts develop. The cysts, which occur suddenly and are associated with pain, tenderness, or burning, are usually three dimensional, smooth, mobile, and well delineated.
- The cause of FBD is unknown but appears to be related to normal fluctuations in progesterone and estrogen levels during the menstrual cycle.

COLLABORATIVE MANAGEMENT

- Hormonal manipulation is the main focus of drug therapy and includes oral contraceptives to suppress oversecretion of estrogen and progestins to correct luteal insufficiency.
- Other interventions include
    1. Vitamins C, E, and B complex
    2. Diuretics to prevent premenstrual breast engorgement
    3. Mild analgesics
    4. Avoidance of excess salt intake before menses
    5. Avoidance of caffeine (not scientifically proven)
    6. Practice of regular breast self-examination
    7. Application of ice or heat
    8. Use of a well-padded, supportive bra to decrease tension on ligaments

Burns

- A burn is an injury to the skin and other epithelial tissues caused by exposure to temperature extremes, radiation, electrical current, mechanical abrasion, or chemical abrasion. Clients who have burns experience a variety of physiologic, metabolic, and psychological changes.
- Burns are classified according to their depth.
  1. *Superficial-thickness* injuries produce the least destruction of all types because the epidermis is the only portion of the skin affected. This type of burn commonly occurs from sunburn or short (flash) exposure to high-intensity heat. Redness with mild edema, pain, and increased sensitivity to heat occur as a result.
  2. *Partial-thickness* injuries involve the entire epidermis and varying depths of the dermis. These injuries are sometimes referred to as second-degree burns. They are subdivided as follows:
     a. *Superficial partial-thickness* wounds are caused by heat injury to the upper third of the dermis, leaving a good blood supply; a vesicle (blister) forms. The wounds are red, moist, and blanch when pressure is applied. Nerve endings are exposed and any touch or temperature change causes intense pain.
     b. *Deep partial-thickness* wounds reach the deeper layers of the dermis and destroy structures within the dermis, such as nerves and hair follicles; blisters are rare in deep partial-thickness burns. The wound surface is red and dry with white areas in deeper parts; edema is present; pain is somewhat less because the nerve endings have been destroyed.
  3. *Full-thickness* burns involve damage to the entire epidermis and dermis, leaving no residual epidermal cells to repopulate; the wound does not re-epithelialize and whatever area of the wound that is not closed by wound contraction will require grafting. Eschar forms and must slough off or be removed from the wound before healing can occur.

> **a.** If the burn completely surrounds an extremity or thorax (circumferential) blood flow and chest movements for breathing may be reduced by tight eschar.
>
> **b.** Escharotomies (incision through eschar) or fasciotomies (incisions through eschar and fascia) are done to relieve pressure and allow normal blood flow and breathing.

4. *Deep full-thickness* burns extend beyond the skin into underlying fascia and tissues; muscle, bone, and tendons are damaged. Wound is blackened and depressed and sensation is completely absent.

- Compensatory responses to burns depend on the depth of the injury. Responses include
  1. Inflammation (immediate response)
  2. Sympathetic nervous system response (stress response)
  3. Vascular changes, including a shift of fluid from the intravascular space into the interstitial space ("third spacing"), which causes extensive edema and weight gain, hypovolemia, metabolic acidosis, hyperkalemia, and hypernatremia (lasts up to 24 to 36 hours); the fluid shifts back into the intravascular space after 48 to 72 hours, causing hyponatremia and hypokalemia
  4. Respiratory insufficiency
  5. Gastrointestinal (GI) changes, such as Curling's ulcer and decreased peristalsis
  6. Metabolic changes, which result in body temperature changes
  7. Immune system compromise
  8. Decreased cardiac output until 18 to 36 hours after the burn
- Common types of burns and emergency interventions limiting the extent of injury include
  1. Dry heat (flame) or moist heat (hot liquids): The client should stop, drop, and roll to smother flames; clothes that are on fire or saturated with hot liquids should be removed.
  2. Contact burns such as hot metal, tar, and grease can cause full-thickness burns.
  3. Chemical: Treatment depends on the type of chemical involved but generally should be flushed with copious amounts of water; agents containing sodium or potassium are covered with mineral oil and are not flushed with water.

4. Electrical: The client should be separated from the electric current by shutting off the source of electricity or using a nonconductive implement, such as wooden poles or ropes made of plant fiber.

5. Radiation: Treatment depends on whether the source is sealed or not sealed (self-contained).

Considerations for Older Adults

- The skin of older adults is thinner and more easily damaged than that of younger persons; therefore burns tend to be more extensive in the older adult.
- Healing time is slower in the older person, increasing the risk for infection and other complications.
- Cardiac changes in older adults limit the amount and types of fluids used in resuscitation; older adults are also more likely than younger persons to experience shock and renal failure.
- The immune responses of older adults may be reduced, increasing the risk of infection and sepsis. In addition, older adults may not have a fever when an infection is present.
- Decreased elasticity of the thoracic cage and decreased number and efficiency of alveoli make older adults more susceptible to hypoxia, hypoventilation, and atelectasis.
- Older adults are more likely to have a pre-existing medical condition that may further compromise vital organ function or interfere with fluid resuscitation and treatment.

COLLABORATIVE MANAGEMENT

Assessment

- During the emergent phase, obtain the following information.
  1. Time of injury
  2. Source of heat or injurious agent
  3. Detailed description of how the burn occurred
  4. Whether the influence of alcohol or drugs may have been a factor
  5. A description of the place or environment where the burn occurred
  6. Events occurring from the time of the burn to admission
  7. Any other events or circumstances contributing to the injury

- Record client information.
  1. Medical history
  2. Current medications
  3. Smoking history and history of drug or alcohol use
  4. Weight, age
- Assess for
  1. Direct airway injury
     a. Changes in the appearance and function of the mouth, nose, pharynx, trachea, and pulmonary mechanisms
     b. Facial injury or singed hair on the head, eyebrows, eyelids, or nasal mucosa
     c. Blisters and soot on the lips and oral mucosa
     d. Alterations in breathing patterns (progressive hoarseness, expiratory wheeze, crowing, and stridor)
  2. Carbon monoxide poisoning
     a. Headache
     b. Decreased cerebral function and visual acuity, coma
     c. Tinnitus
     d. Nausea
     e. Irritability
     f. Pale to reddish-purple skin
  3. Thermal (heat) injury
     a. Ulcerations, erythema, and edema of the mouth and epiglottis
     b. Stridor, hoarseness
     c. Shortness of breath
  4. Smoke poisoning
     a. Atelectasis and pulmonary edema
     b. Hemorrhagic bronchitis 6 to 72 hours after injury
  5. Pulmonary fluid overload
     a. Shortness of breath, hypoxia
     b. Moist breath sounds and crackles
  6. Cardiovascular assessment
     a. Hypovolemic and cardiogenic shock
     b. Rapid, thready pulse
     c. Hypotension and a wide pulse pressure
     d. Diminished peripheral pulses
     e. Slow or absent capillary refill
     f. Edema

    g. Complications that generally develop 48 hours after injury, such as fluid overload, heart failure, and pulmonary edema

7. Renal and urinary assessment
    a. Decreased urinary output
    b. Renal failure

8. Integumentary assessment
    a. Depth of injury
    b. Color and appearance of skin
    c. Estimation of injury size compared with the total body surface area (TBSA)
    d. Evaluation of size of injury using the Lund-Browder and Berkow methods

9. Gastrointestinal (GI) assessment
    a. Paralytic ileus
    b. Gastric dilation and vomiting
    c. GI ulceration
    d. Occult blood in the stool

10. Electrolyte changes

11. Increased white blood cell (WBC) count, followed by a decrease in WBC count

12. Changes in liver enzymes, clotting studies, and urinalysis

Planning and Implementation: Emergent Phase

◆**NDx:** Decreased Cardiac Output; Deficient Fluid Volume; Ineffective Tissue Perfusion

■ The client receives extensive infusion of intravenous fluids; commonly used fluids include Ringer's lactate, normal saline, colloids, and glucose in water.

■ To monitor fluids
    1. Follow facility fluid resuscitation formula and protocol.
    2. Monitor vital signs to determine adequate fluid resuscitation, including
        a. Clear mentation
        b. Normal blood pressure and pulse for the client
        c. Central venous pressure (CVP)
        d. Urinary output equal to 0.5 mL of urine per kilogram of body weight per hour
    3. Take strict measurements of intake and output.

4. Titrate fluids to meet the perfusion needs of the client.
   a. Adjust fluid intake to maintain urinary output at 30 mL/hr.
   b. Record serum electrolyte results.
5. Do not administer diuretics because they decrease circulating volume and cardiac output and may lead to a dangerous reduction in perfusion to other vital organs; however, diuretics may be given to the client with an electrical burn, as ordered.
6. Provide intensive cardiac monitoring such as CVP, pulmonary artery pressures, and cardiac output.
7. Monitor for cardiac dysrhythmias such as atrial fibrillation.
- An escharotomy or fasciotomy may be performed.

NDx: Ineffective Breathing Pattern

- Respiratory management includes
   1. Assessing respiration every hour
      a. Auscultate the lung fields for quality and depth of respirations.
      b. Loosen tight dressings if necessary to facilitate chest expansion.
   2. Turning and encouraging the client to cough and deep breathe at least once every 2 hours
   3. Having intubation equipment readily available (Crowing, stridor, and dyspnea are indications for immediate intubation.)
   4. Assisting the physician with bronchoscopy to examine the vocal cords, accurate diagnosis of the respiratory tract, deep suctioning of the lungs, or removal of sloughing necrotic material
   5. Suctioning the client as clinically indicated; obtaining sputum culture to determine whether an infection is contributing to breathing problems
   6. Performing chest physiotherapy and incentive spirometry
   7. Administering aerosol treatments
   8. Obtaining arterial blood gases and chest x-ray, as indicated
   9. Administering oxygen therapy; intubation, and mechanical ventilation if PaO_2 is less than 60 mm Hg; a tracheostomy may be necessary for long-term intubation

10. Administering antibiotics for pneumonia or other pulmonary infections

- A tracheostomy may be needed for clients who will require long-term intubation.
- Chest tubes may be needed to re-expand the lung when pneumothorax or hemothorax occur.

◆NDx: Acute Pain; Chronic Pain

- Assess the client's pain tolerance, coping mechanisms, and physical status.
- Provide drug therapy.
  1. Administer opioid and non-opioid analgesics, such as morphine, hydromorphone (Dilaudid), and fentanyl.
  2. Monitor the client receiving anesthetic agents, such as ketamine (Ketalar), pentobarbital sodium (Nembutal), and nitrous oxide.
  3. Encourage the client to participate in pain control (e.g., patient-controlled analgesia).
- Provide complementary and alternative therapies such as relaxation techniques, meditative breathing, guided imagery, and music therapy.
- Provide environmental change.
  1. Increase the client's sleep and rest periods to reduce the adverse effects of sleep deprivation, to replenish catecholamine stores, and to restore the diurnal effects of endorphins.
  2. Provide tactile stimulation through frequent position changes and massages; maintain a comfortable room temperature.
- Provide surgical management: Early excision of the burn wound can reduce the pain associated with daily debridement at the bedside or during hydrotherapy.

◆COLLABORATIVE PROBLEM:
Potential for Pulmonary Edema

- Provide drug therapy.
  1. Give digoxin or another inotropic agent to improve left ventricular function and prevent or treat pulmonary edema.
  2. Diuretics may or may not be given based on the client's vascular hydration status and renal function.

◀COLLABORATIVE PROBLEM:

Potential for Acute Respiratory Distress Syndrome (ARDS)

- Combine positive end-expiratory pressure (PEEP) with intermittent mandatory ventilation (IMV).
- Assess and document the client's response so that appropriate ventilator changes can be made.
- Use neuromuscular blocking agents in clients requiring mechanical ventilation to reduce or eliminate spontaneous breathing efforts and to reduce oxygen consumption.

Assessment

- During the acute phase, which begins about 36 to 48 hours after injury and lasts until wound closure is complete, assess for
  1. Cardiopulmonary dysfunction
     a. Pneumonia
     b. Respiratory failure
  2. Neuroendocrine dysfunction
     a. Hypothermia
     b. Weight loss and subsequent negative nitrogen balance
     c. Pseudodiabetes, which causes hyperglycemia and ketosis
  3. Immune system dysfunction
     a. Infections
     b. Sepsis
  4. Musculoskeletal dysfunction
     a. Problems that develop secondary to immobility, healing process, treatment, and other injuries
     b. Decreased range of motion (ROM)
  5. Body image changes
  6. Grieving
  7. Anxiety and fear

Planning and Implementation: Acute Phase

◀NDx: Impaired Skin Integrity

- The health care team performs an in-depth assessment of burned and nonburned skin areas to determine the degree of skin integrity, adequacy of circulation, presence of infection, and effectiveness of therapy.

- Wound debridement procedures can be
  1. *Mechanical,* using hydrotherapy (immersion in tub or showering on a specially designed table, successively washing only small areas of the wound) or using forceps and scissors to remove loose, nonviable tissue
  2. *Enzymatic,* which can occur naturally by autolysis (spontaneous disintegration of tissue by the action of the client's own cellular enzymes) or artificially by application of proteolytic agents such as sutilains (Travase)
  3. *Surgical,* excising the burn wound by either a tangential or a fascial excision technique and covering it with a skin graft or temporary covering. The procedure, performed within the first 5 days after injury, reduces the number of hydrotherapy treatments that are needed, but risks include massive blood loss and complications associated with anesthesia.
- The types of dressings generally used are
  1. *Standard,* involving the application of topical agents on the burn wound, followed by sterile application of multiple layers of gauze. The number of gauze layers used depends on the depth of the injury, the amount of drainage expected, the client's mobility, and the frequency of dressing changes.
  2. *Biologic,* skin or membranes obtained from human tissue donors (homograft or allograft) or animals (heterograft or xenograft)
     a. *Biologic dressings* are used in healing partial-thickness and granulating full-thickness wounds that are clean and free of eschar.
     b. *Heterograft* or xenograft is skin from another species, such as a pig.
     c. *Homograft* or allograft is skin from another human, usually a cadaver.
     d. *Amniotic membrane* is used because it has a low cost, ready accessibility, and large size.
     e. *Artificial skin* is an alternative approach to skin closure; it gradually dissolves as new, healthy skin replaces it.
     f. *Cultured skin* can be grown from a small biopsy specimen of an unburned portion of the client's body; the cells are grown in a laboratory for grafting.

3. *Synthetic and biosynthetic,* such as Op Site, Vigilon, Biobrane, and Tegaderm, are usually in place for 2 to 5 days.

- Surgical excision is used for full-thickness and most deep partial-thickness wounds.
- Wound covering is achieved through the application of an autograft.

NDx: Risk for Infection

- Drug therapy includes
  1. Tetanus toxoid. Additional administration of tetanus immunoglobulin is recommended when the history of tetanus immunity is questionable.
  2. Topical antibiotics or antimicrobials using the open technique (ointment is applied without further dressing of the wound) or closed technique (burn is covered with a dressing after the ointment is applied)
  3. Topical agents commonly used in the treatment of burns including
     a. Silver sulfadiazine (Silvadene, Flamazinel)
        (1) Causes adverse side effects, including local allergic reactions and leukopenia
        (2) Is not consistently effective for burns covering more than 60% of the client's body
     b. Mafenide acetate (Sulfamylon)
        (1) Causes severe pain if used on partial-thickness burns
        (2) Causes adverse side effects, including metabolic acidosis and superinfection
        (3) Is effective against *Pseudomonas* organisms
- Drugs with systemic effects used to treat infections include the aminoglycosides and cephalosporins.
  1. A higher dose than normal is required to maintain therapeutic serum levels; dosage is determined by peak and trough serum levels.
  2. Adverse reactions include ototoxicity and nephrotoxicity.
- Monitor for infection.
  1. Signs of sepsis include altered sensorium, increased respiratory rate, hypothermia or hyperthermia, oliguria, elevated serum glucose, glycosuria, decreased platelet count, and increased WBC count with a left shift.

2. Observe the wound for pervasive odor, exudate, changes in texture, purulent drainage, color changes, and redness at the wound edges.
- Aggressive surgical debridement of the wound may be necessary if the colony count approaches 105 colonies per gram of tissue.
- Provide isolation therapy.
    1. Proper and consistent handwashing is the single most effective technique to prevent the transmission of infection.
    2. The client is isolated according to the specific organism and facility procedure.
    3. Special isolation procedures may be needed if the organism becomes resistant to antibiotic therapy.
    4. Visitors are restricted while the client is immunosuppressed; ill persons and small children should be restricted from visitation.
    5. Wear gloves whenever coming in contact with the burn; change gloves when handling wounds on different areas of the body.
    6. Use disposable equipment as much as possible and do not share equipment among clients.

◆**NDx:** Imbalanced Nutrition: Less than Body Requirements

- Nasoduodenal tube feeding may be initiated until the client has sufficient gastric motility for oral feedings.
- Provide a high-calorie, high-protein diet and offer supplemental feedings as needed.
- Collaborate with the dietitian and client to plan alternatives to conventional nutritional patterns.
- Encourage the client to ingest as many calories as possible and to eat whenever he or she is hungry, not just at the scheduled mealtime.
- Offer frequent high-calorie, high-protein supplemental feedings.
- Record intake, output, and calorie count.
- Total parenteral nutrition (TPN) may be needed.

◆**NDx:** Impaired Physical Mobility

- Interventions include
    1. Maintaining the client in a neutral body position with minimal flexion

2. Using splints and other conforming devices according to the prescribed schedule
3. Performing ROM exercises at least three times a day
4. Assisting the client to ambulate as soon as possible
5. Applying pressure dressings to prevent formation of contractures and tight hypertrophic scars, including
   a. Ace bandages
   b. Custom-fitted elasticized clothing items (Jobst garments), which are worn 23 hours per day, every day, until the scar tissue is mature

◆NDx: Disturbed Body Image

- Interventions include
  1. Reassuring the client that feelings of grief, loss, anxiety, anger, fear, and guilt are normal
  2. Collaborating with other health care team members (e.g., psychiatrist, social worker) to address problems
  3. Accepting the client's physical and psychological characteristics
  4. Providing information and support
  5. Engaging the client in decision making and independent activities
  6. Providing information on and resources for reconstructive and cosmetic surgery, if needed

Community-Based Care

- The rehabilitation phase begins with wound closure and ends when the client returns to the highest level of functioning.
- Emphasis is on psychosocial adjustment of the client, prevention of scars and contractures, and resumption of preburn activity including involvement in work, family, and social roles.
- Explore the client's feelings about the burn injury.
- Begin the discharge process early by assessing the client and family's readiness for discharge and care requirements.
- Needs to be addressed before discharge include
  1. Financial assessment
  2. Evaluation of family resources
  3. Psychological referral
  4. Designation of principal learners (family members or significant others who will help with care)

a. Teach wound care and dressing changes, including use of correct technique, how to dispose of soiled dressings, methods to prevent contamination, and signs and symptoms of infection.
   b. Teach the proper use of prosthetic and positioning devices.
   c. Teach how to apply pressure garments correctly.
   d. Explain the signs and symptoms of infection, drug regimen, and comfort measures to reduce pruritus.
5. Rehabilitation referral
6. Home assessment
7. Medical equipment needed in the home
8. Evaluation of community resources and referral as needed
9. Referral to home health care as needed
10. Re-entry programs for school or work environment
11. Nursing home or transition care placement
12. Prosthetic rehabilitation
- Help the client deal with the reactions of others to the sight of healing wounds and disfigurement.

Cancer

OVERVIEW

- Cancer can develop in any organ or tissue but tends to occur more commonly in some tissues than in others.
- *Neoplasia* is new or continued cell growth not needed for normal development or replacement of dead and damaged tissue; it is always abnormal even if it causes no harm.
- *Benign tumors* are tissues not needed for normal function, growing too much or in the wrong place.
- *Cancer cells* are abnormal, serve no useful function, and are harmful to normal body tissue.
- *Malignant transformation*, the process of changing normal cells into cancer cells, occurs in four stages: initiation, promotion, progression, and metastasis.
- *Primary tumor* is the original tumor that is identified by the tissue from which it arose.

- Primary tumors located in vital organs such as the brain or lungs can grow excessively and either lethally damage the vital organ or "crowd out" healthy organ tissue and interfere with the ability of that organ to perform its vital function.
- Even when the primary tumor occurs in soft tissue or nonvital tissues, it can cause death by spreading into vital organs and disrupting critical physiologic processes.
- In *metastasis,* cancer cells move from the primary location by breaking off from the original group and establishing remote colonies called metastatic or secondary tumors.
  1. Even though the tumor is now in another organ, it is still a cancer from the original tumor.
  2. For example, breast cancer that spreads to the lung and bones is "breast cancer in the lung and bone."
- Three routes of spread of cancer cells are
  1. Local seeding
  2. Bloodborne metastasis
  3. Lymphatic spread
- Grading and staging are used to standardize cancer diagnosis, prognosis and treatment.
- *Grading* of a tumor classifies cellular aspects of cancer; it is a means to evaluate prognosis and appropriate therapy.
- *Staging* classifies the clinical aspects of the cancer by determining the exact location of the cancer and its degree of metastasis at diagnosis.
- Pathologic alterations can occur as a result of treatment regimens and are referred to as *secondary effects.*
- Physiologic dysfunction resulting from cancer may lead to impaired immune and hematopoietic function, altered gastrointestinal (GI) structure and function, motor and sensory deficits, and decreased respiratory function.
  1. Impaired immune and hematopoietic functions
     a. Occur most often in clients with leukemia and lymphoma
     b. Client at risk for infection, anemia, and bleeding
  2. Altered GI structure and function
     a. Reduced ability to absorb nutrients and eliminate waste
     b. Increased metabolic rate and increased need for proteins, carbohydrates, and fat
     c. Liver involvement altering metabolism and leading to malnutrition and death

    d. Anorexia leading to cachexia (profound body wasting and malnutrition)

    e. Change in taste

  3. Motor and sensory deficits

    a. Deficits result from cancers that invade bone or brain, or compress nerves.

    b. Bone metastasis can cause fractures, spinal cord compression, and hypercalcemia.

    c. Pain does not always occur; when present it should be managed aggressively.

    d. Brain metastasis may cause sensory, motor, and cognitive dysfunction.

    e. Sensory changes may occur if the spinal cord is damaged by tumor compression or if nerve ganglia are compressed.

  4. Decreased respiratory function

    a. Results from airway obstruction with tumor, lung tissue involvement, or blockage of blood flow through the chest and lungs

    b. Dyspnea and pulmonary edema

- Therapies for cancer include surgery to remove cancerous tissue; radiation to destroy malignant cells with minimal exposure of normal cells to the cell-damaging actions of the radiation; and chemotherapy, the treatment of cancer through the use of chemical agents.

  1. Surgery

    a. Surgery may be performed for prophylaxis, diagnosis, cure, control, palliation, determination of therapy effectiveness, or reconstruction.

    b. Nursing care depends on the type of procedure performed. The client's ability to cope with the diagnosis, treatment, and changes in body image and role must be assessed and an individualized intervention plan developed by the health care team.

    c. How much function is lost after surgery and how the loss affects the client depends on the location and extent of the surgery.

  2. Radiation

    a. The therapeutic radiation dose varies according to the size, location, and degree of radiation sensitivity of the tumor, as well as the radiation sensitivity of the surrounding normal tissues.

b. Radiation therapy is classified into two categories.

C

(1) *Teletherapy:* the radiation source is external to the client and remote from the tumor site. This type of therapy is called external beam radiation; the client does not emit radiation and poses no hazard to anyone else.

(2) *Brachytherapy:* the radiation source comes into direct continuous contact with the tumor tissue for a specified period of time. It is delivered as an unsealed radiation source (oral, intravenous [IV], or intracavitary) or as a sealed radiation source (implants, interstitial needles, or seeds). Regardless of type, the client emits radiation for a period of time and is a hazard to others.

c. Side effects of radiation therapy vary according to site. Skin irritation and hair loss, fatigue, and altered taste sensation are the most common effects. Some changes are permanent, depending on the dose of the radiation and location of the site.

d. Teach the client

(1) To wash the irradiated area gently each day with either water alone or a mild soap and water

(2) To use his or her hand rather than a washcloth

(3) Not to remove the markings that indicate where the radiation beam is to be focused

(4) To use no powders, ointments, lotions, or creams on the skin unless directed to do so by the radiologist

(5) To wear soft clothing over the skin at the radiation site

(6) To avoid wearing belts, buckles, or any other constrictive clothing over the radiation site

(7) To keep the irradiated area from being exposed to the sun

(8) To avoid heat exposure

(9) To schedule activities to allow for frequent rest periods

      (10) To maintain a balanced diet and provide information on altered taste sensation

  e. Nursing care for clients with sealed radioactive implants includes the following (although hospital protocols vary):

      (1) Assign the client to a private room with a private bath.

      (2) Place a "Caution: Radioactive Material" sign on the door of the client's room.

      (3) Wear a dosimeter film badge at all times while caring for the client to measure exposure to radiation.

      (4) Do not care for the client if you are pregnant; do not allow children younger than 16 years of age or pregnant women to visit.

      (5) Limit each visitor to 30 minutes a day and keep visitors at least 6 feet from the radiation source.

      (6) Never touch the radiation source with bare hands; if it is dislodged, use long-handled forceps to place it into the lead container kept in the client's room.

      (7) Save all dressings and bed linens until after the radiation source is removed, then properly dispose of them.

3. Chemotherapy

  a. Chemotherapy is used to cure, to increase mean survival time, and to decrease the chance of specific life-threatening complications.

  b. Chemotherapeutic agents are administered systemically and exert their cytotoxic (cell-damaging) effects against both healthy and cancerous cells.

  c. The normal cells that undergo frequent cell division are the most profoundly affected, including skin, hair, the epithelial lining of the GI tract, spermatocytes, and hematopoietic cells.

  d. Classifications of chemotherapeutic agents include antimetabolites, antitumor antibiotics, alkylating agents, antimitotic agents, topoisomerase inhibitors, and miscellaneous agents.

  e. Chemotherapy often involves the administration of a combination of agents.

  f. Chemotherapeutic dosing is typically based on the client's total body surface area and the type of cancer.

g. Although the IV route is the most common for drug administration, chemotherapy may also be given by the oral, intra-arterial, isolated limb perfusion, and intracavitary routes.

h. Extravasation is a major complication of IV administration.

 (1) Usually resolves without extensive treatment if less than 0.5 mL of the drug has infiltrated; surgical intervention may be necessary to treat more severe infiltration.

 (2) Immediate treatment depends on the specific agent extravasated.

 (3) Document the event according to institution protocol.

i. Nurses and other health care workers must use caution and wear protective clothing whenever preparing, administering, or disposing of chemotherapeutic agents.

j. The major role of the nurse in caring for clients receiving chemotherapy is management of the symptoms that the client experiences as a result of the therapy; the major side effects include alopecia, nausea and vomiting, mucositis, and immunosuppression.

 (1) For clients with *alopecia*

  (a) Remind the client that hair loss will occur but is temporary.

  (b) Suggest use of caps, scarves, turbans, hats, or wigs.

  (c) Caution the client that when hair grows back, its color, texture, and thickness may be different.

 (2) For clients with *nausea* and *vomiting*

  (a) Administer antiemetics and monitor the client response; drug combinations must be individualized for best effect.

  (b) Promote comfort through anxiety-reducing techniques such as progressive relaxation and imagery.

  (c) Monitor the client for dehydration and electrolyte imbalances.

(3) For clients with *mucositis*

  (a) Perform frequent mouth assessments; document findings.

  (b) Teach the client to avoid traumatizing the oral mucosa and to use a soft-bristled toothbrush or sponge for mouth care. Avoid using dental floss and water-pressure gum cleaners such as a Water Pik. Rinse mouth with water or saline every hour while awake. Avoid alcohol- or glycerin-based mouthwashes.

  (c) Assist the client in menu choices to avoid spicy or hard foods.

  (d) Apply petroleum jelly to the client's lips as needed.

  (e) Administer antimicrobial and analgesic topical medications, as ordered.

  (f) Administer artificial saliva as needed.

  (g) Clean toothbrush with a bleach or peroxide solution or run it through a dishwasher daily.

  (h) Assist the client with mouth care before and after every meal and at bedtime.

(4) For clients with *immunosuppression*, a potentially life-threatening side effect,

  (a) Place the client in a private room if possible.

  (b) Use good handwashing techniques and teach the client to do the same.

  (c) Do not use supplies from common areas.

  (d) Use strict aseptic technique for all invasive procedures.

  (e) Avoid the use of indwelling urinary catheters.

  (f) Monitor the white blood cell count daily.

  (g) Keep fresh flowers and potted plants out of the client's room.

  (h) Teach the client to eat a low-bacteria diet by avoiding salads, raw fruit and vegetables, raw and undercooked meat, pepper, and paprika.

  (i) Teach other infection control measures for the client at home, including avoiding crowds and people who are sick, bathing every day, not sharing personal toilet articles, not drinking water that has been standing for more than

15 minutes, not changing pet litter boxes or animal cages, not digging in the garden or working with houseplants, and taking temperature daily.

(j) Instruct the client to report signs and symptoms of infection immediately.

4. Other drugs used for treating cancer include hormone agonists, hormone antagonists, hormone inhibitors, biologic response modifiers (immunotherapy), gene therapy, targeted therapy, monoclonal antibodies, and antisense drugs.

■ Oncologic emergencies include sepsis and disseminated intravascular coagulation (DIC), superior vena cava (SVC) syndrome, syndrome of inappropriate antidiuretic hormone (SIADH), spinal cord compression, hypercalcemia, and tumor lysis syndrome.

1. Sepsis and DIC

  a. Microorganisms enter the bloodstream; septic shock is a life-threatening result of sepsis.

  b. DIC is a clotting problem caused by sepsis through release of thrombin or thromboplastin (clotting factors); abnormal clot formation occurs in small vessels (using up existing clotting factors and platelets) and is followed by extensive bleeding.

  c. Clots block blood vessels and decrease blood flow to major body organs, resulting in pain, strokelike signs and symptoms, dyspnea, tachycardia, oliguria, and bowel necrosis.

  d. Best treatment is prevention of sepsis through strict adherence to aseptic technique, handwashing, and patient education.

  e. Treatment includes anticoagulants (heparin) followed by cryoprecipitated clotting factors.

2. SVC syndrome

  a. The SVC is compressed or obstructed by tumor growth.

  b. Early signs and symptoms include edema around the face, eyes, arms, and hands, followed by dyspnea, cyanosis, mental status changes, decreased cardiac output, and hemorrhage.

  c. Treatment is high-dose radiation to the mediastinal area; placement of a vena cava stent may be necessary.

3. Tumor lysis syndrome
   a. Large quantities of tumor cells are destroyed rapidly.
   b. Serum potassium levels increase rapidly, and purine release causes hyperuricemia, resulting in cardiac and renal failure.
   c. The best treatment is prevention through hydration with 3 to 5 L of fluid a day if possible. Fluid intake should be consistent throughout the day.
   d. Diuretics, to increase urine flow through the kidneys, and drugs that increase the excretion of purines such as allopurinol (Zyloprim) are given.
   e. IV administration of glucose and insulin may be used to decrease significantly elevated serum potassium levels.
   f. In severe cases, the client may require dialysis.
4. For more information on SIADH, see Syndrome of Inappropriate Antidiuretic Hormone.
5. For more information on spinal cord compression, see Tumors, Spinal Cord.
6. For more information on hypercalcemia, see Hypercalcemia.

Cancer, Bone

OVERVIEW

- Malignant bone tumors may be primary (originate in the bone) or secondary (those that originate in other tissue and metastasize to bone).
- Primary tumors of the prostate, kidney, thyroid, and lung often metastasize to the bone.
- Metastatic tumors greatly outnumber primary malignant bone tumors.
- There are several types of *primary* tumors.
  1. *Osteosarcoma*, or osteogenic sarcoma, is the most common type of primary tumor and is most often found in the distal femur, proximal tibia, and humerus; the lesion typically metastasizes to the lungs within 2 years of treatment and occurs more often in males than in

females (2:1) between 10 and 30 years of age and in older clients with Paget's disease.

   2. *Ewing's sarcoma* is the most malignant type of primary tumor, often extending into soft tissue and metastasizing to the lungs and other bones; it occurs most often in children and adults in their 20s, affecting men more often than women.

   3. *Chondrosarcoma* typically affects the pelvis and proximal femur near the diaphysis; it strikes people who are middle-aged and older.

   4. *Fibrosarcoma* is an uncommon, slow-growing tumor that can metastasize to the lungs; it typically occurs in middle-aged men.

- Primary tumors of the prostate, breast, kidney, thyroid, and lungs are called bone-seeking cancers; they metastasize to the bone more often than do other primary tumors.
- Metastatic bone tumors greatly outnumber primary malignant neoplasms and are found most often in persons older than 40 years of age.

COLLABORATIVE MANAGEMENT

Assessment

- Record client information.
   1. History of radiation therapy for cancer
   2. General health status
   3. Family history of neoplasms
- Assess for
   1. Pain
   2. Swelling
   3. Tender, palpable mass
   4. Ability to perform activities of daily living (ADLs)
   5. Low-grade fever, fatigue, and pallor (seen in Ewing's sarcoma)
   6. Level of support system to help the client cope with the diagnosis and treatment
   7. Anxiety and fear
   8. Elevated serum alkaline phosphatase
   9. Possible elevations of serum calcium level and erythrocyte sedimentation rate
- Bone biopsy determines tumor type, grade, and stage.

Planning and Implementation

◆**NDx:** Acute Pain

- Analgesics and nondrug pain relief measures are used.
- Chemotherapeutic agents, given alone or in combination with radiation therapy and surgery, work best for small, metastatic lesions. The drugs selected are determined in part by the primary source of the tumor.
- Radiation therapy is as effective as surgery for Ewing's sarcoma in reducing the size of the tumor and thereby decreasing pain; radiation is palliative for metastatic bone disease.

SURGICAL MANAGEMENT

- *Wide excision* is the removal of the lesion surrounded by an intact cuff of normal tissue; it leads to cure of low-grade tumors only.
- *Radical resection* includes the removal of the lesion and of the entire muscle, bone, and other tissues directly involved; bone deficits may be corrected with total joint replacements with prosthetic implants, custom metallic implants, and allografts for the iliac crest, tibia, or fibula.
- *Percutaneous cordotomy* may be performed to treat intractable pain.
- Provide preoperative care.
    1. Provide psychological support; answer questions and explain routines and procedures.
    2. Arrange for spiritual assistance if needed.
- Provide postoperative care.
    1. Assess neurovascular status.
    2. Observe and record characteristics of wound drainage.
    3. Maintain pressure dressing and suction.
    4. Encourage muscle-strengthening and range-of-motion exercises as soon as permitted; a continuous passive motion (CPM) machine may be used.
    5. Assist with ADLs as needed.
    6. Observe for complications such as wound infection, loosening of implants, and rapid neurovascular compromise.
- Assist the client to cope with the diagnosis and treatment modalities.

1. Actively listen to the client and encourage the client and family members to verbalize their feelings.
2. Refer questions outside the scope of nursing practice to the physician, spiritual counselor, or other appropriate professional.
3. Encourage the client and family members to write down their questions and have them available when the physician visits.

- Nursing interventions for changes in body image include
  1. Recognizing and accepting the client's view about body image alteration
  2. Developing a trusting relationship with the client
  3. Encouraging the client to verbalize his or her feelings
  4. Emphasizing the client's strengths and remaining capabilities
  5. Assisting the client to set realistic goals regarding lifestyle

◀ **COLLABORATIVE PROBLEM:** Potential for Fractures

- Nursing interventions include
  1. Maintaining a hazard-free environment to prevent falls and minimize trauma (pathologic fracture)
  2. Teaching strengthening exercises
  3. Minimizing pain with treatment of fractures
- Radiation or surgery may be required to reinforce or replace the diseased bone to prevent fractures.

Community-Based Care

- To prepare the client for discharge, the following may be done:
  1. Collaborate with the health care team to ensure that the client can correctly use all adaptive devices ordered for home use.
  2. Instruct the client on the complications and side effects of radiation therapy or chemotherapy as needed.
  3. Teach wound care or how to manage long-term intravenous catheter care as needed.
  4. Develop and reinforce a pain management program, including
     a. Drug information, which includes the importance of taking the correct dosage at the right time
     b. Progressive relaxation techniques and music therapy

5. Review the prescribed exercise regimen.
6. Emphasize the importance of keeping all scheduled appointments with physicians and other members of the health care team.
7. Encourage the client to call the health care provider with questions or to discuss issues regarding medications for pain and nausea, for example.
8. Refer the client to a local cancer support group.

Cancer, Breast

OVERVIEW

- Breast cancer is the leading cause of death in women in the United States, second only to lung cancer. Less than 1% of all cases of breast cancer occur in men.
- Breast cancer is considered noninvasive when it remains within the duct.
- Breast cancer is classified as invasive when it penetrates the tissue surrounding the duct and grows in an irregular pattern.
- The mass is irregular and poorly defined; fibrosis develops around the cancerous tumor and contributes to dimpling, which is characteristically seen in advanced disease.
- The tumor invades the lymphatic channels, blocking skin drainage and causing edema and an orange peel appearance of the skin (peau d'orange).
- Invasion of the lymphatic channels carries tumor cells to the lymphatic nodes in the axilla.
- The tumor replaces the skin, and ulceration of the overlying skin occurs.
- The most common type of breast cancer is *infiltrating ductal carcinoma,* which originates in the epithelial cells lining the mammary ducts.
- *Lobular carcinoma* is more likely to affect both breasts and to have multiple sites within each breast.
- *Medullary carcinoma* occurs more frequently in younger women, especially those who are BRCA1 or BRCA2 positive.
- *Colloid (mucinous) carcinoma* occurs more frequently in older women; soft and slow growing, it may be hard to

distinguish from cysts or benign breast disease on palpation or mammography.

- *Inflammatory carcinoma* is rapidly growing, often with metastasis present at diagnosis; first manifestations are breast skin edema and redness.
- Common sites of metastatic disease are bone, lungs, brain, and liver.
- The stages of breast cancer are

  Stage I: smaller than 2 cm with zero to one lymph node positive and no evidence of metastasis

  Stage II: 2 to 5 cm without lymph node involvement

  Stage III: larger than 5 cm with no lymph node involvement, smaller than 2 cm with axillary node involvement, or 2 to 5 cm with supraclavicular or interclavicular node involvement

  Stage IV: any size, with or without lymph node involvement, but with distant metastasis
- Women who have specific mutations in either the BRCA1 or the BRCA2 gene have a 40% to 89% risk for developing breast cancer; however, only about 5% of all breast cancers are hereditary.
- Risk factors for breast cancer include increased age, family history of breast cancer, exposure to ionizing radiation, early menarche, history of benign breast disease, nulliparity, first birth after age 30, and late menopause. A high alcohol and fat intake may increase the risk of breast cancer.

Considerations for Older Adults

- By 85 years of age, each American woman faces a 1 in 9 risk of being diagnosed with breast cancer.

Cultural Considerations

- Although the incidence of breast cancer is higher in white women, death rates are higher for black women at every stage of the disease.
- Latino/Hispanic women have a lower incidence of breast cancer than white women but have a higher death rate.
- Breast cancer is the most common type of cancer among Asian and Pacific Island women; death rates are higher for Hawaiian women than for all other ethnic groups.

COLLABORATIVE MANAGEMENT

Assessment

- Record client information.
  1. Age, sex, and race
  2. Marital status
  3. Height and weight
  4. Personal and family history of breast cancer
  5. Hormonal history
  6. Age at first menarche
  7. Age at menopause
  8. Age at first child's birth
  9. Number of children
  10. History of breast mass discovery and medical care intervention
  11. Health maintenance, including regularity of breast self-examination and mammography history
  12. Diet history, including alcohol and fat intake
  13. Medications
  14. Other changes in the body within the past year such as bone or joint pain
- Assess for
  1. Location by using the "face of the clock" method
  2. Size, shape, and consistency of mass, and fixation to surrounding tissues
  3. Skin changes, such as dimpling, peau d'orange appearance, increased vascularity, nipple retraction, or ulceration
  4. Enlarged axillary and supraclavicular lymph nodes
  5. Breast pain or soreness
- Mammography, ultrasonography, and biopsy are used to diagnose breast cancer.
- Breast cancer cells that have excessive numbers of (or overexpress) the HER2/neu gene grow more rapidly and are relatively resistant to standard therapies.
- Women with estrogen receptor–positive tumors respond best to adjuvant therapy and have a better overall survival rate than others.
- Three major issues the woman has are
  1. Fear of cancer
  2. Threat to body image and sexuality, intimate relationships, and survival
  3. Decisional conflict related to treatment options

Planning and Implementation

◆NDx: Anxiety

- Interventions to treat the client include
  1. Assessing the client's perceptions and level of anxiety concerning the possible diagnosis
  2. Encouraging the client to ventilate feelings, even if a diagnosis has not been established
  3. Encouraging the client to seek information and outside resources
  4. Adjusting the approach to care as the client's emotional state changes
  5. Contacting resource groups such as Reach to Recovery

◆NDx: Potential for Metastasis

- There are many surgical and nonsurgical options for breast cancer treatment.
- Most women with metastatic breast cancer eventually succumb to the disease. Chemotherapy, radiation, hormonal therapy, and limited surgery are helpful for palliative care, improvement in quality of life, and prolongation of life; these may be used in women with metastatic breast cancer.
- Surgical management includes
  1. Conservative surgical management of breast cancer is used early in the disease and usually involves *lumpectomy with axillary lymph node dissection; sentinel lymph node biopsy,* in which only the tumor and lymph nodes are removed, leaving the breast tissue intact; or a *simple mastectomy,* in which breast tissue and usually the nipple are removed, but the lymph nodes are left intact, followed by radiation therapy.
  2. In a *modified radical mastectomy,* the breast tissue, nipple, and lymph nodes are removed, but muscles are left intact.
- Preoperative care focuses on psychological preparation, as well as the usual preoperative measures, including
  1. Presence of drainage device
  2. Location of incision
  3. Mobility restrictions
  4. Length of hospital stay (if any)
  5. Possibility of additional medical therapy

6. Provision of written material for the client to take home as a reference
- Postoperative care includes
    1. Performing routine postoperative care, including pain management
    2. Placing a sign over the bed to warn staff against taking blood pressure, giving injections, or drawing blood from the affected arm
    3. During dressing changes,
        a. Assessing the incision and flap for signs of infection (excessive redness, drainage, odor)
        b. Assessing the incision and flap for signs of poor tissue perfusion (duskiness, decreased capillary refill)
    4. Avoiding pressure on the flap and suture line by positioning the client on the nonoperative site, or sitting with the head of the bed elevated 30 degrees with the affected arm elevated on a pillow
    5. Recording the amount and color of postoperative drainage and reporting excess. Drains are removed when there is less than 25 mL of drainage in 24 hours (or 1 week after hospital discharge).
    6. Consulting with the physical therapist to recommend and teach the client appropriate postmastectomy exercises (with the physician's consent)
        a. Squeezing the affected hand around a soft, round object and flexion and extension of the elbow
        b. Progression to more strenuous exercises depending on subsequent procedures planned (such as reconstructions) and surgeon preference
    7. Assisting the client to ambulate and begin a regular diet the day after surgery
    8. Supporting the affected arm. Gradually the arm should be allowed to hang straight while the client is walking. Teach the client to avoid the hunched back position with the arm flexed because of the risk of elbow contractures.
- The decision to follow the original surgical procedure with chemotherapy, radiation, stem cell transplantation, or

hormonal therapy is based on the stage of the breast cancer, the age and menopausal state of the client, client preference, pathologic examination, and hormone receptor status.

- Women who have estrogen receptor–positive tumors are given tamoxifen (Nolvadex, Tamofen).
- Client's whose breast cancer cells overexpress the HER2/neu gene product and have large numbers of HER2 receptors may be prescribed targeted therapy with trastuzumab (Herceptin) to slow cancer cell growth.
- Breast reconstruction may begin during the original surgery or may be performed later in one or more stages using skin flaps or prostheses.

Community-Based Care

- Refer the client to home health service for care of drains and dressings and assistance with activities of daily living (ADLs).
- Instruct the client and family on
  1. Measures to take to optimize positive body image after mastectomy
  2. How to enhance interpersonal relationships and roles
  3. Postmastectomy exercises to regain full range of motion
  4. Measures to take to prevent infection of the incision
  5. Measures to take to prevent injury, infection, and swelling of the affected arm, including avoidance of blood pressure measurements, injections, or venipunctures; wearing mitts or gloves for protection when appropriate; and treating cuts and scrapes quickly
  6. The importance of avoiding the use of deodorant, lotion, and ointment on the affected arm
  7. The importance of reporting signs of swelling, redness, increased heat, and tenderness to the physician
  8. The importance of monthly breast self-examination
- Refer the client to community resources, including Reach for Recovery and ENCORE.

Cancer, Cervical

OVERVIEW

- Cervical cancer, a common reproductive cancer, can be preinvasive or invasive.
- *Preinvasive cancer* is limited to the cervix and usually originates in the area called the transformation zone.
- *Invasive cancer* is found in the cervix and other pelvic structures.
- Squamous cell cancers spread by direct extension to the vaginal mucosa, the lower uterine segment, the parametrium, the pelvic wall, the bladder, and the bowel.
- Metastasis is usually confined to the pelvis, but distant metastases occur through lymphatic spread.
- Premalignant changes can be described from dysplasia, the earliest change, to *carcinoma in situ* (CIS), the most advanced premalignant change.
- Preinvasive cancers can also be described using the term *cervical intraepithelial neoplasia* (CIN) and can be classified according to their severity.
- Risk factors associated with cervical cancer include
    1. Low socioeconomic status
    2. Early age at first sexual contact or first pregnancy
    3. Multiple sexual partners
    4. Intrauterine exposure to diethylstilbestrol (DES)

COLLABORATIVE MANAGEMENT

Assessment

- Assess for
    1. Painless vaginal bleeding (the classic symptom)
    2. Watery, blood-tinged discharge that may become dark and foul smelling as the disease progresses
    3. Leg pain or unilateral leg swelling (a late sign)
    4. Weight loss
    5. Flank and/or pelvic pain
    6. Dysuria
    7. Hematuria
    8. Rectal bleeding

9. Chest pain
10. Coughing
11. Abnormal Papanicolaou's stain test (Pap smear) results

Interventions

NONSURGICAL MANAGEMENT OF CIN

- Laser therapy is used when all boundaries of the lesion are visible during colposcopic examination.
- Cryosurgery involves placing a probe against the cervix to cause freezing of the tissues and subsequent necrosis.
- In loop electrosurgical excision procedure (LEEP), a thin loop wire electrode transmits a painless electrical current that is used to cut away or "peel off" affected tissue; spotting after the procedure is common.

NONSURGICAL MANAGEMENT OF INVASIVE CERVICAL CANCER

- Intracavitary and external radiation therapies are used in combination, depending on the extent and location of the lesion.
- For nursing management of clients undergoing radiation therapy, refer to Cancer.
- Chemotherapy has generally performed poorly when used for cervical cancers.

SURGICAL MANAGEMENT

- Conization may be used therapeutically for CIN in women who desire childbearing; it is the definitive treatment for microinvasive cervical cancer.
- A vaginal hysterectomy is commonly performed.
- A radical hysterectomy and bilateral lymph node dissection together are as effective as radiation for cancer that extends beyond the cervix but not to the pelvic wall.
- For preoperative and postoperative care, see Surgical Management under Leiomyoma, Uterine.
- *Pelvic exenteration* is a radical surgical procedure used for recurrent cancers if there is no lymph node involvement.
  1. *Anterior exenteration* is the removal of the uterus, ovaries, fallopian tubes, vagina, bladder, urethra, and pelvic lymph nodes.

2. *Posterior exenteration* is the removal of the uterus, ovaries, fallopian tubes, descending colon, rectum, and anal canal.

3. *Total exenteration* is a combination of the anterior and posterior procedures, with urinary diversion created by an ileal conduit and a colostomy for passage of feces.

- Provide preoperative care.
  1. Assess anxiety, concerns about sexual functioning, and the ability to adjust to altered body image.
  2. Assist in selection of stoma sites.
  3. Provide extensive bowel preparation.
  4. Provide routine preoperative care.

- Inform the client what to expect after surgery with regard to
  1. Transfer to a critical care unit
  2. Multiple intravenous lines
  3. Other invasive lines and monitoring, such as an arterial line
  4. Nasogastric tube

- Refer to Cancer, Colorectal, for preoperative and postoperative care for the client undergoing colostomy and Cancer, Urothelial, for preoperative and postoperative care for the client undergoing ileal conduit.

- After surgery, assess for
  1. Cardiovascular complications, such as hemorrhage and shock
  2. Pulmonary complications, such as atelectasis and pneumonia
  3. Fluid and electrolyte imbalances, such as metabolic acidosis or alkalosis and dehydration
  4. Renal or urinary complications
  5. Gastrointestinal complications, such as paralytic ileus
  6. Pain
  7. Wound infection, dehiscence, or evisceration

- Provide postoperative care.
  1. Assist with coughing and deep breathing.
  2. Observe for dehydration.
  3. Monitor urinary output.
  4. Administer opioid analgesics, as ordered.
  5. Administer and monitor total parenteral nutrition, as ordered.

6. Administer prophylactic heparin; apply antiembolism stockings or sequential compression devices, as ordered, to prevent deep venous thrombosis.
7. Administer antibiotics, as ordered.
8. Perform perineal irrigations.
9. Provide sitz baths.

Community-Based Care

- Implement a teaching plan for the client undergoing exenteration, including
    1. Colostomy or ileal conduit care
    2. Care for perineal drainage (for several months to a year)
    3. Use of sanitary pads
    4. Dietary adjustment to maintain high nutritional intake
    5. Medication effects, dosages, and side effects
    6. Sexual counseling about alternatives to intercourse
    7. Activity modification; walking
    8. Information about complications, including infection and bowel obstruction
    9. Emotional support for changes in body image
    10. Importance of not performing any strenuous activities (which includes most household work) for up to 6 months
    11. Importance of follow-up visits with physicians

Cancer, Colorectal

OVERVIEW

- Colorectal cancer, cancer of the colon or rectum, develops as a multistep process, resulting in loss of key tumor suppressor genes and activation of certain oncogenes that alter colonic mucosa cell division.
- The increased proliferation of the colonic mucosa forms polyps that can be transformed into malignant tumors.
- Tumors occur in all areas of the colon, and most cancers develop from adenomatous polyps, the primary risk factor.
- Tumors spread by direct invasion and through the lymphatic and circulatory systems.

- Complications include bowel perforation with peritonitis, abscess or fistula formation, frank hemorrhage, and complete intestinal obstruction.
- Risk factors include
  1. Genetic predisposition
  2. Personal risk factors such as age and presence of adenomatous polyps
  3. Dietary factors related to high intake of foods such as red meat and animal fat, refined carbohydrates, or fried or broiled meats and fish
  4. History of inflammatory bowel disease
- Black individuals have an increased incidence of colorectal cancer in advanced stages at the time of diagnosis and, consequently, an increased death rate.

COLLABORATIVE MANAGEMENT

Assessment

- Record client information.
  1. Diet history
  2. History of ulcerative colitis or Crohn's disease
  3. Personal history of breast, ovarian, or endometrial cancer; ulcerative colitis; familial polyposis; or adenomas
  4. Change in bowel habits with or without blood in stool
  5. Weight loss, pain, and abdominal fullness (late signs)
  6. Results of barium enema, colonoscopy, computed tomography (CT) scan, sigmoidoscopy, chest x-ray, and liver scan
- Assess for
  1. Rectal bleeding (the most common manifestation)
  2. Change in stool
  3. Anemia (low hemoglobin level and hematocrit; stool positive for occult blood)
  4. Cachexia (a late sign)
  5. Guarding or abdominal distention (a late sign)
  6. Abdominal mass (a late sign)

Planning and Implementation

◆NDx: Grieving
- Observe and identify
  1. The client's and family's current method of coping

2. The client's and family's present perceptions of the client's health problem
3. Effective sources of support used in the past
4. Signs of anticipatory grief such as crying, anger, sadness, and withdrawal from usual relationships

- Encourage the client to verbalize feelings about the diagnosis, treatment, and anticipated changes in body image if an ostomy is planned.
- When the client is physically able, encourage the client to look at the ostomy (if performed) and to participate in colostomy care.
- Invite the client, family, social worker, or religious leader to participate in the discussion and decisions concerning potential lifestyle modifications, treatment, prognosis, and end-of-life decisions.

◀COLLABORATIVE PROBLEM: Potential for Metastasis

NONSURGICAL MANAGEMENT

- Preoperative radiation therapy is effective in providing local or regional control of the disease.
- Radiation is also used postoperatively as a palliative measure to reduce pain, hemorrhage, bowel obstruction, or metastasis.
- Chemotherapy is used postoperatively to interrupt DNA production of cells and improve survival.

SURGICAL MANAGEMENT

- In a colon resection, the bowel segment containing the tumor is resected (removed) along with several inches of bowel beyond the tumor margin and regional lymph nodes; and an end-to-end anastomosis is performed.
- A colectomy (colon removal) with temporary or permanent colostomy may be needed.
- In an abdominal peritoneal (A-P) resection, the sigmoid colon and rectum are removed, the anus is closed, and a permanent colostomy is formed.
- Provide preoperative care.
  1. Reinforce the physician's explanation of the procedure.
  2. If a colostomy is planned, consult the enterostomal therapist (ET) to assist in identifying optimal placement of the ostomy and to instruct the client about the rationale and general principles of ostomies.

3. Instruct the client to consume only clear liquids for a day or more before bowel surgery to minimize colonic contents.

4. Prepare the client for general anesthesia.

5. Administer laxatives, enemas, or GoLYTELY, if ordered, the morning of surgery or the day before surgery to mechanically clean the bowel ("bowel prep").

6. Give oral or intravenous antibiotics preoperatively, as ordered.

- Provide postoperative care.

   1. Give routine postoperative care.

   2. Provide nasogastric tube care, if needed.

   3. Provide pain management.

   4. If an ostomy pouch is not in place, cover the stoma with petroleum gauze to keep it moist, followed by a dry, sterile dressing. If a pouch system is not in place immediately postoperatively

      a. Place a pouch system on the stoma as soon as possible, in collaboration with the enterostomal therapist.

      b. Observe the stoma for

         (1) Necrotic tissue

         (2) Unusual amount of bleeding

         (3) Color changes (The normal color is red-pink, which indicates high vascularity; pale pink indicates low hemoglobin and hematocrit levels; purple-black indicates compromised circulation.)

      c. Check the pouch system for proper fit and signs of leakage.

   5. Assess for functioning of the colostomy 2 to 4 days postoperatively; stool is liquid immediately postoperatively but becomes more solid.

   6. Empty the pouch when excess gas has collected or when it is one-third to one-half full of stool.

   7. Irrigate the perineal wound, if present.

   8. Change the perineal wound dressing as directed.

   9. Assess perineal wound; copious serosanguineous drainage is expected.

   10. Provide comfort measures for perineal itching and pain such as antipruritic medications (benzocaine) and sitz baths.

11. Assess for signs of infection, abscess, or other complications.
12. Instruct the client regarding activities such as assuming a side-lying position, avoiding sitting for long periods, and using a foam pad or pillow when in a sitting position.
13. Administer pain medication.

Community-Based Care

- Provide the client with the following verbal and written instructions.
    1. Avoid lifting heavy objects or straining on defecation to prevent tension on the anastomosis site.
    2. Avoid driving for 4 to 6 weeks.
    3. Note the frequency, amount, and character of the stool.
    4. For colon resection, watch for and report clinical manifestations of bowel obstruction and perforation (cramping, abdominal pain, nausea, and vomiting).
    5. Resume normal diet but avoid gas-producing foods and carbonated beverages.
- Teach the client and family colostomy care, including
    1. Normal appearance of stoma
    2. Signs and symptoms of complications
    3. How to measure the stoma
    4. How to protect the skin adjacent to the stoma
    5. Dietary measures to control gas and odor
- Other discharge preparation includes
    1. Inspection of the abdominal incision (and perineal wound if an A-P resection was performed) for redness, tenderness, swelling, and drainage
    2. Pain management, including medications
    3. Tips on how to resume normal activities, including work, travel, and sexual intercourse
    4. Psychosocial preparation
- Provide the following contacts for community and health resources as needed.
    1. Social services
    2. Enterostomal therapist
    3. United Ostomy Association
    4. American Cancer Society
    5. Home health services
    6. Pharmacy or other medical supply source

Cancer, Endometrial

OVERVIEW

- Endometrial cancer (cancer of the uterus) is the most frequently occurring reproductive organ cancer.
- It is a slow-growing tumor associated with menopause and arises from the glandular component of the endometrial mucosa.
- Its initial growth is within the uterine cavity, followed by extension into the myometrium and cervix.
- The spread occurs through the lymphatics to the ovaries and parametrial, pelvic, inguinal, and para-aortic lymph nodes; by hematogenous metastasis to the lungs, liver, or bone; and by transtubal or intra-abdominal spread to the peritoneal cavity.
- Risk factors associated with endometrial cancer include
  1. Obesity
  2. Diabetes mellitus
  3. History of uterine polyps
  4. History of infertility
  5. Nulliparity
  6. Polycystic ovarian disease
  7. Estrogen stimulation, including unopposed menopausal estrogen replacement therapy (ERT)
  8. Late menopause
  9. Family history of uterine cancer

COLLABORATIVE MANAGEMENT

Assessment

- Record client information.
  1. Family history of endometrial cancer
  2. History of uterine cancer, diabetes, and hypertension
  3. Age
  4. Race
  5. History of obesity
  6. Childbearing status
  7. Prolonged estrogen use

- Assess for
  1. Postmenopausal bleeding (the primary symptom)
  2. Watery, serosanguineous vaginal discharge
  3. Low back pain
  4. Abdominal pain
  5. Low pelvic pain
  6. Enlarged uterus

Interventions

NONSURGICAL MANAGEMENT

- Radiation therapy (external and internal) is used alone or in combination with surgery, depending on the stage of the cancer.
- If intracavity radiation therapy (IRT) is performed, an applicator is positioned within the uterus through the vagina.
  1. Maintain strict isolation and radiation precautions.
  2. Provide bedrest, laying the client on her back, with her head either flat or elevated less than 20 degrees.
  3. Restrict active movement to prevent dislodgment.
  4. Insert a Foley catheter.
  5. Assess for skin breakdown.
  6. Provide a low-residue diet.
  7. Encourage fluid intake.
  8. Administer antiemetics, broad-spectrum anti-infectives, tranquilizers, analgesics, heparin, and antidiarrheal medications.
  9. Restrict visitors.
- Nurses who are pregnant or attempting pregnancy are usually not assigned clients undergoing IRT.
- Instruct the client undergoing external radiation to
  1. Observe for signs of skin breakdown.
  2. Avoid sunbathing.
  3. Avoid bathing over the markings that outline the treatment site.
  4. Recognize the complications of treatment, including cystitis, diarrhea, and nutritional alterations.
  5. Recognize that reactions to radiation therapy vary among clients and that some may feel unclean or radioactive after treatments.

- Chemotherapy is used as an adjuvant treatment when the risk for distant spread exceeds 20%. (See discussion of nursing care under Cancer.)
- Hormone therapy may be used for stages I and II cancers, which are estrogen dependent, and for stage IV cancer as palliative treatment. Hormones commonly used are medroxy-progesterone (Depo-Provera) and megestrol acetate (Megace).
- Tamoxifen citrate (Nolvadex, Tamofen), an antiestrogen, is also used.

SURGICAL MANAGEMENT
- Total abdominal hysterectomy and bilateral salpingo-oophorectomy are performed for stage I tumors; a radical hysterectomy with node dissection is performed for stage II tumors and above.
- For the client undergoing hysterectomy, refer to preoperative and postoperative care under Cancer, Cervical.
- Nursing interventions include
  1. Providing emotional support
  2. Creating an atmosphere that encourages the client to ask questions and express fears and concerns

Community-Based Care

- Provide verbal and written instructions on
  1. Side effects that should be reported to the physician, including vaginal bleeding, rectal bleeding, foul-smelling discharge, abdominal pain or distention, and hematuria
  2. Medication use
- Inform the client that
  1. High-dose radiation causes sterility.
  2. Vaginal shrinkage occurs.
  3. Sexual partners cannot "catch" cancer.
  4. The client is not radioactive.
  5. Vaginal douching may decrease inflammation.
  6. A normal diet may be resumed.
- After an abdominal hysterectomy, give the following instructions and information to the client as discussed under Leiomyoma, Uterine.
- Refer the client to the local chapter of the American Cancer Society.

Cancer, Liver

- Primary hepatic carcinoma is rare in the United States but is one of the most common cancers in other parts of the world.
- Liver cancer usually develops as a metastatic process from primary cancer sites such as the esophagus, stomach, colon, rectum, breasts, lungs, or skin (malignant melanoma).
- Initial symptoms are epigastric or right upper-quadrant abdominal pain, fatigue, anorexia, and weight loss. Later symptoms include jaundice, ascites, bleeding, and encephalopathy.
- Nuclear radioisotope liver scan detects metastasis; a needle biopsy confirms the metastasis.
- Surgery is indicated for the client with a single metastatic lesion; a hepatic lobe resection is performed.
- High-dose hepatic chemotherapy may be given; other interventions include: hepatic artery embolization, alcohol ablation, and ultrasound-guided cryoablation.
- A newer procedure, RF ablation, uses a radiofrequency generator as a heat source to "burn" a tumor in a percutaneous procedure.

Cancer, Lung

OVERVIEW

- Lung cancers metastasize by direct extension through the blood and invading lymph glands and vessels.
- The four major types of lung cancer are
  1. Small cell lung cancer (SCLC)
  2. Epidermoid (squamous cell)
  3. Adenocarcinoma
  4. Large cell carcinoma
- The last three types are referred to as non–small cell lung cancers (NSCLCs).

- Lung cancers occur as a result of repeated exposure to inhaled substances that cause chronic tissue irritation or inflammation (e.g., smoking or exposure to "passive" smoke).
- People with a mutated CYP 2D6 gene do not activate the tobacco carcinogen and are less susceptible to lung cancer even if they smoke.
- People, particularly women, who are missing glutathione S transferase are less able to detoxify and clear carcinogens from the body and are at a greater risk for lung cancer if they are exposed to tobacco smoke.

COLLABORATIVE MANAGEMENT

Assessment

- Record client information.
  1. Smoking history
  2. Environmental exposure to carcinogens
  3. Chest pain
     a. Localized or unilateral pain
     b. Sensations of fullness, tightness, or pressure
     c. Piercing chest pain or pleuritic pain on inspiration
     d. Pain radiating to the arm
  4. Dyspnea, wheezing: Record the level of dyspnea at rest, with activity, and supine.
- Assess for
  1. Hoarseness
  2. Wheezing, dyspnea
  3. Decreased or absent breath sounds
  4. Abnormal retractions, stridor, or use of accessory muscles
  5. Asymmetry of diaphragmatic movement
  6. Decreased tactile fremitus when the bronchus is obstructed
  7. Increased vibrations felt on the chest wall indicating areas of the lung in which air spaces are replaced with tumor or fluid
  8. Tracheal deviation
  9. Blood-streaked sputum
  10. Rust-colored or purulent sputum
  11. Hemoptysis
  12. Pleural friction rub
  13. Distant heart sounds

14. Cardiac dysrhythmias

15. Cyanosis of the lips or fingertips, or clubbing

16. Lethargy, fatigue, recent weight loss, anorexia

17. Persistent chills, fever, and cough, which may be related to pneumonitis or bronchitis and are associated with obstruction of the bronchi

18. Fear, anxiety

19. Diagnostic test results

   a. Cytology results of early morning sputum specimen

   b. Chest x-ray, computed tomography (CT) scan, magnetic resonance imaging (MRI) study, positron emission tomography

   c. Fiberoptic bronchoscopy

   d. Thoracoscopy

   e. Pulmonary function and arterial blood gases

   f. Other diagnostic tests to determine whether the cancer has metastasized

NONSURGICAL MANAGEMENT

- Chemotherapy
  1. Exact combination of chemotherapeutic agents depends on the type of cancer and the overall health of the client.
  2. Side effects include
     a. Alopecia. Hair loss is temporary and the client can disguise hair loss by use of wigs, caps, scarves, and turbans.
     b. Nausea and vomiting. Administer antiemetics before and after chemotherapy; drug combinations must be individualized for best effect.
     c. Open sores on mucous membranes. Treat with frequent oral hygiene and instruct the client to use a soft toothbrush or disposable mouth sponge and to avoid the use of dental floss and water pressure gum cleaners.
     d. Immunosuppression, which is medically managed by the administration of biological response modifiers. Instruct the client and significant others what precautions to take to reduce client's chances of developing an infection.
- Gefitinib (Iressa), an oral medication, is an experimental treatment for advanced NSCLC.

- Radiation therapy
    1. Therapy is usually performed daily for 5 to 6 weeks.
    2. Immediate side effects include skin irritation and peeling.
    3. Instruct the client not to wash off dye marks, which indicate the area of radiation; not to use lotions or ointments on the skin unless prescribed by the radiologist; and to avoid direct skin exposure to sun during treatment and for 1 year after radiation therapy is completed.

SURGICAL MANAGEMENT

- Preoperative care includes
    1. Providing routine preoperative care
    2. Teaching the client shoulder exercises and about the chest tube and drainage system (except after pneumonectomy)
- Operative procedures include
    1. *Thoracotomy,* an opening into the thoracic cavity to locate tumors, perform a biopsy, or identify sites of bleeding or injury
    2. *Lobectomy,* the removal of an entire lung lobe
    3. *Resection,* which is any surgical removal of part of the lung that does not involve a complete lobectomy
        a. Limited resection is performed for clients unable to tolerate lobectomy or pneumonectomy.
        b. Segmental resection (segmentectomy) is a lung resection that includes the bronchus, pulmonary artery and vein, and tissue of the involved lung segments.
        c. Wedge resection is the removal of the peripheral portion of a small localized area of disease.
    4. *Pneumonectomy,* the removal of an entire lung, including all blood vessels. The bronchus to that lung is severed and sutured.
- Postoperative care includes
    1. Providing routine postoperative care
    2. Maintaining chest tubes, which drain air and blood that accumulate in the pleural space
    3. Taping tubing junctions to prevent accidental disconnections
    4. Keeping sterile gauze at the bedside to cover the insertion site immediately if the chest tube becomes dislodged
    5. Keeping padded clamps at the bedside for use if the drainage system is interrupted

6. Positioning the drainage tubing to prevent kinks and large loops of tubing
7. Monitoring for excess bleeding in the drainage system and recording output every 4 hours
8. Checking the water seal chamber for continuous bubbling, which indicates an air leak
9. Checking for the rise and fall of fluid in the column as the client breathes in and out
10. Assessing for the absence or presence of lung sounds
11. Positioning the client after a pneumonectomy according to surgeon preference

Interventions for Palliation

- Oxygen therapy or supplemental oxygen with humidification is administered for the client who is hypoxemic or needs it to relieve dyspnea and anxiety.
- Drug therapy includes
    1. Bronchodilators and corticosteroids, which are prescribed for the client with bronchospasms to decrease bronchospasm, inflammation, and edema
    2. Mucolytics, which may be used to ease removal of thick mucous and sputum
    3. Antibiotics, which treat bacterial infections
- Radiation therapy is used to relieve hemoptysis, obstruction of the bronchi and great veins, dysphagia, and pain from bone metastasis.
- Laser therapy is used to relieve bronchial obstructions when tumors are accessible by bronchoscopy.
- Thoracentesis and pleurodesis
    1. *Thoracentesis* is the placement of a large needle or catheter into the intrapleural space and application of suction to rapidly remove fluid.
    2. A chest tube is inserted to drain the fluid and a sclerosing agent is instilled to create a *pleurodesis,* an inflammation that causes the pleura to stick to the chest wall and prevent formation of effusion fluid.
- To manage dyspnea
    1. Position client: Client fatigues easily and is often most comfortable resting in a semi-Fowler's position, sitting in a lounge chair or a reclining chair.

2. Administer supplemental oxygen.
3. Morphine drip may be prescribed.
- To manage pain
  1. Perform a complete pain assessment with attention to onset, intensity, quality, duration, and client description of the pain.
  2. Give analgesics (parenteral, oral, transdermal opioids) around the clock.
  3. Document the client's response to pain and collaborate with the health care team to make adjustments as necessary to the pain management protocol.
  4. Intervene with nonpharmacologic measures such as positioning, hot or cold compresses, distractions, and guided imagery.
- Refer the terminally ill client to hospice.
- Refer the client to community health agencies, as needed.

Cancer, Nasal and Sinus

OVERVIEW

- Tumors of the nose and sinuses are uncommon; they may be benign or malignant.
- Symptoms mimic sinusitis and include persistent nasal obstruction, drainage, bloody discharge, pain, and lymph node enlargement.

COLLABORATIVE MANAGEMENT

- Treatment includes
  1. Radiation therapy (primary treatment)
  2. Surgical resection of the tumor or insertion of a tracheostomy tube
- Postoperative care includes
  1. Routine postoperative care
  2. Maintaining a patent airway (tracheostomy care may be required)
  3. Monitoring for hemorrhage
  4. Providing wound care

5. Strict attention to the client's nutritional needs
6. Providing meticulous mouth care and maxillary cavity care using saline irrigations
7. Managing pain and monitoring the client for infection

C

Cancer, Oropharyngeal

OVERVIEW

- Tumors of the oral cavity are classified as premalignant, malignant, or benign; the focus herein is on premalignant and malignant lesions.
- *Premalignant* lesions include
  1. *Leukoplakia,* which presents as slowly developing changes in the oral mucous membranes that are characterized by thickened, white, firmly attached patches and can be caused by mechanical factors such as poorly fitting dentures, cheek nibbling, malocclusion, or smoking; by familial factors; or by poor nutrition
  2. *Erythroplakia,* a red, velvety-appearing patch in the mouth that is usually asymptomatic; 90% of all lesions are early squamous cell carcinoma
- The types of oral cancer include
  1. Squamous cell carcinoma, which grows slowly and is associated with tobacco and alcohol use and poor nutrition
  2. Basal cell carcinoma, which occurs primarily on the lips and which usually does not metastasize
  3. Kaposi's sarcoma, which appears as painless red-purple oral plaques and is associated with acquired immuno-deficiency syndrome (AIDS) (see AIDS)

||| Cultural Considerations

- The relative survival rate for Caucasians with oral cancer and pharyngeal cancer is 55%, compared with a relative 5-year survival rate of 33% for black individuals with oral cancer.
- Clients who work outdoors are more likely than others to have basal cell carcinomas, especially fair-skinned individuals.

COLLABORATIVE MANAGEMENT

Assessment

- Record client information.
  1. Employment history and history of exposure to known carcinogens or irritants such as tobacco and alcohol
  2. Family history of cancer, especially oral cancer
  3. Oral hygiene practices
  4. Past and current nutritional status
  5. Report of pain, soreness, or burning sensation of the mouth or lip
  6. Use of alcohol or tobacco products
- Assess for
  1. Lesions in the oral cavity: lumps or thickening of the buccal mucosa, or red or white patches appearing on the gums, tongue, or oral mucous membranes
  2. Difficulty chewing or swallowing
  3. Alteration in speech
  4. Enlarged cervical lymph nodes (indicate metastasis)
  5. Fear of cancer
  6. Disturbed body image

Planning and Implementation

◀**NDx:** Ineffective Breathing Pattern

- Maintain airway patency, which is the goal of nursing interventions and is centered on decreasing the tenacity of oral secretions, enabling the client to expectorate secretions and decreasing edema of the head and neck.
  1. Place client in semi-Fowler's or high Fowler's position.
  2. Encourage fluid intake to help liquefy secretions.
  3. Perform chest physiotherapy.
  4. Encourage the client to cough and deep breathe.
  5. Provide oral suction with a Yankauer catheter as needed.
  6. Administer steroids and antibiotics as prescribed.
- Assess risk for aspiration and implement precautions as needed.

SURGICAL MANAGEMENT

- A tracheostomy may be needed for the client to sustain normal breathing.

- Teach good oral hygiene.
  1. Because of oral pain, bleeding, or edema, suggest modifications in oral hygiene practice such as use of a Water Pik (at lowest pressure setting) or gauze sponges
  2. Instruct the client to avoid the use of commercial mouthwashes, which contain alcohol, and instead to use a solution of $1/2$ teaspoon of baking soda in 8 ounces of water or a solution of half hydrogen peroxide and half normal saline.
- The two standard nonsurgical therapies for clients with cancer of the oral cavity are radiation therapy and chemotherapy.
  1. Radiation therapy can be administered by external beam to the tumor site or by implantation of radioactive substances directly into the tumor area (interstitial radiation therapy).
  2. Methotrexate, bleomycin, cisplatin, cyclophosphamide, and doxorubicin are some of the chemotherapeutic agents that may be used to treat oral cancers.

SURGICAL MANAGEMENT

- Small, noninvasive lesions can be excised using carbon dioxide laser therapy or cryotherapy (extreme cold application) in a surgical center. Clients with more invasive or extensive lesions require more radical surgical excision.
- Preoperative care includes
  1. Assessing the client's understanding of the surgical procedure
  2. Reviewing preoperative and postoperative expectations with the client and family or other support persons
     a. For small lesion excision: liquid to soft food diet after surgery, no activity limitations, and analgesic therapy
     b. For large lesion excision (composite resection): probable tracheostomy, oxygen therapy, temporary speech loss (from the tracheostomy), frequent vital sign monitoring, nothing by mouth (NPO) status for 7 to 10 days, and placement of intravenous lines
  3. Assessing the client's ability to read and write and select a method of communication to use postoperatively.
- Postoperative care includes
  1. After local excision, teaching the client routine gentle oral hygiene and advising him or her to avoid extremely

hot foods and beverages, spicy foods, hard or crisp foods, and alcohol until the area is completely healed

2. Maintaining airway patency after extensive excision or composite resection (this is the most important intervention)
3. Providing tracheostomy care; suctioning as needed
4. Giving humidified oxygen
5. Protecting the surgical incision site from mechanical damage and infection
6. Assessing for the presence of unusual odor from the mouth, which can indicate infection
7. Assessing the need for a speech-language pathologist
8. Providing gentle mouth care when permitted
9. Elevating the head of the bed to at least 30 degrees
10. Administering analgesics for pain, as ordered
11. Maintaining enteral or parenteral nutrition while the client is on NPO status
12. Monitoring for difficulty in swallowing, aspiration, or leakage of saliva or fluids from the suture line

Community-Based Care

- Plan for ongoing nutritional management.
  1. Inform the client that the effects of radiation include treatment-related mucositis, stomatitis, xerostomia, dental decay, and alterations in taste, such as an aversion to meat (usually beef or pork) and a metallic taste in the mouth.
  2. Collaborate with the dietitian to meet the client's nutritional needs.
  3. Instruct the client with dysphagia on swallowing exercises, the use of thickened liquids, and dietary supplements.
  4. Soft diet may be encouraged to prevent injury to the mucous membranes.
- Plan for discharge.
  1. Assess the client's need for equipment, such as that required for oral suctioning and nasogastric (enteral) feedings at home.
  2. Provide instructions regarding medications, dressing changes, early symptoms of infection, and special treatments such as tracheostomy care.
  3. Reinforce oral hygiene routine, putting particular emphasis on the need for frequent rinsing of the oral

cavity and changing toothbrush weekly; use of saliva substitutes may be needed.
4. Refer the client and family to home health services, if needed, for treatments, pain control, nutritional support, and emotional support.
5. Assess the client for disturbed body image.
6. Inform the client that people who undergo total glossectomy (removal of the tongue) can be fitted with a special maxillofacial prosthesis to allow speech.
7. Refer the client to the case manager to assess financial needs.

Cancer, Ovarian

OVERVIEW

- Ovarian cancer is the leading cause of death from female reproductive organ malignancies.
- The most common tumor is the serous adenocarcinoma.
- Serous adenocarcinoma tumors grow rapidly, spread quickly, and are often bilateral, with the worst prognosis of all epithelial tumors.
- Ovarian cancer spreads by several mechanisms: direct spread to other organs in the pelvis, distal spread through lymphatic drainage, and peritoneal seeding.

COLLABORATIVE MANAGEMENT

- Record client information.
  1. Family history of ovarian cancer
  2. History of breast, bowel, or endometrial cancer
  3. Nulliparity
  4. Infertility
  5. History of dysmenorrhea or heavy bleeding
  6. Diet history, including intake of animal fat
- Assess for
  1. Abdominal pain or swelling
  2. Dyspepsia
  3. Indigestion

4. Gas and distention
   5. Heavy menstrual flow
   6. Dysfunctional bleeding
   7. Premenstrual tension
   8. Abdominal mass
- Exploratory laparotomy is performed to diagnose and stage ovarian tumors.
- For nursing care, see discussions under Cancer, Cervical, and Cancer, Endometrial.
- The options for treatment depend on the stage of the cancer and include
   1. Chemotherapy: used postoperatively for all stages, although its purpose is usually palliative for stage IV tumors; it is usually given every 3 to 4 weeks for six cycles
   2. Intraperitoneal chemotherapy: involves the instillation of chemotherapy agents into the abdominal cavity; it is used less often because of the inconvenience to the client and risk of complications
   3. Immunotherapy: alters the immunologic response of the ovary and promotes tumor resistance
   4. External radiation therapy: used if the tumor has invaded other organs
   5. Total abdominal hysterectomy and bilateral salpingo-oophorectomy: the surgical procedure for all stages of ovarian cancer
- Nursing interventions include
   1. Routine postoperative care for any client having abdominal surgery
   2. Encouraging the client to express feelings about the disease
   3. Providing information about ovarian cancer and treatment options
   4. Providing encouragement and support to the client and family
- A second-look procedure (laparoscopy or laparotomy) may be performed after 1 year of chemotherapy to confirm the absence or presence of tumor and to remove any new or residual tumor.

Cancer, Pancreatic

OVERVIEW

- Pancreatic tumors are highly malignant and originate in the epithelial cells of the pancreatic ductal system.
- Primary tumors are generally adenocarcinomas and grow in well-differentiated glandular patterns.
- Pancreatic adenocarcinomas grow rapidly and spread to surrounding organs (stomach, duodenum, gallbladder, and intestine) by direct extension and invasion of the lymphatic and vascular system.
- Pancreatic cancer may result from metastasis from cancer of the lung, breast, thyroid, or kidney, or from skin melanoma.

COLLABORATIVE MANAGEMENT

Assessment

- Assess for
    1. Jaundice (yellow discoloration associated with obstruction) and pruritus (itching)
    2. Clay-colored stool and dark, frothy urine
    3. Abdominal pain, described as a vague, constant dullness in the upper abdomen and nonspecific in nature, or pain related to eating or activity; back pain
    4. Weight loss
    5. Anorexia accompanied by early satiety, nausea, flatulence, and vomiting
    6. Glucose intolerance
    7. Splenomegaly
    8. Gastrointestinal bleeding
    9. Leg or calf pain (from thrombophlebitis)
    10. Fatigue and weakness
    11. Dull sound on abdominal percussion indicating ascites
    12. Body image change and fear
    13. Elevated serum lipase, amylase, alkaline phosphatase, and bilirubin levels

Planning and Implementation

- Drug therapy includes
  1. High doses of opioid analgesia; dependency is not a consideration because of the poor prognosis
  2. Chemotherapy, which has limited success
- External beam radiation therapy to shrink pancreatic tumor cells, alleviating obstruction and improving food absorption may provide pain relief but has not increased survival rates.
- Implantation of radon seeds, in combination with systemic or intra-arterial administration of floxuridine (FURD), has also been used.
- Biliary stent may be inserted to relieve biliary obstruction.

SURGICAL MANAGEMENT

- Surgery is the most effective form of management for pancreatic cancer.
- The classic surgery, the Whipple procedure, entails extensive surgical manipulation, including resection of the proximal head of the pancreas, the duodenum, a portion of the jejunum, the stomach (partial or total gastrectomy), and the gallbladder, with anastomosis of the pancreatic duct (pancreatojejunostomy), the common bile duct (choledochojejunostomy), and the stomach (gastrojejunostomy) to the jejunum; the spleen may also be removed (splenectomy).
- Palliative measures to relieve obstruction, such as cholecystojejunostomy, may be performed as a bypass procedure.
- Preoperative care and monitoring includes
  1. Inserting the nasogastric tube for decompression
  2. Starting intravenous fluids or total parenteral nutrition to improve the client's nutritional status before surgery
- Postoperative care and monitoring includes
  1. Monitoring the drainage tubes placed during surgery to remove drainage and secretions from the area and to prevent stress on the anastomosis site
  2. Assessing the tubes and drainage devices for undue stress or kinking; maintaining tubes in a dependent position
  3. Monitoring drainage for color, consistency, and amount
  4. Observing for fistula formation (Drainage of pancreatic fluids are corrosive and irritating to the skin, and internal leakage causes peritonitis.)

5. Placing the client in a semi-Fowler's position to reduce stress on the suture line and anastomosis and to optimize lung expansion
6. Maintaining fluid and electrolyte balance
7. Closely monitoring vital signs for decreased blood pressure and increased heart rate, decreased vascular pressures, decreased hemoglobin levels and hematocrit, and electrolyte imbalances
8. Assessing blood glucose levels for transient hyperglycemia or hypoglycemia resulting from surgical manipulation of the pancreas
9. Monitoring the client for pitting edema of the extremities and dependent edema in the sacrum and back

- Enteral feeding with commercially prepared tube feeding is used while intestinal function is intact.
- A jejunostomy tube is inserted for late stages of pancreatic carcinoma; this method is preferred for lessening reflux and facilitating absorption.
- Hyperalimentation by total parenteral nutrition to optimize nutrition may be used as a single measure or in combination with tube feedings; a Hickman or other type of catheter may be required for long-term use.

Community-Based Care

- Many of the care measures are palliative and aimed at providing relief of symptoms.
- Many clients are diagnosed just a few months before death occurs.
- Special home care preparations depend on the client's physical and activity limitations.
- Regular home care nursing and assistive nursing personnel are scheduled to assist the client and family.
- Help the client identify what needs to be done to prepare for death such as write a will, see family members and friends, make requests for memorial service or funeral known.
- Refer the client to religious leader or support services.

Cancer, Prostatic

OVERVIEW

- Prostatic cancer is the most common type of cancer among American men and the second most deadly.
- Of prostatic tumors, 95% are adenocarcinomas arising from the epithelial cells of the prostate and are usually located in the posterior lobe or outer portion of the gland.
- A prostatic tumor is a slow-growing malignancy with a predictable metastatic pattern to the nearby lymph nodes; bone marrow; and bones of the pelvis, sacrum, and lumbar spine.
- Spread to visceral organs occurs late in the course of the disease; common sites of metastasis include the lungs, liver, adrenals, and kidneys.

COLLABORATIVE MANAGEMENT

- Clinical manifestations include
  1. Symptoms related to bladder neck obstruction
     a. Difficulty in initiating urination
     b. Recurrent bladder infections
     c. Urinary retention
     d. Gross, painless hematuria
  2. Bone pain (advanced disease)
  3. Elevated serum acid phosphatase in clients with advanced cancer
- Prostate cancer screening includes
  1. Digital rectal examination for a stony hard prostate gland with irregularities or indurations
  2. Prostate-specific antigen (PSA) level as a screening test only
     a. Normal level of PSA is less than 4 ng/mL.
     b. PSA levels are elevated in clients with increased prostatic tissue as a result of various conditions, including cancer of the prostate, benign prostatic hyperplasia, prostatic infarction, and prostatitis.
     c. PSA levels are slightly higher in older adults and black individuals than in others.
  3. Biopsy of prostatic tissue

- Older adult clients who are asymptomatic and have other illnesses may choose management by observation without immediate active treatment, especially if the cancer is early stage.
- Surgical intervention includes
  1. Prostatectomy
  2. Radical prostatectomy
  3. Cryosurgical ablation
  4. Bilateral orchiectomy
- Nursing care of the client after a radical prostatectomy includes
  1. Encouraging the client to use patient-controlled analgesia (PCA) as needed
  2. Monitoring the client for bladder spasms induced by the indwelling catheter and administering antispasmodics if prescribed
  3. Monitoring drainage of nasogastric tube, which is usually removed the day after surgery
  4. Keeping the client on nothing by mouth (NPO) status (Solid food is introduced when bowel sounds return.)
  5. Maintaining the sequential compression device until the client begins to ambulate
     a. Ambulation usually begins the second day after surgery; assist as needed and encourage the client to ambulate at least twice a day.
  6. If scrotal or penis swelling occurs, elevate and apply ice to the area intermittently (20 minutes on and 20 minutes off) for the first 24 to 48 hours.
  7. Keeping an accurate record of intake and output, including for Jackson-Pratt or other drainage device
  8. Monitoring the client for complications of a radical prostatectomy
     a. Deep vein thrombosis
     b. Pulmonary embolus
  9. Teaching the client how to care for the urinary catheter because client will be discharged with the catheter in place
- Discharge planning includes
  1. Teaching the client how to use a leg bag
  2. Emphasizing the importance of not straining during a bowel movement; advising the client not to use suppositories or enemas

3. Educating the client on the complications of radical prostatectomy, which include urinary incontinence and erectile dysfunction
   a. Teach the client to perform Kegel perineal exercises.
   b. Biofeedback has been used successfully as a non-invasive treatment for urinary incontinence.
   c. An artificial sphincter may be surgically implanted to treat urinary incontinence.
4. Instructing the client to avoid vigorous exercise, to avoid lifting heaving objects, and to take a shower rather than a tub bath
5. Instructing the client to inspect incision site daily for signs of infection
6. Emphasizing the importance of follow-up appointments with the health care provider to monitor progress

- Cryosurgical ablation of the prostate is a minimally invasive procedure used as an alternative to radical prostatectomy. Advantages of this procedure are minimal blood loss, minimal postoperative pain, decreased risk for postoperative urinary incontinence, a 1- to 2-day hospital stay, and earlier than otherwise return to activities such as work.
- Bilateral orchiectomy is palliative surgery to arrest cancer spread.
- Interstitial radiation therapy or radioactive seed implantation is used to treat localized disease.
- External beam radiation is performed as an alternative curative treatment to surgery for locally contained tumors, as an adjunct to radical prostatectomy, or for palliation of the client's symptoms.
- Hormone therapy is with estrogens such as diethylstilbestrol (DES) and a gonadotropin-releasing hormone agonist or androgen-blocking agent such as flutamide.
- Systemic chemotherapy has not proved effective as a main treatment; it may be used for the client who fails to respond to hormonal manipulation.
- Targeted therapies take advantage of one or more differences in a cancer cell that is either not present or only slightly present in normal cells.
- Health teaching includes a discussion of quality-of-life issues, including sexuality, body image, and the impact of a cancer diagnosis on life.

Cancer, Renal

OVERVIEW

- Renal cell carcinoma is also referred to as adenocarcinoma of the kidney.
- The healthy functional tissue of the kidney is damaged and replaced by cancer cells.
- Systemic effects include anemia, erythrocytosis, hypercalcemia, liver dysfunction with elevated liver enzymes, increased sedimentation rate, hypertension, and other miscellaneous hormonal effects.
- Complications of renal tumors include metastasis through the blood or lymph to the liver, lungs, and long bones, and other kidney and urinary tract infections.

COLLABORATIVE MANAGEMENT

Assessment

- Assess the client for
  1. Risk factors, such as smoking or environmental exposures (lead, phosphate, cadmium)
  2. Weight loss
  3. Changes in urine color
  4. Abdominal or flank pain
  5. Asymmetry or obvious protrusion in the flank area
  6. Hematuria (late sign)
  7. Renal bruit
  8. Skin pallor
  9. Increased pigmentation of the nipples and gynecomastia
  10. Muscle wasting, weakness, generally poor nutritional status
  11. Anxiety and fear
  12. Red blood cells (RBCs) in the urine
  13. Decreased hemoglobin level and hematocrit
  14. Increased sedimentation rate, adrenocorticotropic hormone, cortisol, and renin
  15. Hypercalcemia

Interventions

- Treatment consists of
    1. Chemotherapy
    2. Radiofrequency ablation, which has shown some promise in treating renal cancer
    3. Radical nephrectomy, which may be followed by radiation therapy
- Postoperative care includes
    1. Observing the abdomen for distention resulting from bleeding
    2. Observing for adrenal insufficiency. Large urinary output with subsequent loss of sodium and water leads to hypotension, which is followed by oliguria.
    3. Administering intravenous fluids and packed RBCs, as ordered
    4. Monitoring intake and output hourly
    5. Weighing the client daily
    6. Monitoring vital signs and neurologic signs every 4 hours
    7. Administering pain medication, as ordered: Acute pain control is most effectively achieved when sedatives are used in combination with the opioid analgesic.
    8. Administering antibiotics or steroids, as ordered

Cancer, Skin

OVERVIEW

- Overexposure to sunlight is the major cause of skin cancer.
- The most common skin cancers include
    1. Actinic or solar keratoses: premalignant lesions involving the keratinocytes of the epidermis; common in chronic sun-damaged skin and may progress to squamous cell carcinoma
    2. Squamous cell carcinomas: malignant neoplasms of the epidermis characterized by local invasion and risk for metastasis; predisposed by sun exposure and chronic epithelial damage from repeated injury or irritation
    3. Basal cell carcinomas: lesions that arise in the basal cell layer of the epidermis, resulting primarily from ultraviolet

light radiation exposure, genetic predisposition, and chronic irritation
   4. Melanomas: highly metastatic pigmented malignant lesions originating in the melanin-producing cells of the epidermis

- Risk factors include genetic predisposition and precursor lesions, which resemble unusual moles.

COLLABORATIVE MANAGEMENT

Assessment

- Record client information.
   1. Risk factors
   2. Age and race
   3. Family history of skin cancer
   4. Past surgical removal of skin growths
   5. Changes in size, color, or sensation of any mole, birthmark, wart, or scar
   6. Sunlight exposure
   7. Exposure to chemical carcinogens
   8. Skin lesions subjected to repeated irritation
- Assess for
   1. Skin lesions in sun-exposed areas and the entire skin surface
   2. Unusual appearance of moles, warts, birthmarks, and scars
   3. Associated symptoms, such as tenderness and itching

Interventions

- Treatment consists of
   1. Topical chemotherapy with 5-fluorouracil cream for multiple actinic keratoses or for widespread superficial basal cell carcinoma
   2. *Interferon*, a biologic response modifier, for stage III or higher melanomas
   3. *Radiation therapy* for older clients who are poor surgical risks with large, deeply invasive basal cell tumors
   4. *Immunotherapy*, an experimental treatment for clients with melanoma that has metastasized to distant sites
   5. *Cryosurgery* with liquid nitrogen for isolated lesions
   6. Procedures used for small lesions with well-defined borders: *curettage*, to scrape away the cancerous tissue,

followed by *electrodesiccation,* which involves place-ment of an electric probe on the wound surface to destroy the malignant tissue remnants by thermal and electrical energy
7. *Excision* for large or poorly defined cancers
8. *Mohs' surgery* for basal and squamous cell carcinoma
9. Plastic and reconstructive surgery to correct functional defects and alter physical appearance

Cancer, Stomach

OVERVIEW

- Malignant neoplasms found in the stomach develop in the mucosal cells that form the innermost lining of any portion or all of the stomach.
- Adenocarcinomas are the most common type, followed by lymphomas and sarcomas.
- In advanced disease, invasion extends to the stomach muscle or beyond.
- Most stomach cancers develop in the pylorus and antrum.
- Methods of extension include extension through the gastric wall into the regional lymphatics and direct organ invasion.

COLLABORATIVE MANAGEMENT

Assessment

- Assess for *early* symptoms of disease.
  1. Indigestion
  2. Abdominal discomfort
  3. Feeling of fullness
  4. Epigastric, back, or retrosternal pain
- Assess for *late* symptoms of disease.
  1. Nausea and vomiting
  2. Obstructive symptoms
  3. Iron deficiency anemia
  4. Palpable epigastric mass
  5. Enlarged lymph nodes
  6. Weakness and fatigue

7. Progressive weight loss
8. Signs of distant metastasis
9. Virchow's nodes (enlarged supraventricular lymph nodes)
10. Blumer's shelf (firm mass palpable on vaginal or rectal examination)
11. "Sister Mary Joseph's nodes" (subcutaneous periumbilical deposits)
12. Krukenberg's tumor (metastatic ovarian nodules)
13. Hypoalbuminemia, elevated carcinoembryonic antigen (CEA) level, anemia

Planning and Implementation

- Combination drug chemotherapy including 5-fluorouracil, doxorubicin, and mitomycin C has proved more effective than single-agent chemotherapy.
- Radiation therapy is used in conjunction with surgery.
- Surgical management is usually curative in *early* disease and involves distal subtotal gastrectomy.
- Palliative surgical resection in *late* disease may improve the client's quality of life.
- Surgical procedures include
  1. Subtotal gastrectomy is done for tumors in the mid or distal (lower) portions of the stomach, combined with lymph node dissection and removal of the omentum and spleen.
  2. Total gastrectomy is performed for cancer in the upper portion of the stomach; the entire stomach, lymph nodes, and omentum are removed. The esophagus is sutured to the duodenum or jejunum to re-establish continuity of the gastrointestinal tract.
  3. Gastroenterostomy is performed for tumors at the gastric outlet.
- Routine postoperative care includes care of the nasogastric tube (see also Surgical Management under Ulcers, Peptic), pain management, and antiemetics, if needed.
- Total parenteral nutrition (TPN) may be required immediately after surgery and in the later recovery period if oral intake is poorly tolerated.
- Postoperative oral intake progresses from oral liquids to small, frequent solid food feedings; milk and dairy products are often eliminated because of lactose intolerance.

- Teach relaxation techniques, cutaneous stimulation, and visual imagery.
- Observe the client for postoperative complications such as
    1. Anastomotic leak
    2. Pneumonia
    3. Hemorrhage
    4. Reflux aspiration
    5. Sepsis
    6. Reflux gastritis
    7. Paralytic ileus
    8. Bowel obstruction
    9. Wound infection
    10. Dumping syndrome
- In collaboration with the dietitian, counsel the client and family about methods of food preparation and types of food that increase caloric and protein intake.

Community-Based Care

- Provide verbal and written postoperative instructions on
    1. Dietary restrictions individualized to the client
    2. Pain management techniques, including medications
    3. Inspection of incision for redness, tenderness, swelling, and drainage
    4. Dressing change procedures, if necessary
    5. Side effects of chemotherapy or radiation treatments
- Refer the client and family to home health services, hospice services, and appropriate support groups, such as I Can Cope, provided by the American Cancer Society.

Cancer, Testicular

- Testicular cancer is the most common malignancy in males 15 to 35 years of age.
- Primary testicular cancers fall into two groups:
    1. *Germinal* tumors arise from the sperm-producing germ cells and include seminoma and nonseminoma tumors (embryonal, teratoma, and choriocarcinoma).

2. *Nongerminal* tumors arise from other structures in the testicles and include interstitial cell tumors and androblastoma.

C

COLLABORATIVE MANAGEMENT

Assessment

- Record client information.
  1. Age and race
  2. History or presence of undescended testes
  3. Family history of testicular cancer
  4. Family situation
     a. Desire for children
     b. Interest in sperm storage in a sperm bank
- Assess for
  1. Palpable lymphadenopathy
  2. Abdominal masses
  3. Gynecomastia
  4. Psychological ramifications of the disease
  5. Increased alfa-fetoprotein and the beta subunit of human chorionic gonadotropin

Planning and Implementation

NDx: Risk for Sexual Dysfunction

- Health teaching before surgery includes
  1. Normal reproduction and possible effects of cancer and its treatment on reproductive function
  2. Reproductive options
  3. Fertility
  4. Sexuality

COLLABORATIVE PROBLEM: Potential for Metastasis

NONSURGICAL MANAGEMENT

- Chemotherapy and radiation therapy may be used alone or in combination.

SURGICAL MANAGEMENT

- *Unilateral orchiectomy* (removal of the testis) is performed for diagnosis and primary surgical management.

- *Radical retroperitoneal lymph node dissection* is used to stage the disease and to reduce tumor volume so that chemotherapy or radiation therapy is more effective.
- Provide preoperative care.
    1. Provide routine preoperative care.
    2. Prepare the client for an extensive surgical procedure and a large incision if radical retroperitoneal lymph node dissection is to be performed.
- Provide postoperative care.
    1. Provide routine postoperative care.
    2. Assess the client for any complications of major abdominal surgery.
    3. Administer pain medication, as ordered.
    4. Monitor the client for complications of immobility.
- Combination chemotherapy is dramatically effective for treating nonseminomatous testicular cancer, especially the use of cisplatin (Platinol) in combination with other agents.
- Radiation therapy is the treatment of choice for clients with a pure seminoma after orchiectomy.
- Stem cell transplantation with high-dose chemotherapy is under investigation for treatment in men with advanced germ cell cancer.

Community-Based Care

- Postoperative instructions for the client include
    1. Notifying the physician of chills, fever, increasing tenderness or pain around the incision, drainage, or dehiscence of the incision
    2. Resuming normal activities except lifting objects heavier than 15 pounds or stair climbing
    3. Performing monthly testicular self-examination on the remaining testis
    4. Following instructions for radiation therapy and chemotherapy
    5. Following up with visits to the physicians for at least 3 years

Cancer, Thyroid

OVERVIEW

- The four types of thyroid cancer are
  1. *Papillary* carcinoma
     a. A slow-growing tumor found more often in women than in men
     b. Good prognosis if localized to the thyroid gland
  2. *Follicular* carcinoma
     a. Primarily affects older clients
     b. Invades blood vessels and metastasizes to bone and lung tissue
     c. Can adhere to the trachea, neck muscles, great vessels, and skin, resulting in dysphagia and dyspnea
     d. Fair prognosis if metastasis is minimal at the time of diagnosis
  3. *Medullary* carcinoma
     a. Primarily affects clients over 50 years of age
     b. Involves metastasis that occurs via regional lymph nodes and invades surrounding structures
     c. May occur as part of multiple endocrine neoplasia type II, a familial endocrine disorder
     d. Possible excessive secretion of calcitonin, adrenocorticotropic hormone, prostaglandins, and serotonin
  4. *Anaplastic* carcinoma
     a. A rapidly growing, extremely aggressive tumor
     b. Directly invades adjacent structures, causing stridor, hoarseness, and dysphagia
     c. Poor prognosis

COLLABORATIVE MANAGEMENT

- The treatment of papillary, follicular, and medullary carcinoma includes
  1. Total *thyroidectomy* with a modified radical neck dissection if regional lymph nodes are involved
  2. Postoperative suppressive doses of thyroid hormone for 3 months, followed by a radioactive iodine (RAI) uptake

study; if there is RAI uptake, clients are treated with ablative amounts of RAI

   3. A course of chemotherapy if recurrent thyroid cancer does not respond to RAI

- The treatment for anaplastic carcinoma is palliative surgery, radiation, or chemotherapy. For nursing care, see both Cancer and Hyperthyroidism.

Cancer, Urothelial

OVERVIEW

- Urothelial cancers are malignancies of the urothelium, which is the lining of transitional cells in the renal pelvis, ureters, urinary bladder, and urethra.
- Most tumors occur in the urinary bladder; consequently, *bladder cancer* is a general term used to describe urothelial cancer.
- The urothelium is described initially in terms of cellular dysplasia.
- Effects of tumors include local inflammation, ischemia, hemorrhage, and urinary obstruction.

COLLABORATIVE MANAGEMENT

Assessment

- Record client information.
   1. Active and passive exposure to cigarette smoke
   2. Employment history to determine exposure to harmful environmental agents
- Assess for
   1. Abdominal tenderness or discomfort
   2. Bladder distention
   3. Abdominal asymmetry
   4. Changes in color, frequency, or amount of urine
   5. Painless hematuria
   6. Dysuria
   7. Frequency

8. Urgency
9. Anxiety, fear

Planning and Implementation

NONSURGICAL MANAGEMENT

- Prophylactic immunotherapy with intravesical instillation of bacille Calmette-Guérin (BCG) is used to prevent tumor recurrence of superficial cancer.
- Multiagent systemic chemotherapy may be used.
- Radiation therapy may be performed in combination with chemotherapy.

SURGICAL MANAGEMENT

- Cystectomy, or surgical removal of the cancerous bladder with urinary diversion, is performed.
- Preoperative care includes
  1. Routine preoperative care
  2. Educational counseling about the urinary diversion and postoperative care requirements
  3. Assisting in the selection of the stoma site (with the enterostomal therapist)
  4. Ensuring an accurate understanding of self-care practices, methods of pouching, control of urinary drainage, and minimization of odor
- Surgical techniques include
  1. Transurethral resection of the bladder tumor
  2. Partial cystectomy
     a. *Ureterostomy* diverts urine directly to the skin through a ureteral skin opening (stoma). After the procedure, the client must wear a pouch (bag) to collect the urine. Types of ureterostomy include
        (1) Cutaneous ureterostomy
        (2) Cutaneous ureteroureterostomy
        (3) Bilateral cutaneous ureterostomy
     b. *Conduits* collect urine in a portion of the intestine, which is then opened onto the skin surface as a stoma. The client must wear a pouch to collect the urine. Types of conduits include
        (1) Ileal (Bricker's) conduit
        (2) Colon conduit

    c. *Sigmoidostomy* diverts urine to the large intestine, so no stoma is required; the client excretes urine during bowel movements, and bowel incontinence may occur. Types of sigmoidostomy include

        (1) Ureterosigmoidostomy

        (2) Ureteroileosigmoidostomy

    d. *Ileal reservoir* diverts urine into a surgically created pouch or pocket that functions as a bladder. The stoma is continent, and the client removes urine by regular self-catheterization. One type is the continent internal ileal reservoir (the Kock pouch)

- Postoperative care depends on the type and extent of the surgical procedure.
  1. Provide routine postoperative care.
  2. Maintain drainage tubes.
  3. Collaborate with the enterostomal therapist to provide wound and skin care and to manage the urinary drainage system.
  4. Monitor urinary output and characteristics of the urine.
  5. Administer analgesics, antispasmodics, and antibiotics, as ordered.

Community-Based Care

- Health teaching includes
  1. Providing dietary instructions, including the avoidance of gas-forming foods if urinary diversion is into the gastrointestinal tract
  2. Teaching care of the external pouch, including application, skin care, pouch care, methods of adhesion, and drainage mechanisms
  3. Instructing the client on catheterization techniques following the Kock pouch procedure
  4. Providing educational and psychological counseling for the impact of urinary diversions on self-image and self-esteem
  5. Referring the client to local, state, and national support groups

Cancer, Vaginal

OVERVIEW

- Primary vaginal cancer, a rare disease, usually occurs as an extension of cervical, endometrial, or vulvar cancer.
- Most vaginal cancers are squamous cell carcinomas that develop in the upper third of the vagina.
- Adenocarcinomas are associated with intrauterine exposure to diethylstilbestrol as a result of maternal ingestion during pregnancy.
- The spread of vaginal cancer depends on the tumor location; upper vaginal lesions spread in the same manner as cervical cancer, whereas the spread of lower lesions is similar to that of vulvar cancer.
- Early metastasis occurs.
- Predisposing factors associated with development of vaginal cancer include
  1. Repeated pregnancies
  2. Sexually transmitted diseases, such as herpesvirus and papillomavirus infection
  3. Prior radiation therapy
- Both nonsurgical and surgical interventions may be used to treat women with vaginal cancer.

COLLABORATIVE MANAGEMENT

Nonsurgical Management

- Laser therapy is performed after iodine staining of the vagina to identify the affected areas. Close follow-up is necessary: a Papanicolaou (Pap) smear and colposcopic examination once every 4 months for 1 year and then once every 6 to 12 months.
- Local application of 5-fluorouracil (5-FU) cream to the vagina daily for 1 week is another treatment.
- Intracavitary radiation therapy (IRT) is used alone for treatment of cancer limited to the vaginal wall.
- External radiation therapy is used in combination with IRT for treatment of cancer that extends beyond the vaginal wall.

- Complications of radiation therapy include vaginal stenosis, adhesions, and drainage.
  1. Teach the client to use a vaginal dilator.
  2. Assess for sexual dysfunction.
- Chemotherapy is used for recurrent disease, but no effective therapy is known.

Surgical Management

- Local wide excision is performed for localized lesions.
- Partial or total vaginectomy (removal of part or all of the vagina) is performed for invasive disease.
  1. Inform the client that vaginectomy affects sexual function.
  2. Counsel the client on alternative sexual activities.
- Radical hysterectomy or pelvic exenteration may also be performed, depending on the extent of the cancer.

Cancer, Vulvar

OVERVIEW

- Vulvar cancer is slow growing, stays localized for a long period, and metastasizes late. More than 50% of vulvar cancer occurrences are in women older than 65 years of age.
- Most vulvar cancers are squamous cell carcinomas and develop in the absence of premalignant changes in the epithelium.
- The first change is usually vulvar atypia or mild dysplasia.
- The cancer can spread directly to the urethra, the vagina, and the anus and through the lymphatic system to the inguinal, femoral, and deep iliac pelvic nodes.

COLLABORATIVE MANAGEMENT

Assessment

- Record client information.
  1. Age
  2. Family history of cervical cancer or diabetes

3. Obesity

4. Possible sexually transmitted diseases

- Assessment findings include

    1. Irritation or itching in the perineal area

    2. Bleeding (a late sign)

    3. Multifocal lesions on the labia

Interventions

- Management depends on the extent of the spread.
- Laser therapy is performed for premalignant vulvar lesions.
- Chemotherapy, in the form of a topical application of 5-fluorouracil, is used for carcinoma *in situ*.
- External radiation therapy follows surgery for deep pelvic node involvement.
- Surgical interventions include

    1. Local wide *excision* of the lesion

    2. Simple vulvectomy: the removal of the vulva, the labia majora, the labia minora, and possibly the clitoris (not commonly performed)

    3. Skinning vulvectomy: the removal of the superficial skin of the vulva, without removal of the clitoris, and replacement of the skin with a split-thickness skin graft

    4. *Modified radical* or *radical vulvectomy* for invasive cancer: the removal of the entire vulva—skin, labia, clitoris, subcutaneous tissues, and possibly inguinal and femoral node dissection

- Provide postoperative care.

    1. Maintain patency of drainage tubes.

    2. Provide an egg crate mattress or air mattress and a bed cradle to increase the client's comfort.

    3. Apply antiembolism stockings or sequential compression devices to prevent thromboembolism and leg edema.

    4. Provide wound care and change dressings over the incision frequently because of the amount of wound drainage and risk for infection.

    5. Monitor the client for indications of infection.

    6. Sitz bath or whirlpool bath may be prescribed.

    7. Encourage the client to eat a diet rich in vitamin C, iron, and protein to promote wound healing.

    8. Provide care of the Foley catheter according to institutional policy.

9. Administer analgesics, as ordered.
10. Explain changes in sexual functioning that occur as a result of the surgery.
11. Refer the client for counseling as needed.
- Health teaching is focused on
  1. Relief of postoperative discomfort, including medications
  2. Diet instructions, including intake of vitamin C, iron, and protein
  3. Change in body image and sexual functioning
  4. Wound care that may be ordered at home, including
     a. Sitz bath, using a squeeze bottle or squirt gun to pour/squirt over the wound area
     b. Tub bath: teach the client to meticulously clean the tub before and after use; $1/2$ cup of salt may be added to the warm bath water

Carditis, Rheumatic (Rheumatic Endocarditis)

- Rheumatic carditis (rheumatic endocarditis) is a sensitivity response that develops after an upper respiratory tract infection with group A beta-hemolytic streptococci and is a major indicator of rheumatic fever.
- Inflammation is evident in all layers of the heart, which results in impaired contractile function of the myocardium, thickening of the pericardium, and valvular damage.
- Common clinical manifestations include
  1. Tachycardia
  2. Cardiomegaly
  3. Development of a new murmur or change in existing murmur
  4. Pericardial friction rub
  5. Precordial pain
  6. Electrocardiogram (ECG) changes (prolonged PR interval)
  7. Indications of heart failure
  8. Evidence of an existing streptococcal infection

- Treatment includes
  1. Give antibiotics, usually penicillin or erythromycin (Eryc, Erythromid).
  2. Manage fever by maintaining hydration, administering antipyretics.
  3. Encourage the client to obtain adequate rest.
  4. Teach the client that antibiotic prophylaxis is necessary for the rest of his or her life to prevent infective endocarditis.

Cardiomyopathy

OVERVIEW

- Cardiomyopathy is a subacute or chronic heart muscle disease of unknown cause; it is not a common disorder.
- Cardiomyopathy is divided into three categories on the basis of abnormalities in structure and function:
  1. *Dilated cardiomyopathy* (DCM), the most common type, involves extensive damage to the myofibrils and interference with myocardial metabolism; it is characterized by dilation of both ventricles and impairment of systolic function.
  2. Asymmetric ventricular hypertrophy and disarray of the myocardial fibers are cardinal features of *hypertrophic cardiomyopathy* (HCM). Left ventricular (LV) hypertrophy leads to a stiff LV that results in diastolic filling abnormalities. In about 50% of clients, HCM is transmitted as a single gene autosomal dominant trait.
  3. *Restrictive cardiomyopathy* (RCM), the least common of the three cardiomyopathies, results in restriction of filling of the ventricles. It is caused by endocardial or myocardial disease and produces a clinical picture similar to that of constrictive pericarditis.
- Sudden death may be the first and only manifestation of cardiomyopathy.

COLLABORATIVE MANAGEMENT

Assessment

- Assess for clinical manifestations of *DCM*.
  1. Left ventricular failure
  2. Progressive dyspnea on exertion
  3. Orthopnea
  4. Palpitations
  5. Activity intolerance
  6. Right-sided heart failure late in the disease
  7. Atrial fibrillation
- Assess for clinical manifestations of *HCM*.
  1. Exertional dyspnea (90% of clients)
  2. Angina (75% of clients)
  3. Syncope
  4. Atypical chest pain that occurs at rest, is prolonged, has no relation to exertion, and is not relieved by nitrates
  5. Ventricular dysrhythmias
- Assess for clinical manifestations of *RCM*.
  1. Exertional dyspnea
  2. Weakness
  3. Exercise intolerance
  4. Palpitations
  5. Syncope

Interventions

NONSURGICAL MANAGEMENT

- Care of the client with DCM or RCM is the same as that for clients with heart failure (see Heart Failure).
- Treatment includes
  1. Diuretics, vasodilators, and cardiac glycosides to increase cardiac output
  2. Antidysrhythmics or implantable cardiac defibrillator to control ventricular dysrhythmias, including tachycardia
  3. Teaching the client to abstain from alcohol because of its cardiac depressant effects
  4. Teaching the client to report any palpitations, dizziness, or fainting, which might indicate a dysrhythmia
- Management of HCM includes beta-adrenergic blocking agents (carvedilol) and calcium antagonists (diltiazem); strenuous exercise is prohibited.

SURGICAL MANAGEMENT

- The type of surgery performed depends on the type of cardiomyopathy.
- The most commonly performed surgery for HCM is excision of a portion of the hypertrophied ventricular septum to create a widened outflow tract.
- Cardiomyoplasty is used when cardiac transplantation is not an option and the client is asymptomatic at rest.
- *Heart transplantation* is the treatment of choice for clients with severe DCM; a donor heart from a person with a comparable body weight and ABO compatibility is transplanted into a recipient within 6 hours of procurement.
- Criteria for candidates for heart transplantation include
  1. Life expectancy less than 1 year
  2. Age younger than 65 years (variable)
  3. New York Heart Association class III or IV (poor functional status)
  4. Normal or only slightly increased pulmonary vascular resistance
  5. Absence of active infection
  6. Stable psychosocial status
  7. No evidence of drug or alcohol abuse
- Nursing interventions include
  1. Providing postoperative care similar to that provided for clients having open heart surgery (see Coronary Artery Disease, Surgical Management)
  2. Monitoring carefully for occult bleeding into the pericardial sac with the potential for cardiac tamponade
  3. Teaching the client to change positions slowly due to the potential of orthostatic hypotension
  4. Teaching the client the importance of taking immunosuppressants for the duration of his or her life to prevent transplant rejection
  5. Monitoring closely for infection
- Discharge teaching includes
  1. Teach the client to report signs and symptoms of rejection, such as hypotension, dysrhythmias, weakness, fatigue, and dizziness (initial episode of acute rejection usually occurs in the first 3 months after transplantation).
  2. Inform the client that the surgeon will perform endomyocardial biopsy at regularly scheduled intervals to detect rejection.

3. Encourage the client to follow a lifestyle similar to that of clients with coronary artery disease.
4. Encourage the client to participate in an exercise program, allowing at least 10 minutes of warm-up and cooldown for the denervated heart to adjust to changes in activity level.
5. Provide information about discharge medications and diet.

Carpal Tunnel Syndrome

OVERVIEW

- Carpal tunnel syndrome (CTS) is a condition in which the median nerve in the wrist is compressed, causing pain and numbness.
- Risk factors include synovitis, hand or wrist trauma from repetitive activities, and congenital or familial problems.
- CTS typically occurs in women 30 to 60 years of age.

COLLABORATIVE MANAGEMENT

Assessment

- Assess for
  1. Nature, location, and intensity of the pain and numbness
  2. Time that day pain usually occurs (CTS pain is usually worse at night)
  3. Paresthesia
  4. Positive results for Phalen's maneuver, which produces paresthesia in the median nerve distribution within 60 seconds (the client is asked to relax the wrist into flexion or place the backs of both hands together and flex both wrists simultaneously)
  5. Positive Tinel's sign, which is the same response as for the Phalen's maneuver (elicited by tapping lightly over the area of the median nerve)
  6. Weak pinch, clumsiness, and difficulty with fine movements
  7. Muscle weakness and wasting

8. Wrist swelling
9. Autonomic changes manifested by skin discoloration, nail changes such as brittleness, and increased or decreased swelling of the hand and wrist
10. Fear that the symptoms are related to a spinal problem or that job or lifestyle changes may have to be made

Interventions

NONSURGICAL MANAGEMENT

- Nonsurgical management includes the use of
  1. Analgesics such as aspirin and nonsteroidal anti-inflammatory drugs
  2. Direct injection of corticosteroids into the carpal tunnel to relieve inflammation
- Wrist immobilization is tried before surgical intervention.

SURGICAL MANAGEMENT

- Surgery is performed to relieve compression on the median nerve; it may be performed as an endoscopic procedure using a laser to free the trapped nerve or as an open carpal tunnel release.
- If CTS is a complication of rheumatoid arthritis, a *synovectomy,* or removal of excess synovium, may resolve the problem.
- Provide postoperative care.
  1. Check pressure dressing carefully for drainage and tightness.
  2. Elevate the hand and arm per surgeon's order.
  3. Check the client's neurovascular status during the immediate postoperative period.
  4. Encourage the client to move all fingers of the affected hand frequently.
  5. Administer pain medication as needed.
  6. Explain to the client the importance of not lifting heavy objects for 4 to 6 weeks.
  7. Remind the client that weakness and discomfort can occur for weeks or months after surgery.
  8. Teach the client how to assess for neurovascular status.
  9. Ensure that assistance (family or significant others) is available in the home for routine daily tasks as needed.

Cataracts

OVERVIEW

- A cataract is an opacity of the lens that distorts the image projected onto the retina.
- Types of cataracts include
  1. Age-related: generally affecting persons older than 65 years of age
  2. Traumatic: caused by blunt trauma, penetrating blows, or overexposure to excessive heat, x-rays, or radioactive material
  3. Toxic: seen after ingestion of or exposure to certain chemicals such as extended use of corticosteroids, chlorpromazine, or miotic agents
  4. Associated: seen with other diseases such as diabetes mellitus, hypoparathyroidism, Down syndrome, and atopic dermatitis
  5. Complicated: develops as a result of ocular disorders such as retinitis pigmentosa, glaucoma, and retinal detachment

COLLABORATIVE MANAGEMENT

Assessment

- Record client history.
  1. Age
  2. History of trauma
  3. Exposure to radioactive materials or x-rays
  4. Current medical problems, especially systemic diseases such as diabetes mellitus, hypoparathyroidism, Down syndrome, or atopic dermatitis
  5. Medication history
  6. History of intraocular disease
- Assess for
  1. Blurred vision
  2. Decrease in color vision: blue, green, and purple appear gray
  3. Diplopia
  4. Reduced visual acuity progressing to blindness

5. Presence of white pupil (late stage)
6. Anxiety and fear

Planning and Implementation

NDx: Disturbed Sensory Perception (Visual)

- Surgery is the only treatment for cataracts. Two extraction procedures are commonly performed.
  1. Extracapsular: removal of the anterior portion of the capsule
  2. Intracapsular: removal of the lens completely within the capsule
- Most often a clear plastic lens is implanted at the same time of cataract removal to resolve issues related to loss of accommodation refractive ability.
- Provide preoperative care.
  1. Provide routine preoperative care and teaching.
  2. Assess how client's vision affects activities of daily living (ADLs), especially eating, dressing, and ambulation.
  3. Review the procedure for local and retrobulbar anesthesia, which is generally used.
  4. Teach the client how to instill eye drops.
  5. Administer preoperative medications, if ordered.
- Provide postoperative care.
  1. Provide routine postoperative care.
  2. Administer antibiotics immediately after surgery subconjunctivally as an antibiotic plus steroid ointment; both are used for several days after surgery.
  3. Report drainage on the eye pad to the surgeon.
  4. Apply cool compresses if the eye itches.
  5. Administer analgesics such as acetaminophen.
  6. Recommend eyeglasses, sunglasses, or an eye shield during the day and an eye shield at night.
  7. Observe for and report complications of surgery, including
     a. Increased intraocular pressure, manifested by severe pain, nausea, and vomiting
     b. Infection
     c. Bleeding into the anterior chamber of the eye, manifested by a change in vision

- Before discharge, review the signs and symptoms of complications.
  1. Sharp, sudden pain
  2. Bleeding or increased drainage
  3. Lid swelling
  4. Decreased vision
  5. Flashes of light or floating shapes
- Teach the client required self-care activities, including
  1. Personal care
  2. Shield application
  3. Eyedrop instillation
  4. Activities permitted and restricted
  5. Medication
- Reinforce activity restrictions such as no coughing, bending at the waist, sneezing, lifting of objects that weigh more than 15 pounds (6.8 kg), and sleeping or lying on the operative side (which increases intraocular pressure).
- Inform the client that hair washing is allowed several days after surgery if it can be done with the head tilted back, such as in a hair salon.
- Advise the client to stand in the shower with the face turned away from the shower head.
- Advise the client not to drive, operate machinery, or participate in sports until given specific permission to do so.
- Advise the client that light housekeeping is permitted but vacuuming should be avoided for several weeks.
- Emphasize the importance of follow-up visits with the physicians.

Chancroid

- Chancroid is most common in tropical and subtropical countries.
- Recent spread of the causative organism *Haemophilus ducreyi* has made chancroid an important sexually transmitted disease in the United States.
- The incubation period varies from 3 to 10 days.

- Genital lesions and inguinal lymphadenopathy without systemic illness are the usual symptoms.
- Lesions rapidly break down to form irregularly shaped, deep ulcers that have purulent discharge and bleed easily.
- Complications include inguinal adenopathy, balanitis, phimosis, and urethral fistulas.
- Transmission is through contact with the ulcer or with discharge from the infected local lymph glands during sexual intercourse.
- Treatment includes antibiotics such as azithromycin (Zithromax), erythromycin (E-Mycin, Apo-Erythro), or ceftriaxone sodium (Rocephin).
- Health teaching is similar to that for syphilis.

Cholecystitis

OVERVIEW

- Cholecystitis is an inflammation of the gallbladder that can occur as an acute or chronic process.
- *Acute* cholecystitis (inflammation) usually develops in association with cholelithiasis (gallstones).
- *Acalculous* cholecystitis occurs in the absence of gallstones and is associated with biliary stasis caused by any condition that affects the regular filling or emptying of the gallbladder such as decreased blood flow to the gallbladder or anatomic problems such as kinking of the gallbladder neck or cystic duct that can result in pancreatic enzyme reflux into the gallbladder and cause inflammation.
- *Chronic* cholecystitis results when repeated episodes of cystic duct obstruction results in chronic inflammation, and the gallbladder becomes fibrotic and contracted, resulting in decreased motility and deficient absorption.
- Complications of cholecystitis include *pancreatitis* and *cholangitis* (inflammation/inflection of the common bile ducts).
- Cholangitis is usually associated with choledocholithiasis (common bile duct stones).

- *Jaundice* (yellow discoloration of body tissues) and *icterus* (yellow discoloration of the sclera) can occur in acute disease but are most commonly seen in the chronic phase of cholecystitis. Jaundice results from increased bilirubin in the body that collects in the skin and sclera. Itching and a burning sensation result.

COLLABORATIVE MANAGEMENT

Assessment

- Record client information.
    1. Height and weight
    2. Sex, age, race, and ethnic group
    3. Food preferences, including excess fat and cholesterol intake
    4. Food intolerances and related gastrointestinal (GI) symptoms, including flatulence, dyspepsia (indigestion), eructation (belching), anorexia, nausea, vomiting, and abdominal pain in relation to fatty food intake
    5. Exercise routine or daily activities
    6. Family history of gallbladder disease
    7. In women, history of estrogen replacement therapy
- Assess for
    1. Abdominal pain of varying intensity in the right upper abdominal quadrant, including radiation to the right upper shoulder; ask the client to describe the intensity, duration, precipitating factors, and relief measures
    2. Other GI symptoms, including nausea, vomiting, dyspepsia, flatulence, eructation, and feelings of abdominal heaviness
    3. With right subcostal palpation, increasing pain with deep inspiration (Murphy's sign)
    4. Guarding, rigidity, and rebound tenderness (Blumberg's sign)
    5. Sausage-shaped mass in the right upper quadrant
    6. Late symptoms seen in chronic cholecystitis, such as jaundice, clay-colored stools, and dark urine
    7. Steatorrhea (fatty stools)
    8. Elevated temperature with tachycardia and dehydration from fever and vomiting

9. Results of serum liver enzyme and bilirubin tests (may be elevated)
10. Increased white blood cell (WBC) count
11. Elevated serum and urine amylase levels (if pancreas is affected)

 Considerations for Older Adults

- Older adults and client with diabetes mellitus have atypical manifestations, including the absence of pain and fever. Localized tenderness may be the only presenting sign.
- The older adult may become acutely confused.
- Older adults should not be given meperidine (Demerol) for pain because it can cause acute confusion and nausea.

Planning and Implementation

NONSURGICAL MANAGEMENT

- Clients with chronic cholecystitis are encouraged to consume frequent small, low-fat meals.
- If gallstones are causing an obstruction of bile flow, fat-soluble vitamins and bile salts may be prescribed to facilitate digestion and vitamin absorption.
- Food and fluids are withheld during nausea and vomiting episodes; nasogastric decompression is initiated for severe vomiting.
- Drug therapy includes
  1. Opioid analgesics such as meperidine (Demerol), to relieve pain and reduce spasm
  2. Antispasmodic agents or anticholinergics to relax the smooth muscle
  3. Antiemetics to provide relief from nausea and vomiting

SURGICAL MANAGEMENT

- A percutaneous transhepatic biliary catheter may be inserted to decompress obstructed extrahepatic ducts so bile can flow.
- Cholecystectomy (removal of the gallbladder) is the usual surgical treatment. One of two procedures may be performed:
  1. Traditional open surgical approach
  2. Laparoscopic laser procedure (performed more often than traditional surgical approach)

- A T-tube drain is surgically inserted when the common bile duct is explored to ensure patency of the duct.
- Provide the following preoperative care for clients having *traditional* surgery.
  1. Stress the importance of deep breathing, coughing, and turning, as well as early ambulation after surgery.
  2. Teach how to use sustained maximal inspiration (SMI) devices.
  3. Teach how to use a folded blanket or pillow as a splint for the abdomen to prevent jarring during coughing.
- Laparoscopic laser cholecystectomy is commonly performed by making several small punctures, through which the laparoscope is inserted. A laser dissects the gallbladder before removal through a puncture site. This procedure is less invasive than traditional surgery and is performed on an outpatient (ambulatory) basis.
- No special preoperative care is required for the laparoscopic procedure.
- Provide postoperative care for laparoscopic clients as follows:
  1. Teach the client the importance of early ambulation to absorb the carbon dioxide that is retained in the abdomen
  2. Inform the client that he or she can return to usual activities 1 to 3 weeks after the procedure.
- Provide postoperative care for traditional surgery clients as follows:
  1. Administer intravenous (via patient-controlled analgesia) meperidine (Demerol) for pain relief, as ordered; morphine is not given because it can constrict the sphincter of Oddi and cause biliary ductal spasm.
  2. Administer antiemetics for relief of postoperative nausea and vomiting, as ordered.
  3. Ensure that the client receives nothing by mouth (NPO) for 8 to 24 hours.
  4. Advance the diet from clear liquids to solid foods, as tolerated by the client.
  5. Maintain the client's T-tube.
     a. Keep the drainage system below the level of the gallbladder.
     b. Assess the amount, color, consistency, and odor of drainage (bile output is approximately more than 400 mL per day).

c. Administer synthetic bile salts such as dehydrocholic acid (Decholin), as ordered.

d. Report to the physician sudden increases or output of more than 1000 mL in 24 hours in bile output.

e. Assess for foul odor and purulent drainage and report changes in drainage to the physician.

f. Inspect the skin around the T-tube insertion site for signs of inflammation.

g. Place the client in a semi-Fowler's position.

h. Never irrigate, aspirate, or clamp the T-tube without a physician's order.

i. Assess the drainage system for pulling, kinking, or tangling of the tubing.

j. Assist the client with early ambulation.

k. Teach client to observe stools for brown color 7 to 10 days postoperatively.

Community-Based Care

- If traditional surgery is performed, give the client written postoperative instructions on
  1. Inspection of the abdominal incision for redness, tenderness, swelling, and drainage
  2. Dressing change, wound care, and T-tube drain care instructions
  3. Pain management, including prescriptions
  4. Signs and symptoms of infection, including when to call the physician (elevated temperature and increased pain)
  5. Activity limitations
- Provide diet therapy instructions based on the client's tolerance of fats. Instruct the client to eat a low-fat diet that includes small, frequent meals; instruct on what foods to avoid, as well as weight reduction if indicated.
- Provide information to the client and family about the potential for postcholecystectomy syndrome manifested by jaundice of the skin or sclera, darkened urine, light colored stools, pain, fever, chills.
- Refer to home health nursing if needed.

Cholesteatoma

- A cholesteatoma is a benign growth of squamous cell epithelium and is most common in clients who have chronic otitis media with a perforated tympanic membrane that fails to heal.
- A cholesteatoma appears as a grayish white, shiny mass behind or involving the tympanic membrane and is often described as having a cauliflower-like appearance.
- Clinical management depends on structures that are damaged by the tumor; effects include decreased hearing, chronic otitis media, vertigo, and facial paralysis.
- Treatment includes
  1. Antibiotics if an infection is present
  2. Surgical removal of the tumor:
     a. *Myringoplasty* to repair the tympanic membrane
     b. *Tympanoplasty* to repair or replace the ossicles to improve conductive hearing
     c. *Mastoidectomy* for more extensive growths

Chronic Obstructive Pulmonary Disease (COPD)

OVERVIEW

- Chronic obstructive pulmonary disease (COPD) is a chronic lung disease that includes emphysema and chronic bronchitis and is characterized by bronchoconstriction and dyspnea.
- Characteristics of *emphysema* are as follows:
  1. Primary pathologic changes are loss of lung elasticity and hyperinflation of the lung.
  2. Classifications are panlobular, centrilobular, or paraseptal:
     a. Panlobular disease involves destruction of entire alveolus uniformly and is more diffuse and more severe in the lower lung areas.

b. In centrilobular disease, openings occur in the bronchioles, allowing spaces to develop as tissue wall breaks down. Disease is diffuse and more severe in the upper lung areas; it is often seen in long-time cigarette smokers.

c. Paraseptal disease is confined to only the alveolar ducts and alveolar sacs; bullae form and the upper half of the lungs are affected.

- *Chronic bronchitis* is characterized by inflammation of the bronchi and bronchioles caused by chronic exposure to irritants, especially tobacco smoke. Thickening of the bronchial wall along with excessive thick mucus, blocks some of the smaller airways and narrows larger ones, hindering airflow and gas exchange.
- Risk factors for COPD include cigarette smoking, alpha-1 antitrypsin deficiency, and air pollution.
- Complications of COPD include
  1. Hypoxemia and acidosis
  2. Respiratory infections
  3. Cardiac failure
  4. Cardiac dysrhythmias

COLLABORATIVE MANAGEMENT

Assessment

- Record client information.
  1. Age, gender, occupational history, ethnic/cultural background, and family history
  2. Smoking history, including length of time client has smoked and number of packs smoked daily
  3. Current breathing problem
     a. Does the client have difficulty breathing when talking? Can the client speak in complete sentences or does the client take a breath every one to two words?
     b. Is there presence, duration, or worsening of wheezing, coughing, and shortness of breath and what activities trigger these problems?
     c. If the cough is productive, what is the sputum color and amount, and has the amount increased or decreased? Record these findings.

    d. What is the relationship between activity tolerance and dyspnea?

    e. Is it difficult for the client to eat, sleep, or perform other activities of daily living (ADLs)?

    f. Has the client lost weight as the COPD becomes more severe?

4. General appearance: The client is usually thin, has a loss of muscle mass in the extremities (although the neck muscles may be enlarged), has a barreled chest, and is slow moving and slightly stooped.

- Assess for
  1. Rapid, shallow respirations; limited diaphragm movement; crackles
  2. Decreased vibrations when the client says "99"
  3. Hyperresonance on chest percussion
  4. Dyspnea
  5. Cardiac manifestations
     a. Heart rate and rhythm, swelling of feet and ankles, symptoms of right-sided heart failure
     b. Cyanosis or pallor of the nail beds, oral mucous membranes, or both
  6. Social isolation
  7. Economic status
     a. The client may not be able to work or may have had to change jobs, which could affect income and health insurance.
     b. The client may be unable to pay for expensive medications; the client may use medications only during exacerbations and not as prescribed.
  8. Diagnostic test results
     a. Serial arterial blood gases (ABG)
     b. Pulse oximetry: results lower than 90% require immediate medical attention
     c. Sputum culture
     d. Hemoglobin and hematocrit to determine polycythemia
     e. Serum electrolytes because hypophosphatemia, hyperkalemia, hypocalcemia, and hypomagnesemia cause muscle weakness
     f. Serum alpha-antitrypsin deficiency (if suspected)
     g. Chest x-ray

h. Pulmonary function tests (PFTs)

i. Peak expiratory flow meter results

Planning and Implementation

C

<u>**NDx:** Impaired Gas Exchange</u>

NONSURGICAL MANAGEMENT

- Maintain a patent airway.
    1. Maintain the client's head, neck, and chest in alignment
    2. Assist the client in liquefying secretions
    3. Clear the airway of secretions
- Provide oxygen therapy.
    1. Provide prescribed humidified oxygen usually 2 to 4 L/min via nasal cannula or up to 40% via Venturi mask. The client who is hypoxemic and also has chronic hypercarbia requires a lower level of oxygen delivery, usually 1 to 2 L/min via nasal cannula.
    2. Assess the client's response to treatment and intervene to prevent complications.
- Drug therapy includes
    1. Beta-adrenergic agents
    2. Cholinergic antagonists
    3. Methylxanthines
    4. Corticosteroids
    5. Cromolyn sodium/nedocromil
    6. Leukotriene modifiers
    7. Mucolytics
    8. Stepped therapy, which is recommended to enable the client to have more awareness of the disease and to increase participation in symptom management, including
        a. Pharmacologic therapy
        b. Monitoring of the disease
        c. Control of environmental irritants and allergens

SURGICAL MANAGEMENT

- Lung reduction surgery may be performed to improve gas exchange through removal of hyperinflated lung tissue, which is useless for gas exchange.
- Lung transplantation
- Preoperative care includes
    1. Standard preoperative care and teaching

2. Pulmonary rehabilitation to maximize lung and muscle function
3. Tests to determine the location of the greatest hyper-inflation and poorest perfusion
   a. Pulmonary plethysmography
   b. Gas dilution
   c. Perfusion scans
- Postoperative care includes
  1. Routine postoperative care
  2. Management of the chest tube
  3. Pain management, usually with opioids
  4. Pulmonary hygiene including incentive spirometer, chest physiotherapy, and frequent pulmonary assessment

◆NDx: Ineffective Breathing Pattern

- Assess the client to determine the breathing pattern, especially the rate, rhythm, depth, and use of accessory muscles.
- Identify factors that may contribute to the increased work of breathing such as a respiratory tract infection.
- Aim interventions at improving the client's breathing efforts and decreasing the work of breathing.
  1. Teach breathing techniques.
     a. Diaphragmatic or abdominal breathing
     b. Pursed lip breathing
  2. Elevate the head of the bed.
  3. Teach exercise conditioning of larger muscle groups through pulmonary rehabilitation.
  4. Teach energy conservation to plan and pace activities for maximal tolerance and minimal discomfort.
     a. Collaborate with the client to develop a personal chart of the day's activities and rest periods.
     b. Instruct the client to avoid working with the arms raised.
     c. Adjust work heights to reduce back strain and fatigue.
     d. Organize workspaces so that items used most often are in easy reach.
     e. Instruct the client not to talk when engaged in activities that require energy, such as walking.

◆NDx: Ineffective Airway Clearance

- Assess breath sounds routinely and before and after interventions.

- Teach the client to cough on arising in the morning, before meals, and at bedtime.
  1. Record the color, consistency, odor, and amount of secretions.
  2. Assist the client with mouth care after coughing exercises.
- Perform chest physiotherapy and postural drainage.
- Suction only when abnormal breath sounds are present.
- For clients who can tolerate sitting in a chair, assist the client out of bed for 1 hour two to three times per day.
- Unless hydration is contraindicated for other health problems, encourage the client to drink 2 to 3 L/day.

NDx: Imbalanced Nutrition: Less than Body Requirements

- Clients with COPD often have food intolerance, nausea, early satiety, loss of appetite, and meal-related dyspnea.
- The increased work of breathing raises calorie and protein requirements.
- Encourage the client to perform coughing exercises and then allow for rest times before meals. Use of a bronchodilator 30 minutes before meals may be helpful.
- Plan the largest meal for when the client is most hungry and well rested. Four to six small meals may be preferable to three large meals per day.
- Request a dietary consult and assist the client to select high-calorie, high-protein, easy-to-chew, and non–gas forming foods.
  1. Dry foods stimulate coughing.
  2. Chocolate and milk may increase the thickness of saliva and secretions.
  3. Dietary supplements such as Pulmocare are designed to provide nutritional supplementation with reduced CO_2 production.
  4. The client should avoid caffeinated beverages because they promote diuresis and contribute to dehydration.
- Provide assistance with feeding as needed.

NDx: Anxiety

- Collaborate with the client to develop a written plan that states exactly what to do to control anxiety, such as using pursed-lip and diaphragmatic breathing techniques.
- Collaborate with the health care team to see whether a referral to a professional counselor is needed.

- Explore with the client other approaches to control dyspneic episodes and anxiety attacks, such as relaxation techniques, hypnosis, and biofeedback.

◆**NDx:** Activity Intolerance

- Assist with activities of daily living (ADLs) based on the assessment of the client's needs and fatigue level.
- Instruct the client to pace activities and not to rush.
- Assess the client's physiologic response to activity by noting skin color changes, pulse rate and regularity, blood pressure, and work of breathing.

◆**NDx:** Potential for Pneumonia or Other Respiratory Infection

- Teach the client to avoid large crowds.
- Stress the importance of receiving a pneumonia vaccination and annual influenza vaccination.

Community-Based Care

- Coordinate plans for the client discharged to the home setting.
  1. It may be unrealistic to cover all of the topics needed for client education; coordination with home health or clinic staff may be needed.
  2. Refer to pulmonary rehabilitation program.
  3. Provide the client and significant others with education about management of COPD, including
     a. Medications
     b. Signs and symptoms of infections
     c. Respiratory therapy interventions and bronchial hygiene
     d. Management of dyspnea
     e. Diet and nutrition
     f. Adaptation of daily routine and activity progression
     g. Control of environment
     h. Relaxation techniques
     i. Energy conservation
     j. Body image and human sexuality
  3. Collaborate with the case manager and/or social worker to obtain needed services at home, such as
     a. Oxygen and nebulizer
     b. Home health nurse or aide
     c. Hospital bed or other assistive equipment

4. Collaborate with the social worker to make referrals to community agencies as needed for
   a. Financial assistance for disability benefits through Social Security or private disability insurance
   b. Meals on Wheels
   c. Support groups such as the American Lung Association, Better Breathing Groups, or the American Heart Association

Cirrhosis

OVERVIEW

- Cirrhosis is a chronic, progressive liver disease characterized by diffuse fibrotic bands of connective tissue that distort the normal architectural anatomy of the liver.
- Cirrhosis is essentially an irreversible reaction to hepatic inflammation and necrosis.
- *Compensated cirrhosis*: the liver has significant scarring but is still able to perform essential functions without causing significant symptoms.
- *Decompensated cirrhosis*: Liver function is significantly impaired with obvious signs and symptoms of liver failure.
- The main causes of cirrhosis are
  1. Alcohol
     a. Alcohol has a direct toxic effect on liver cells, causing liver inflammation (alcoholic hepatitis).
     b. The liver becomes enlarged with cellular infiltration by fat, leukocytes, and lymphocytes.
     c. Early scar formation is caused by fibroblast infiltration and collagen formation.
     d. Damage to the liver progresses, and widespread scar tissue forms with fibrotic infiltration of the liver as a result of cellular necrosis.
  2. Viral hepatitis
     a. Inflammation caused by hepatitis infection over time leads to progressive scarring of the liver.

b. Alcohol accelerates the process in the presence of hepatitis C; Hepatitis B causes low-grade damage over decades that can lead to cirrhosis.

3. Autoimmune hepatitis
   a. Host's immune system produces a high level of circulating autoantibodies, causing inflammation of the liver.

4. Steatohepatitis
   a. Fat and cholesterol deposits in the liver cause chronic inflammation.
   b. Risk factors are obesity and elevated lipid profile.

5. Drugs and toxins
   a. Medications, herbal supplements, and environmental exposure to toxins may damage the liver so significantly that cirrhosis occurs.

6. Biliary disease
   a. Chronic biliary obstruction, bile stasis, and inflammation result in severe obstructive jaundice.
   b. Primary biliary cirrhosis (PBC) results from intrahepatic bile stasis.
   c. Primary sclerosing cholangitis (PSC) is characterized by diffuse inflammation and fibrosis that involves the biliary system.

7. Cardiovascular disease
   a. Severe right-sided congestive heart failure results in an enlarged, edematous, congested liver.
   b. The liver serves as a reservoir for a large amount of venous blood that the failing heart is unable to pump into circulation.
   c. The liver becomes anoxic, resulting in liver cell necrosis and fibrosis.

8. Various metabolic and genetic disorders can cause cirrhosis.

- Complications of cirrhosis include
  1. Portal hypertension. A persistent increase in pressure within the portal vein developing as a result of increased resistance or obstruction to flow. Blood flow backs into the spleen causing splenomegaly. Veins in the esophagus, stomach, intestines, abdomen, and rectum become dilated.
  2. Ascites. Free fluid containing almost pure plasma accumulates within the peritoneal cavity. Increased hydrostatic

pressure from portal hypertension results in venous congestion of the hepatic capillaries, causing plasma to leak directly from the liver surface and portal vein. Other contributing factors include reduced circulating plasma protein and increased hepatic lymphatic formation.

3. Bleeding esophageal varices. Fragile, thin-walled, distended esophageal veins become irritated and rupture. Varices occur most frequently in the lower esophagus and in the proximal esophagus and stomach.

4. Coagulation defects. Decreased synthesis of bile fats in the liver prevent the absorption of fat-soluble vitamins. Without vitamin K and clotting factors II, VII, IX, and X, the client is susceptible to bleeding and easy bruising.

5. Jaundice is caused by one of two mechanisms:
   a. Hepatocellular jaundice. The liver is unable to effectively excrete bilirubin.
   b. Intrahepatic obstruction. Edema, fibrosis, or scarring of the hepatic bile duct channels and bile ducts interferes with normal bile and bilirubin excretion.

6. Portal systemic encephalopathy (also known as hepatic encephalopathy and hepatic coma). End-stage hepatic failure and cirrhosis is manifested by neurologic symptoms and characterized by altered level of consciousness, impaired thinking processes, and neuromuscular disturbances.

7. Hepatorenal syndrome. Progressive, oliguric renal failure is associated with hepatic failure, resulting in functional impairment of kidneys with normal anatomic and morphologic features. It is manifested by a sudden decrease in urinary flow and elevated serum urea nitrogen and creatinine levels, with abnormally decreased urine sodium excretion and increased urine osmolarity.

8. Spontaneous bacterial peritonitis manifestations include fever, chills, and abdominal pain and tenderness.

COLLABORATIVE MANAGEMENT

Assessment

- Record client information.
  1. Age, sex, and race
  2. Employment history, including working conditions exposing the client to harmful chemical toxins

3. History of individual and family alcoholism
4. Previous medical conditions, including jaundice, acute viral hepatitis, biliary tract disease, viral infections, blood transfusions, autoimmune disorders, and history of heart disease or respiratory disorders
5. Sexual history
6. History of or present substance use

■ Assess for
1. Generalized weakness, fatigue
2. Weight loss
3. Gastrointestinal (GI) symptoms, including loss of appetite, early morning nausea and vomiting, dyspepsia, flatulence, and changes in bowel habits
4. Abdominal pain or tenderness
5. Jaundice of the skin and sclera
6. Dry skin, rashes, pruritus
7. Petechiae or ecchymosis
8. Palmar erythema
9. Spider angiomas on the nose, cheeks, upper thorax, and shoulders
10. Hepatomegaly palpated in the right upper quadrant
11. Ascites revealed by bulging flanks and dullness on percussion of the abdomen
12. Protruding umbilicus
13. Dilated abdominal veins *(caput medusae)*
14. Presence of blood in vomitus or nasogastric drainage
15. Fetor hepaticus, the fruity, musty breath odor of chronic liver disease
16. Amenorrhea in women
17. Testicular atrophy, gynecomastia, and impotence in men
18. Changes in mentation and personality
19. Asterixis (liver flap), a coarse tremor characterized by rapid, nonrhythmic extension and flexions in the wrist and fingers
20. Elevated serum liver enzyme and serum bilirubin levels
21. Decreased total serum protein and albumin levels
22. Elevated serum globulin level
23. Prolonged prothrombin time
24. Elevated serum ammonia level
25. Enlarged liver seen on x-ray

Planning and Implementation

◆**NDx:** Excess Fluid Volume

NONSURGICAL MANAGEMENT

- Provide diet therapy.
    1. Provide a low-sodium diet initially, restricting sodium to 500 mg to 2 g/day.
    2. Suggest alternatives to salt such as lemon, vinegar, parsley, oregano, and pepper.
    3. Collaborate with the dietitian to explain purpose of diet and meal planning; suggest elimination of table salt, salty foods, canned and frozen vegetables, and salted butter and margarine.
    4. Restrict fluid intake to 1000 to 1500 mL/day if the serum sodium level falls.
    5. Supplement vitamin intake with thiamine, folate, and multivitamin preparations.
- Provide drug therapy.
    1. Give diuretics to reduce fluid accumulations and to prevent cardiac and respiratory impairment.
    2. Monitor intake and output carefully.
    3. Weigh the client daily.
    4. Measure abdominal girth daily.
    5. Monitor electrolyte balance.
    6. Administer low-sodium antacids.
- Paracentesis may be indicated if dietary restrictions and drug administration fail to control ascites.
    1. Explain the procedure.
    2. Obtain vital signs and weight.
    3. Measure the client's abdominal girth.
    4. Assist the client to an upright position at the side of the bed.
    5. Monitor vital signs every 15 minutes during the procedure; rapid, drastic removal of ascitic fluid leads to decreased abdominal pressure, which may contribute to vasodilation and shock.
    6. Measure and record drainage.
    7. Position the client in bed and maintain bedrest until vital signs are stable.

- Provide comfort measures.
  1. Elevate the head of the bed to minimize shortness of breath.
  2. Encourage the client to sit up in a chair with his or her feet elevated.
- Monitor the client's fluids and electrolytes.

SURGICAL MANAGEMENT

- A peritoneovenous shunt may be placed for severe ascites. Ascites are drained through a one-way valve into a silicone rubber tube that terminates in the superior vena cava.
- Preoperative care is aimed at optimizing the client's physical state.
- Provide preoperative care by treating underlying medical conditions.
  1. Treat abnormal coagulation with fresh frozen plasma or vitamin K.
  2. Correct electrolyte imbalances.
  3. Ensure that packed red blood cells (RBCs) are available for surgery.
  4. Provide routine preoperative care.
- Provide postoperative care.
  1. Provide routine postoperative care.
  2. Auscultate breath sounds for the presence of crackles, indicating excessive lung fluid.
  3. Assess for excess fluid volume and hemodilution.
  4. Administer diuretics for volume excess.
  5. Monitor coagulation study results.
  6. Perform daily abdominal girth measurements.
  7. Record accurate fluid intake and output daily.
  8. Weigh the client daily.

◄**COLLABORATIVE PROBLEM:** Potential for Hemorrhage

- Esophageal bleeding is controlled by
  1. *Gastric intubation* to lavage the stomach until the fluid returned is clear
  2. *Esophagogastric balloon tamponade* to compress bleeding vessels with a tube called a tamponade tube
     a. The tube is inserted through the nose and into the stomach. The large esophageal balloon compresses

the esophagus; a smaller gastric balloon helps anchor the tube and exerts pressure against bleeding varices at the distal esophagus and the cardia of the stomach; a third limen terminates in the stomach and is connected to suction, allowing the aspiration of gastric contents and blood.

   b. Check balloons for integrity and leaks; label each lumen to prevent errors in adding or removing pressure and volume.

   c. Keep tube taped and secure.

   d. Keep an extra tube and scissors at the bedside.

   e. Monitor the client for respiratory distress caused by obstruction from the esophageal balloon or aspiration; if distress occurs, cut both balloon ports to allow for rapid balloon deflation and tube removal.

3. *Administering blood products* (RBCs and fresh frozen plasma) and intravenous fluids

4. *Giving vasopressin intra-arterially or intravenously* to lower pressures in the portal venous system to decrease bleeding

5. *Injection sclerotherapy,* which may be performed to sclerose bleeding esophageal varices

   a. Monitor the client's vital signs and assess for chest pain.

   b. Administer pain medication and report severe pain to the physician.

   c. Assess lung sounds to determine presence of pneumonia or pleural effusion.

6. *Endoscopic band ligation* procedure, which uses bands to ligate the bleeding varices

7. *Transjugular intrahepatic portal-systemic shunt,* a nonsurgical procedure whereby the physician implants a shunt, passed through a catheter, between the portal vein and the hepatic vein to reduce portal venous pressure and therefore control the bleeding

SURGICAL MANAGEMENT

- Surgical management of portal hypertension and esophageal varices are a last resort intervention associated with high mortality secondary to coagulation abnormalities, infection, poor tolerance to anesthesia, and ascites.

COLLABORATIVE PROBLEM:

Potential for Portal-Systemic Encephalopathy (PSE)

NONSURGICAL MANAGEMENT

- Provide diet therapy.
  1. Client has increased nutritional requirements: high-carbohydrate, moderate-fat, and high-protein foods.
  2. Clients with PSE usually have protein intake limited in the diet to reduce excess protein breakdown by intestinal bacteria and thus decrease ammonia formation.
  3. Clients with cirrhosis who have had a gastrointestinal bleed are given nothing by mouth (NPO), and a nasogastric tube may be inserted.
  4. Total parenteral nutrition may be needed.
- Provide drug therapy.
  1. Administer lactulose to promote excretion of fecal ammonia.
     a. When giving orally, dilute it with fruit juice to help the client tolerate the sweet taste.
     b. The desired effect of lactulose is 2 to 5 soft stools per day; watery diarrheal stools may signify excessive lactulose administration.
  2. Neomycin sulfate acts as an intestinal antiseptic to destroy normal flora in the bowel, diminishing protein breakdown, and decreasing ammonia production.
  3. Metronidazole (Flagyl, Novonidazol) is a broad-spectrum antibiotic with similar action to neomycin but has less potential for renal toxicity.
  4. Administer stool softeners, as ordered, to prevent constipation in long-term therapy.
  5. Restrict drugs such as opioids, sedatives, and barbiturates.

Community-Based Care

- Health teaching is individualized for the client, depending on the cause of the disease.
- Identify if the client needs a family member or friend to help with medications, a home health care nurse or aide.
- Teach the client and family to
  1. Follow the prescribed diet.
  2. Restrict sodium intake if ascites occur.
  3. Restrict protein intake if susceptible to encephalopathy.

4. Take diuretics as prescribed, report symptoms of hypokalemia, and consume foods high in potassium.
5. Take H_2-receptor antagonist agent of proton pump inhibitor for GI bleeding.
6. Avoid all nonprescription medications.
7. Avoid alcohol (refer to Alcoholics Anonymous if client is an alcoholic).
8. Recognize signs and symptoms of PSE.
9. Notify their health care provider immediately in case GI bleeding or PSE.
10. Keep follow-up visits with the physicians.

Colitis, Ulcerative

OVERVIEW

- Ulcerative colitis is a chronic inflammatory process affecting the mucosal lining of the colon or rectum. It can affect absorption of vital nutrients.
- Classified as an inflammatory bowel disease, ulcerative colitis is characterized by diffuse inflammation of the intestinal mucosa, resulting in loss of surface epithelium, causing ulceration and abscess formation.
- Ulcerative colitis typically begins in the rectum and proceeds in a uniform, continuous manner proximally toward the cecum.
   1. Epithelial cell damage and loss, areas of ulceration, redness, and bleeding occur in the *acute stage*.
   2. *Chronic* changes in the colon lead to fibrosis and retraction of the bowel resulting in muscle hypertrophy, deposits of fat and fibrous tissue, and a narrower and shorter colon.
- Complications of the disease include intestinal perforation with peritonitis and fistula formation, toxic megacolon, hemorrhage, increased risk of colon cancer, abscess formation, bowel obstruction, malabsorption, and extraintestinal clinical manifestations.

COLLABORATIVE MANAGEMENT

Assessment

- Record client information.
  1. Family history of inflammatory bowel disease
  2. Previous and current therapy for illnesses
  3. Diet history, including usual patterns and intolerances of milk products and greasy, fried, or spicy foods
  4. History of weight loss
  5. Presence of abdominal pain, cramping, urgency, and diarrhea
  6. Bowel elimination patterns; color, consistency, and character of stools and the presence or absence of blood
  7. Relationship between the occurrence of diarrhea and the timing of meals, pain, emotional distress, and activity
  8. Extraintestinal symptoms such as arthritis, mouth sores, vision problems, and skin disorders
- Assess for
  1. Abdominal cramping, pain and distention
  2. Bloody diarrhea, tenesmus (uncontrollable straining)
  3. Low-grade fever, tachycardia
  4. Client's understanding of the disease process
  5. Psychosocial impact of the disease
     a. Relationship of life events to disease exacerbations
     b. Stress factors that produce symptoms
     c. Family and social support systems
     d. Concerns regarding the possible genetic basis and associated cancer risks of the disease
  6. Abnormal laboratory values: hematocrit, hemoglobin, white blood cell (WBC) count, erythrocyte sedimentation rate, electrolytes

Planning and Implementation

◆**NDx:** Diarrhea

NONSURGICAL MANAGEMENT

- Management of ulcerative colitis is aimed at relieving the symptoms and reducing intestinal motility, decreasing inflammation, and promoting intestinal healing.
- At the onset of treatment, activity is restricted to promote comfort and intestinal healing.

- Diarrhea management is as follows:
  1. Record the color, volume, frequency, and consistency of stools.
  2. Monitor the skin in the perianal area for irritation and ulceration resulting from loose, frequent stools.
  3. Stool cultures may be ordered.
- Drug therapy is as follows:
  1. Salicylate compounds may be prescribed.
     a. Sulfasalazine (Azulfidine, PMS-Sulfasalazine) is used to prevent reoccurrence, as well as to treat acute exacerbations; the drug should be taken after meals with a full glass of water.
     b. Oral mesalamine (Asacol, Pentasa, Salofalk ✳) is used for its anti-inflammatory effect.
     c. Olsalazine (Dipentum) is used for maintenance therapy.
  2. Corticosteroids may be prescribed during acute exacerbations.
  3. Immunosuppressants in combination with steroids may be given; observe for side effects such as thrombocytopenia, leukopenia, anemia, renal failure, infection, headache, gastrointestinal (GI) ulceration, stomatitis, and hepatotoxicity.
  4. Antidiarrheal drugs are given to provide symptomatic management of diarrhea; they are given cautiously because they can precipitate colonic dilation and toxic megacolon.
  5. Infliximab (Remicade) may be refractory disease or for severe complications, such as toxic megacolon.
- Diet therapy may include
  1. Nothing by mouth (NPO) for the client with severe symptoms
  2. Total parenteral nutrition (TPN)
  3. Elemental formulas, which are absorbed in the upper bowel, thereby minimizing bowel stimulation
  4. Low-fiber diet; teach client to avoid foods such as whole wheat grains, nuts, and fresh fruits or vegetables
  5. Avoidance of caffeinated beverages, pepper, and alcohol
- Encourage the client to avoid smoking.
- Ensure that the client has easy access to the bedside commode or bathroom.

- Complementary and alternative therapies used as a supplement to traditional therapies may include herbs such as flaxseed, selenium, vitamin C, biofeedback, yoga, acupuncture and Ayurveda (combination of diet, herbs, breathing exercises).

SURGICAL MANAGEMENT

- The need for surgery is based on the client's response to medical interventions.
- Surgical procedures include
  1. Total proctocolectomy with permanent ileostomy. The colon, rectum, and anus are removed and the anus closed. The end of the terminal ileum forms the stoma, which is located in the right lower quadrant. Postoperatively, the nurse provides skin and ostomy care.
     a. Oral or parenteral antibiotics may be given preoperatively as a bowel antiseptic.
     b. Generally the client wears an ostomy patch at all times.
     c. Initial output from the ileostomy is a loose, dark green liquid; over time the volume decreases, becomes thicker, and turns yellow-green or yellow-brown.
     d. Any foul or unpleasant odor may be a symptom of some underlying problem (blockage or infection).
  2. Total colectomy with a continent ileostomy, (Kock ileostomy) or ileal reservoir. An intra-abdominal pouch or reservoir is constructed from the terminal ileum where stool can be stored until the pouch is drained by the nurse or client. The pouch is connected to the stoma with a nipple-like valve constructed from an intussuscepted portion of the ileum; the stoma is flush with the skin.
     a. Immediately postoperatively, a Foley catheter is placed in the pouch and connected to low intermittent suction and irrigated, as ordered.
     b. Monitor character and quality of drainage.
     c. Teach the client to drain the stoma. When the pouch needs to be emptied, the client experiences a sense of fullness.
  3. Total colectomy with ileoanal anastomosis (two stages): In the first stage, the surgeon excises the rectal mucosa, performs an abdominal colectomy, constructs the reservoir

or pouch to the anal canal, and creates a temporary loop ileostomy. After 3 to 4 months the loop ileostomy is closed.

4. Creation of an ileoanal reservoir, also known as a J-pouch: The colon is removed and the ileum is sutured into the rectal stump to form a reservoir.

- If the procedure involves an ostomy, an enterostomal therapist is consulted for recommendations on the location.
- Specific nursing care interventions are determined by the procedure performed, including ostomy or perineal wound care.

◆NDx: Chronic Pain

- Pain management includes
  1. Assessing the client for changes in complaints and responses to pain that may indicate disease complications, such as increased inflammation, obstruction, hemorrhage, or peritonitis
  2. Assessing for pain, including its character, pattern of occurrence (such as before or after meals, during the night, or before or after bowel movements), and duration
  3. Assisting the client to reduce or eliminate factors that can precipitate or increase the pain
  4. Using antidiarrheal drug with caution to control diarrhea; toxic megacolon can develop
  5. Giving anticholinergic drugs, if prescribed, before meals to provide relief from the pain and cramping that may occur with diarrhea
  6. Referring to a dietitian for diet teaching and meal planning
  7. Taking measures to relieve irritated skin caused by frequent contact with diarrheal stool
  8. Assisting the client to use other pain relief measures such as biofeedback and music therapy

◆COLLABORATIVE PROBLEM:
Potential for Gastrointestinal Bleeding

- Monitor the client for signs and symptoms of internal bleeding.
- Check all stools for blood, using both gross and occult examination.
- Monitor hemoglobin, hematocrit, and electrolyte levels.

- Observe for fever, tachycardia, fluid volume depletion, severe abdominal pain, and change in mental status (especially in older adults).
- Notify the health care provider immediately of GI bleeding, because surgical interventions may be necessary.

Community-Based Care

- Health teaching includes
  1. Providing information on the nature of the disease, including acute episodes, remissions, and symptom management
  2. Teaching dietary measures to reduce bloating and cramping
  3. Providing information on medication
  4. Teaching the client and family members symptoms that should be reported immediately to the health care provider
  5. Teaching the client to include adequate amounts of salt and water in their diet because the ileotomy promotes the loss of these elements
  6. Teaching the necessity for using caution in situations that promote profuse sweating or fluid loss such as
     a. During strenuous physical activities
     b. In high environmental temperature
     c. During episodes of diarrhea or vomiting
  7. Providing additional information for the client with an ostomy regarding
     a. Ostomy care
     b. Pouch care
     c. Skin care
     d. Special issues related to medications (e.g., to avoid taking enteric-coated medications and capsule medications); client should inform health care providers and pharmacist that he or she has an ostomy
     e. Symptoms to watch for, such as increased or no drainage and stomal swelling
     f. Activity limitations, including avoidance of heavy lifting
- Refer the client to home heath care ostomy outpatient clinics if needed.

- Refer the client to support groups such as the United Ostomy Association and the Crohn's and Colitis Foundation of America.

Conjunctivitis

- Conjunctivitis is an inflammation or infection of the conjunctiva of the eye.
- Types of conjunctivitis and their treatment include
  1. *Allergic* or *inflammatory* conjunctivitis
     a. Associated with a sensitivity to pollens, animal protein, feathers, certain foods or materials, insect bites, and drugs
     b. Manifested by edema of the conjunctiva, burning and itching sensation, excessive tearing, and engorgement of blood vessels
     c. Treated with instillation of vasoconstrictors and corticosteroid eyedrops; the client is instructed to avoid using makeup until all symptoms have subsided
  2. *Infectious* conjunctivitis (bacterial or viral)
     a. Referred to as "pink eye" and easily transmitted; often caused by *Staphylococcus aureus, Haemophilus influenzae,* or *Pseudomonas aeruginosa*
     b. Manifested by blood vessel dilation, mild conjunctival edema, tearing, and watery discharge, which becomes purulent
     c. Treated with rest and a broad-spectrum antibiotic ointment until the causative organism is identified
- Health teaching consists of
  1. Hygienic principles to prevent spread of the infection
  2. The importance of handwashing before and after instilling eyedrops
  3. How to instill eyedrops
  4. The importance of not rubbing the eye or carelessly disposing of tissues

Contusions, Pulmonary

- Pulmonary contusion most often follows injuries caused by rapid deceleration. Hemorrhage occurs in and between the alveoli. The resulting edema decreases pulmonary compliance and reduces the area for gas exchange.
- After a contusion, respiratory failure develops over time rather than instantaneously.
- Manifestations include
  1. Hypoxemia
  2. Dyspnea
  3. Irritated bronchial mucosa
  4. Increased bronchial secretions
  5. Hemoptysis
  6. Decreased breath sounds, crackles, and wheezes
  7. Hazy opacity in the pulmonary lobes or parenchyma
- Treatment is aimed at maintenance of ventilation and oxygenation.
  1. Closely monitor central venous pressure.
  2. Fluid intake is restricted as necessary.
  3. The client may require mechanical ventilation with positive end-expiratory pressure (PEEP).
  4. The major complication is adult respiratory distress syndrome (ARDS).

Corneal Disorders

- There are several types of corneal problems.
  1. Keratoconus: degeneration of the cornea
  2. Dystrophies: characterized by deposits in the cornea, reducing the refractory power
  3. Keratitis: inflammation of the cornea caused by infection or irritation
  4. Corneal ulcer: break in the normally intact corneal epithelium, which can provide an entrance for bacteria, viruses, and fungi

COLLABORATIVE MANAGEMENT

Assessment

- Assess for
  1. Location, quantity, quality, timing, and setting
     a. Eye pain
     b. Reduced vision
     c. Eye secretions
     d. Photophobia
  2. Hazy or cloudy-looking cornea
  3. Altered corneal light reflex

Interventions

NONSURGICAL MANAGEMENT

- Drug therapy includes
  1. Antibiotics, antifungal agents, and antiviral agents depending on the causative organism
  2. Steroids for selected causes of ocular herpes to reduce the inflammatory response in the eye
  3. Timing ophthalmic administration of drugs carefully so that if two medications must be administered at the same time, 5 minutes separates their instillation
  4. Using separate, clearly labeled bottles of medication if the same medication is used for both eyes, one of them infected
  5. Assisting the client in using his or her functional vision, suggesting sunglasses and indirect lighting

SURGICAL MANAGEMENT

- *Keratoplasty,* or corneal transplant, is used to restore vision.
- Tissue for a keratoplasty is obtained from a local eye bank or tissue bank. An eye bank obtains corneal tissue from deceased volunteer donors.
- Provide preoperative care.
  1. Provide routine preoperative care.
  2. Inform the client that regional anesthesia is typically used.
- Provide postoperative care.
  1. Leave the pressure dressing and eye shield in place until a specific order for removal is written by the surgeon.
  2. Notify the physician of any significant drainage.

3. Observe for and report complications of surgery.
   a. Bleeding
   b. Infection
   c. Graft rejection
   d. Wound leakage
4. Instruct the client to lie on the nonsurgical side to reduce intraocular pressure.

- Graft rejection is possible. Vision is reduced and the cornea becomes cloudy; it is treated with frequent applications of topical corticosteroids.
- Severe pain or pain accompanied by nausea is indicative of increased intraocular pressure; notify the physician immediately and elevate the head of the bed 30 degrees.
- Before discharge, show the client how to apply the patch.

Coronary Artery Disease

OVERVIEW

- Coronary artery disease (CAD) is a broad term that includes stable angina pectoris and acute coronary syndromes.
- CAD affects the arteries that provide blood, oxygen, and nutrients to the myocardium.
- Ischemia occurs when insufficient oxygen is supplied to meet the requirements of the myocardium. Infarction (necrosis or cell death) occurs when severe ischemia is prolonged, resulting in irreversible damage to tissue.
- The most common cause of CAD is atherosclerosis, which is characterized by a fibrous plaque lesion that narrows the vessel lumen or obstructs blood flow (see Atherosclerosis).
- Other causes include increased myocardial oxygen requirements (e.g., exercise or aortic stenosis) and transient reductions in blood flow (e.g., hypotension or coronary artery spasm).
- *Angina pectoris* is a temporary imbalance between the ability of the coronary arteries to supply oxygen and the demand of the myocardium for it.
  1. *Stable* angina is chest discomfort that occurs with exertion in a pattern that is familiar to the client and that has

not increased in frequency, duration, or intensity of symptoms during the past several months; it is usually associated with a stable atherosclerotic plaque.

2. *Unstable* angina is chest pain or discomfort that occurs at rest or with minimal exertion; it is characterized by an increase in the number of episodes ("attacks") and the intensity of pain; the pain may last longer than 15 minutes or be poorly relieved by rest or nitroglycerin.

☀ Women's Health Considerations

- ◆ Many women experience atypical angina; described as a choking sensation that occurs with exertion, indigestion, pain between the shoulders, or an aching jaw.
- ◆ Angina is more likely to be the primary presenting symptom of CAD in women than in men.
- ◆ Angina is twice as common as myocardial infarction (MI) in women.

Myocardial Infarction

- ■ MI occurs when the myocardial muscle is abruptly and severely deprived of oxygen. Ischemia and necrosis (infarction) of the myocardial tissue result if blood flow is not restored.
- ■ The client's response to an MI depends on which coronary arteries were obstructed and which part of the left ventricular wall was damaged: anterior, lateral, septal, inferior, or posterior.
  1. Clients with obstruction of the left anterior descending artery have anterior or septal MIs, or both; clients with anterior MIs are most likely to experience left ventricular heart failure and ventricular dysrhythmias.
  2. Clients with obstruction of the circumflex artery may experience a posterior wall or a lateral wall MI and sinus dysrhythmias.
  3. Clients with obstruction of the right coronary artery often have inferior MIs; these clients are likely to experience bradydysrhythmias or atrioventricular conduction defects, especially transient second-degree heart block.
- ■ Women have higher morbidity and mortality rates after MI than men do.
- ■ Nonmodifiable risk factors include age, gender, family history, and ethnic background.

- Modifiable risk factors include elevated serum cholesterol levels, cigarette smoking, hypertension, impaired glucose tolerance, obesity, physical inactivity, and stress.

COLLABORATIVE MANAGEMENT

Assessment

- Collection of historical data is delayed until interventions for pain, vital sign instability, and dysrhythmias are initiated and the discomfort resolves.
- Record the client's family history and risk factors.
- Assess for clinical manifestations of MI.
  1. Chest, epigastric, jaw, back, or arm discomfort (often described as tightness, burning, pressure, or indigestion)
  2. Nausea and vomiting
  3. Diaphoresis
  4. Dizziness
  5. Weakness
  6. Palpitations
  7. Shortness of breath
  8. Diminished or absent pulses
  9. Sinus tachycardia with premature ventricular contractions
  10. Abnormal blood pressure
  11. S_3 gallop or S_4 heart sound
  12. Increased respiratory rate
  13. Crackles or wheezes (if heart failure occurs)
  14. Elevated temperature
  15. Denial (early reaction to chest discomfort)
  16. Fear and anxiety
  17. Elevated serum cardiac enzyme levels
     a. Creatine kinase (CK-MB isoenzyme) and myoglobin
     b. Lactate dehydrogenase (LDH) (LDH1 isoenzyme rises higher than LDH2 in the presence of an MI)
     c. Troponins T and I are more sensitive and specific than LDH
     d. Elevated white blood cell (WBC) count
  18. Electrocardiography changes
     a. In angina, ST depression or elevation or T-wave inversion
     b. In MI, ST elevation, T-wave inversion, and an abnormal Q wave

19. Results of exercise tolerance test (stress test), thallium scan, contrast-enhanced magnetic resonance (CMR) multigated acquisition (MUGA) scan, and cardiac catheterization, if performed

Considerations for Older Adults

- About 25% of older adults and clients with diabetes who experience MI complain primarily of shortness of breath; chest discomfort may be mild or absent.
- Many older clients do not typically experience chest discomfort but have disorientation or confusion as the primary manifestation.

☀ Women's Health Considerations

- Chest discomfort is often not the initial symptom.
- Women may initially have atypical symptoms such as heart "flutters" without pain, shortness of breath, fatigue, and depression.
- As the MI progresses, women usually report typical chest discomfort; arm and shoulder pain; back pain; or an aching jaw, neck, or tooth.

Planning and Implementation

◀NDx: Acute Pain

- Drug therapy includes
  1. Nitroglycerin (sublingually), used for angina, to increase collateral blood flow, redistributing blood flow toward the subendocardium; if three repeated doses do not relieve discomfort, the client may be experiencing an MI
  2. Nitroglycerin (intravenously [IV]), administered in a specialized unit to carefully monitor the client's blood pressure; hypotension is a serious side effect of this drug
  3. Morphine sulfate (IV) for clients unresponsive to nitroglycerin
  4. Aspirin 325 mg (chewed), which may be administered immediately
- Other interventions include
  1. Providing supplemental oxygen
  2. Placing the client in a semi-Fowler's position for comfort

3. Maintaining a quiet, calm environment to the extent possible
4. Providing acetaminophen (Tylenol, Exdol) for headaches caused by nitroglycerin

◆**NDx:** Ineffective Tissue Perfusion: Cardiopulmonary

- Thrombolytic agents are given IV or by intracoronary route during cardiac catheterization to dissolve thrombi in the coronary arteries and to restore myocardial blood flow. Examples include tissue plasminogen activator (t-PA; alteplase, Activase), anisoylated plasminogen-streptokinase activator complex (APSAC), reteplase (Retavase), and tenecteplase (TNKase).
- Thrombolytic agents are most effective when used within 6 hours of a coronary event.
- Interventions following administration of thrombolic agents include monitoring the client for signs of obvious and occult bleeding and reporting indications of bleeding immediately to the physician (most common in women who receive thrombolytic therapy).
  1. Monitor the client for indications of cerebrovascular bleeding.
  2. Observe all IV sites for bleeding and patency.
  3. Monitor clotting studies.
  4. Observe for signs of internal bleeding (watching hematocrit and hemoglobin).
  5. Test stool, urine, and emesis for occult blood.
- Glycoprotein (GP) 11a/111b inhibitors prevent fibrin from attaching to activated platelets at the site of a thrombus.
  1. GP 11a/111b is used particularly in unstable angina and non–Q-wave MI and before and during percutaneous transluminal coronary angioplasty (PTCA) to ensure patency of the newly opened artery.
  2. If GP 11a/111b inhibitors are used with fibrinolytic agent, then the dose of the thrombolytic should be reduced.
- Monitor for indications of coronary artery reperfusion, including abrupt cessation of chest pain or discomfort, sudden onset of ventricular dysrhythmias, and resolution of ST segment depression, a peak at 12 hours of markers of myocardial damage.

- IV heparin and aspirin may be given after thrombolytic therapy to maintain the patency of the coronary artery; monitor activated partial thromboplastin time (aPTT).
- PTCA may be used to reopen the thrombosed coronary artery.
- After an MI, the following medications are often prescribed:
  1. One enteric-coated aspirin daily or every other day to prevent platelet aggregation at the site of obstruction
  2. Beta-adrenergic agents
     a. Monitor heart rate.
     b. Check blood pressure.
     c. Check client's level of consciousness.
     d. Monitor for any chest discomfort.
     e. Assess lung sounds for crackles and wheezes.
     f. Monitor the client for hypoglycemia, depression, nightmares, and forgetfulness.
  3. Angiotensin-converting enzyme (ACE) inhibitors prevent ventricular remodeling and the development of heart failure.
     a. Monitor for decreased urinary output, hypotension, cough, and changes in serum potassium, creatinine, and blood urea nitrogen.
  4. Calcium channel blockers for clients with variant angina or for those who are hypertensive and continue to have angina despite therapy with beta blockers

NDx: Activity Intolerance

- Cardiac rehabilitation is divided into three phases.
  1. Phase 1 begins with acute illness and ends with discharge from the hospital.
  2. Phase 2 begins after discharge and continues through convalescence at home.
  3. Phase 3 involves long-term conditioning.
- Nursing interventions include
  1. Promoting rest and assisting with activities of daily living (ADLs)
  2. Progressing client mobility gradually, starting with having the client dangle the legs at the side of the bed and proceeding to ambulation
  3. Assessing the client's vital signs and level of fatigue with each higher level of activity

4. Notifying the health care provider if there are indications of activity intolerance: decreases greater than 20 mm Hg in the systolic blood pressure, changes of 20 beats/min in the pulse rate, or complaints of dyspnea or chest pain

◆NDx: Ineffective Coping

- Direct interventions toward assisting the client to take personal actions to manage stressors related to CAD.
  1. Assess the client's understanding of the disease process.
  2. Assess the client's coping mechanisms (commonly denial, anger, and depression) and level of anxiety.
  3. Provide simple, repeated explanations of therapies, expectations, and surroundings.
  4. Help the client identify the information that is most important to obtain.
  5. Denial that results in a client's "acting out" and refusing to follow treatment regimen can be harmful.
     a. Remain calm and avoid confronting the client.
     b. Clearly indicate when a behavior is not acceptable and is potentially harmful.
  6. Anger may be the result of a client's attempt to regain control of his or her life.
     a. Encourage client to verbalize frustrations.
     b. Provide opportunities for decision making and control.
  7. Depression may be a client's response to grief.
     a. Listen to the client and do not offer false or general reassurances.
     b. Acknowledge depression but expect the client to perform ADLs and other activities within restrictions.

◆COLLABORATIVE PROBLEM:
Potential for Dysrhythmias

- If a dysrhythmia occurs, the following actions are taken.
  1. Identify the dysrhythmia.
  2. Assess the client's hemodynamic status.
  3. Evaluate the client for chest discomfort.
- Dysrhythmias are treated when they are causing hemo-dynamic compromise, are increasing myocardial oxygen requirements, or are predisposing the client to lethal ventricular dysrhythmias.

COLLABORATIVE PROBLEM:
Potential for Heart Failure

- Heart failure is a relatively common complication following MI; the most severe form of heart failure, cardiogenic shock, accounts for most in-hospital deaths following MI.

NONSURGICAL MANAGEMENT

- Decreased cardiac output related to heart failure is a common complication after MI.
- Assess the client with left ventricular failure and pulmonary edema by auscultating for crackles and identifying their location within the lungs.
- Assess for
  1. Tachypnea, wheezing
  2. Frothy sputum
  3. Change in client's orientation or mental status
  4. Urine output less than 30 mL/hr
  5. Cold, clammy skin with poor peripheral pulses
  6. Unusual fatigue
  7. Recurrent chest pain
  8. Changes in right atrial pressure, pulmonary artery pressure, systolic and diastolic pressures, pulmonary wedge pressure, systemic vascular resistance, cardiac output, and cardiac index
- Classification of post-MI heart failure is as follows:
  1. Class I post-MI heart failure often responds well to reduction in preload with IV nitrates and diuretics. Monitor hourly the urine output and vital signs; review serum potassium levels; and assess for signs of heart failure.
  2. Class II and class III post-MI heart failure may require diuresis and more aggressive medical intervention such as reduction of afterload (IV nitroglycerin or nitroprusside) or enhancement of cardiac contractility (dopamine, dobutamine, or amrinone).
- Class IV cardiogenic shock is manifested by tachycardia, hypotension, blood pressure less than 90 mm Hg systolic or 30 mm Hg less than client's baseline, cold and clammy skin with poor peripheral pulses, agitation, pulmonary congestion, and continued chest pain.

- Medical management may include
  1. IV morphine to decrease pulmonary congestion and relieve pain
  2. Oxygen therapy (intubation and mechanical ventilation may be necessary)
  3. Information from hemodynamic monitoring, which is used to titrate drug therapy
  4. Diuretics, nitroglycerin, or nitroprusside
- Clients who do not respond to drug therapy may require an *intra-aortic balloon pump* (IABP), which is inserted to improve myocardial perfusion, reduce afterload, and facilitate ventricular emptying.
- Immediate reperfusion may be performed on clients with cardiogenic shock. A left-sided cardiac catheterization is performed. If the client has a treatable lesion, the surgeon performs a PTCA or the client undergoes a coronary artery bypass graft (CABG).
- The goal of medical management of right-side heart ventricular failure is to improve right ventricular stroke volume.
  1. Provide IV fluids (as much as 200 mL/hr) to increase right atrial pressure to 20 mm Hg.
  2. Monitor pulmonary artery wedge pressure (attempting to maintain it below 15 to 20 mm Hg).
  3. Auscultate the lungs to ensure left-sided heart failure does not develop.
  4. Monitor cardiac output to ensure that fluid administration has the desired effect.

COLLABORATIVE PROBLEM:
Potential for Recurrent Chest Discomfort and Extension of Injury

- Recurrent chest pain despite medical therapy is a major indicator of surgery.

SURGICAL MANAGEMENT

- *Percutaneous transluminal coronary angioplasty (PTCA)*, an invasive but technically nonsurgical technique, is performed to provide symptom reduction for clients with chest discomfort without a significant risk of complications. PTCA is performed by introducing a balloon-tipped catheter into the area of the coronary artery occlusion. When the balloon is inflated, it presses the atherosclerotic plaque against the vessel wall to reduce or eliminate the occlusion.

- Techniques used to ensure patency of the vessel are laser angioplasty, stents, and atherectomy devices.
- Nursing interventions include
  1. Monitoring for potential problems after the procedure, including acute closure of the vessel, bleeding from the insertion site, reaction to the dye used in angiography, hypotension, hyperkalemia, and dysrhythmias
  2. Instructing the client to report the development of chest pain immediately
  3. Frequently monitoring circulation to the limb where the catheter was inserted and reporting changes immediately to the physician
  4. Maintaining immobilization of the affected limb for at least 6 hours
  5. Maintaining pressure dressing and sandbag over the insertion site
  6. Elevating the head of the bed slowly, per hospital protocol
  7. Instructing the client to
     a. Return to usual activities in 1 to 2 weeks or when instructed by the physician.
     b. Avoid heavy lifting for several weeks.
     c. Apply manual pressure if there is bleeding from the insertion site and notify the physician if the bleeding is extensive or if oozing persists for more than 15 minutes.
     d. Take long-term nitrates, calcium channel blockers, and aspirin, as prescribed.
- *Coronary artery bypass graft (CABG)* surgery is indicated when other treatments have been unsuccessful. This procedure is performed while the client is under general anesthesia and undergoing cardiopulmonary bypass (CPB). The graft, to either the saphenous vein or the internal mammary artery, bypasses the occluded vessel to restore blood supply to the myocardium.
- Preoperative care includes
  1. If surgery is performed as an elective procedure, familiarizing the client and family with the cardiac surgical critical care environment

2. Teaching the client how to splint the chest incision, cough and deep breathe, perform arm and leg exercises, what to expect during the postoperative period, and how pain will be managed

- Provide immediate postoperative care in a specialized unit.
  1. Maintain mechanical ventilation for 3 to 6 hours.
  2. Monitor chest tube drainage system.
  3. Monitor pulmonary artery and arterial pressures.
  4. Frequently assess vital signs and cardiac rate and rhythm.
  5. Ensure that pain is appropriately managed.
  6. Treat symptomatic dysrhythmias according to unit protocols or physician order.
  7. Monitor for complications of CABG surgery, including
     a. Fluid and electrolyte imbalances
     b. Hypotension
     c. Hypothermia
     d. Hypertension
     e. Bleeding
     f. Cardiac tamponade
     g. Altered cerebral perfusion

- Provide continued postoperative care.
  1. Encourage deep breathing and coughing every 2 hours while splinting incision.
  2. Assist the client in slowly resuming activity and ambulation.
  3. Monitor for dysrhythmias, especially atrial fibrillation, which occurs on the second or third postoperative day.
  4. Assess for wound or sternal infection (mediastinitis), such as prolonged fever (more than 4 days), reddened sternum, purulent incisional drainage, and elevated white blood cell (WBC) count.
  5. Observe for indications of postpericardiotomy syndrome: pericardial and pleural pain, pericarditis, friction rub, elevated temperature and WBC count, and dysrhythmias; problem may be self-limiting or may require treatment for pericarditis.

- Minimally invasive direct coronary arterial bypass (MIDCAB) is indicated for clients with a lesion of the left anterior descending artery. Cardiopulmonary bypass is not required.
  1. Assess the client for postoperative chest pain and electrocardiographic changes because occlusion of the

internal mammary artery graft occurs acutely in 10% of clients.

2. Encourage the client to cough and deep breathe (chest tube and thoracotomy incision).

■ Transmyocardial laser revascularization, for clients with unstable angina and inoperable CAD with area of reversible myocardial ischemia, involves the creation of 20 to 24 long, narrow channels through the left ventricular muscle to the left ventricle, which eventually allows oxygenated blood to flow and nourish the muscle.

■ Off-pump coronary artery bypass is open heart surgery performed without the use of a heart-lung bypass machine.

■ Robotic heart surgery allows surgeons to operate endoscopically through 8- to 10-mm long incisions in the chest wall, eliminating tremors that can exist with human hands, increasing the ability to reach inaccessible sites, and improving depth perception and visual acuity.

Community-Based Care

■ The client should be assigned to a case manager at the beginning of the hospitalization to provide constant care and assist with the transition to home or subacute care center.

■ Most clients are still recovering from their illness or surgery when discharged from the hospital; home health services may be required.

■ Teach the client and family about
1. The pathophysiology of angina and MI
2. Risk factor modification
   a. Smoking cessation
   b. Dietary changes (decreasing fat intake)
   c. Blood pressure control
   d. Blood glucose control
3. Gradual increase in physical and sexual activity, according to cardiac rehabilitation protocol
4. Cardiac medications
5. Occupational considerations, if any
6. Complementary and alternative therapies such as progressive relaxation, guided imagery, music therapy, pet therapy

■ Teach the client to seek medical assistance if they experience
1. Pulse rate that remains 50 or less while awake
2. Wheezing or difficulty breathing

3. Weight gain of 3 pounds in 1 week, or 1 to 2 pounds overnight
4. Slow, persistent increase in nitroglycerin use
5. Dizziness, faintness, or shortness of breath with activity

- Clients should call for emergency transportation to the hospital if they experience the following:
    1. Chest discomfort that does not improve after 20 minutes or after taking three nitroglycerin tablets
    2. Extremely severe chest or epigastric discomfort with weakness, nausea, or fainting
    3. Other symptoms that are particular to the client such as fatigue or nausea
- Other important discharge plans include
    1. Referring the client to the American Heart Association for information
    2. Referring the client for continued cardiac rehabilitation
    3. Referring the client who has had CABG surgery to Mended Hearts, a nationwide program that provides education and support to clients and their families

Crohn's Disease

OVERVIEW

- Crohn's disease, or regional enteritis, is an idiopathic inflammatory disease that occurs anywhere in the gastrointestinal (GI) tract but most often affects the terminal ileum with patchy lesions that extend through all bowel layers.
- Chronic nonspecific inflammation of the entire intestinal tract occurs, and eventually deep fissures and ulceration develop and often extend through all bowel layers, predisposing the client to development of bowel fistulas.
- Chronic pathologic changes include thickening of the bowel wall, resulting in narrowing of the bowel lumen and strictures.
- Complications of Crohn's disease include malabsorption, fistulas, hemorrhage, abscess formation, bowel obstruction, and cancer (usually after the client has the disease for 15 to 40 years).

COLLABORATIVE MANAGEMENT

Assessment

Assess for

1. Fever, abdominal pain, loose stools
2. Frequency, consistency, and presence of blood in the stool
3. Periumbilical pain before and after bowel movements
4. Weight loss (indicates serious nutritional deficiencies)
5. Family history of the disease
6. Distention, masses, or visible peristalsis
7. Ulcerations or fissures of the perianal area
8. Bowel sounds diminished or absent in the presence of severe inflammation
9. High-pitched or rushing sounds over the areas of narrowed bowel loops
10. Diarrhea with steatorrhea (the stool does not usually contain blood)
11. Psychosocial issues related to coping skills and support systems
12. Results of barium enema and upper GI series that show narrowing, ulcerations, strictures, and fistulas consistent with Crohn's disease
13. Results of laboratory studies

Interventions

- The care of the client with Crohn's disease is similar to care for the client with ulcerative colitis (see Colitis, Ulcerative).
- Drug therapy includes
    1. Sulfasalazine, used as an anti-inflammatory
    2. Metronidazole (Flagyl, Novonidazol), used for clients with fistulas
    3. Immunosuppressive therapy, used for clients with refractory disease or fistulas
    4. Infliximab (Remicade), an anti–tumor necrosis factor, used for active disease and fistulas
- Malnutrition can result in poor fistula and wound healing, loss of lean muscle mass, decreased immune system response, and increased morbidity and mortality.
    1. Monitor tolerance to diet.

2. Assist the client to select high-calorie, high-protein, high-vitamin, low-fiber meals.
3. Offer enteral supplements such as Ensure and Vivonex.
4. Record food intake and accurate calorie count.
5. Total parenteral nutrition (TPN) may be needed for severe exacerbations.

- Electrolyte therapy includes
  1. Fluid and electrolyte replacement by oral liquids and nutrients, as well as intravenous fluids
  2. Cautious use of antidiarrheal agents to decrease fluid loss
  3. Strict monitoring of intake and output
- Impaired skin integrity results from fistula formation. The degree of associated problems is related to the location of the fistula, the client's general health status, and the character and amount of fistula drainage.
  1. In collaboration with the enterostomal therapist, apply a pouch to the fistula to prevent skin irritation and to measure the drainage.
  2. Cover the area around the fistula with skin barriers, such as Stomahesive or DuoDerm, and apply a wound drainage system over the fistula, securing it to the protective barriers.
  3. Clean adjacent skin and keep it dry. The wound drainage should *never* be allowed to have direct skin contact without prompt cleaning because intestinal fluid enzymes are caustic.
- Observe for subtle signs of infection or sepsis such as fever, abdominal pain, or change in mental status.
- Some clients with Crohn's disease require surgery such as a bowel resection and anastomosis with or without a colon resection to improve the quality of life (see Surgical Management under Cancer, Colorectal).
- Stricturoplasty may be performed for bowel strictures.

Community-Based Care

- See Community-Based Care under Colitis, Ulcerative.

Cystitis (Urinary Tract Infection)

OVERVIEW

- Cystitis is an inflammation of the urinary bladder with both infectious and noninfectious causes. Infectious causes are bacteria, viruses, fungi, and parasites. Noninfectious causes are chemical exposure and radiation therapy.
- Interstitial cystitis is a chronic inflammation of the entire lower urinary tract (bladder, urethra, and adjacent pelvic muscles) that is not the result of infection and can lead to pyelonephritis and sepsis.
- Urosepsis is the spread of infection from the urinary tract to the bloodstream.
- Coliform bacteria, especially *Escherichia coli* normally found in the gastrointestinal tract, account for most cases of bacterial cystitis.
- Other factors that contribute to the development or recurrence of cystitis, or urinary tract infections (UTIs), include
    1. Structural or functional abnormalities of the urinary tract
    2. Use of indwelling urinary catheters
    3. Sexual intercourse, diaphragm use, and pregnancy in women (women are at a higher risk then men)
    4. Prostate disease or structural abnormality of the urinary tract in men

Considerations for Older Adults

- UTIs occur more often in older adults than in younger adults, with females more commonly affected than men.
- Elderly clients are at greater risk than others of having an overwhelming and generalized infection, known as urosepsis, caused by a gram-negative bacteremia.

COLLABORATIVE MANAGEMENT

Assessment

- Record client information.
    1. History of UTIs
    2. History of renal or urologic problems, such as kidney stones
    3. History of health problems, such as diabetes mellitus

- Assess for
    1. Pain or discomfort on urination
    2. Urgency to void
    3. Difficulty in initiating urination
    4. Feelings of incomplete bladder emptying
    5. Voiding in small amounts
    6. Increased frequency of voiding
    7. Complete inability to urinate
    8. Change in urine color, clarity, or odor; presence of white or red blood cells
    9. Abdominal or back pain
    10. Bladder distention
    11. Urinary meatus inflammation
    12. Prostate gland changes or tenderness
    13. Positive urine culture
    14. Elevated white blood cell (WBC) count (occasional)

Considerations for Older Adults

- The only symptoms may be as vague as increasing mental confusion or frequent unexplained falls.
- A sudden onset of or worsening of incontinence may be an early symptom.
- Fever, tachycardia, tachypnea, and hypotension even without any urinary symptoms may be signs of urosepsis.
- Loss of appetite, nocturia, and dysuria are common symptoms.

Planning and Implementation

- Drug therapy includes
    1. Analgesics to promote comfort
    2. Urinary antiseptics such as nitrofurantoin (Macrodantin, Nephronex) and trimethoprim (Proloprim, Trimpex)
    3. Antispasmodics to decrease bladder spasm and promote complete bladder emptying
    4. Antibiotics for systemic infection. Antibiotics may be given in daily bladder instillations or in oral or parenteral form. In simple, acute bacterial cystitis in healthy, ambulatory clients, a 1- to 3-day course of antibiotic treatment may be adequate; long-term antibiotics may be needed for clients with chronic recurring infections.

5. Antifungal agents such as amphotericin B in daily bladder instillations and ketoconazole (Nizoral) in oral form
- Diet therapy includes
  1. Ensuring that the client maintains an adequate caloric intake
  2. Ensuring a fluid intake of 2 to 3 L/day unless contra-indicated
- Other therapy includes providing warm sitz baths to relieve local symptoms.

SURGICAL MANAGEMENT

- Surgical interventions for management of cystitis include endourologic procedures with stone manipulation or pulverization for the management of urinary retention if bladder or urethral calculus is the cause.

Community-Based Care

- Teach the client to
  1. Self-administer medications and complete all of the prescribed medication.
  2. Expect changes in color of urine as appropriate.
  3. Use appropriate techniques to prevent discomfort with sexual activities and how to prevent postcoital infections.
  4. Consume liberal fluid intake of at least 2 to 3 L/day.
  5. Clean the perineum properly after urination.
  6. Empty the bladder as soon as the urge is felt.
  7. Obtain adequate rest, sleep, and nutrition.
  8. Avoid known irritants such as bubble baths, nylon underwear, and scented toilet tissue.
  9. Wear cotton underwear.
  10. Seek prompt medical care if recurrences are suspected.
- Refer clients to the National Kidney Foundation as appropriate.
- Refer clients with interstitial cystitis to the Interstitial Cystitis Foundation.

Cystocele

- A cystocele is a protrusion of the bladder through the vaginal wall resulting from weakened pelvic structures.
- Causes include obesity, advanced age, childbearing, and genetic predisposition.

COLLABORATIVE MANAGEMENT

- Assess for
  1. Difficulty emptying the bladder
  2. Urinary frequency and urgency
  3. Urinary tract infections (UTIs)
  4. Stress urinary incontinence
  5. Significant bulging of the anterior vaginal wall during pelvic examination
- Management is conservative with mild symptoms and includes
  1. Use of a pessary for bladder support
  2. Estrogen therapy for the postmenopausal client to prevent atrophy and weakening of vaginal walls
  3. Kegel exercises to strengthen perineal muscles
- Surgical intervention (anterior colporrhaphy or anterior repair) is recommended for severe symptoms. (Care is similar to that for other vaginal surgeries.)
- Postoperatively, the client should
  1. Limit her activities
  2. Not lift anything heavier than 5 pounds
  3. Avoid strenuous exercise
  4. Avoid sexual intercourse for 6 weeks
  5. Notify her physician if she has signs of infection, including fever, persistent pain, and purulent, foul-smelling discharge

Cysts, Bartholin's

- Bartholin's cysts are one of the most common disorders of the vulva.
- The cysts result from obstruction of a duct; the secretory function of the gland continues, and the fluid fills the obstructed duct.
- The cause of the obstruction may be infection, congenital stenosis or atresia, thickened mucus near the ductal opening, or mechanical trauma.
- Ranging in size from 1 to 10 cm, cysts usually appear unilaterally.
- Assessment for *small cysts* may reveal no symptoms, or the client may complain of dyspareunia, of inadequate genital lubrication, or of feeling a mass in the perineal area.
- Assessment for *large cysts* includes assessing for
  1. Constant, localized pain
  2. Difficulty walking or sitting
  3. Swelling immediately beneath the skin in the posterior vulva
  4. Brown or sanguineous cyst
- If the cyst is draining, the fluid is sent for culture and sensitivity testing.
- A specimen of the cyst is sent for pathologic examination if the client is older than 40 years of age.
- For symptomatic cysts, surgical treatment with incision and drainage may provide temporary relief.
- Marsupialization (the formation of a pouch that serves as a new duct opening) may be performed to prevent recurrence.
- Local comfort measures and prophylactic antibiotics may be provided.
- If the cyst becomes infected, an *abscess* can form, which usually ruptures spontaneously within 72 hours.
- Interventions for abscess include bedrest, analgesics, moist heat, antibiotics, and an incision and drainage.
- Total excision of the Bartholin's gland is performed for women over 40 years of age when cancer is suspected or if repeated infections with abscess formation occur.

Cysts, Ovarian

OVERVIEW

- There are several types of ovarian cysts.
  1. Follicular cysts
     a. Follicular cysts occur in young menstruating females, are not malignant, and do not grow without hormonal influences.
     b. Cysts develop when a mature follicle fails to rupture or an immature follicle fails to reabsorb follicular fluid.
     c. Follicular cysts are usually small (6 to 8 cm) and may be asymptomatic unless they rupture, causing acute, severe pelvic pain, which usually resolves with bedrest and administration of mild analgesics.
     d. If cysts do not rupture, they usually disappear in two or three menstrual cycles without medical intervention.
     e. Oral contraceptives may be prescribed for one or two menstrual cycles to depress ovulation, resulting in cyst shrinkage.
     f. Surgery is recommended only before puberty, after menopause, or when cysts are larger than 8 cm.
     g. Cystectomy (removal of cyst) is recommended instead of oophorectomy (removal of an ovary).
  2. Corpus luteum cysts
     a. Corpus luteum cysts occur after ovulation and are often associated with increased secretion of progesterone.
     b. The cysts are small, averaging 4 cm, and are purplish red as a result of hemorrhage within the corpus luteum.
     c. Corpus luteum cysts are associated with delay in the onset of menses and irregular or prolonged flow, and may be accompanied by unilateral, low abdominal, or pelvic pain.
     d. Cyst rupture may cause intraperitoneal hemorrhage.
     e. Corpus luteum cysts may disappear in one or two menstrual cycles or with suppression of ovulation.
     f. The treatment is the same as that for follicular cysts.
  3. Theca-lutein cysts
     a. Theca-lutein cysts, the least common of the functional ovarian cysts, are associated with hydatidiform mole

and develop as a result of prolonged stimulation of the ovaries by excessive amounts of human chorionic gonadotropin (hCG).

    b. The cysts regress spontaneously within 3 months with the removal of the molar pregnancy or source of the excess hCG.

- *Polycystic ovary (Stein-Leventhal) syndrome* results when elevated levels of luteinizing hormone cause hyperstimulation of the ovaries; endometrial hyperplasia or carcinoma may result.
  1. The typical client is obese, is hirsute, has irregular menses, and may be infertile because of anovulation.
  2. The best treatment is administration of oral contraceptives because of lutein production inhibition.
  3. Bilateral salpingo-oophorectomy (removal of both tubes and ovaries) and hysterectomy (removal of uterus) are advised for women over 35 years of age who no longer desire childbearing.
  4. Women desiring fertility can be treated with drugs to stimulate ovulation.

Degeneration, Macular

- Macular degeneration, deterioration of the macula, can be atrophic (age related or dry) or exudative (wet).
- Macular degeneration is characterized by sclerosing of the retinal capillaries, decrease in central vision, mild blurring, and distortion of vision.
- Loss of central vision may interfere with the client's ability to read, write, drive, and recognize safety hazards.
- Management of exudative macular degeneration is directed toward treating the underlying cause and preventing further deterioration of vision.
- Laser therapy or photodynamic therapy may be used to seal leaking blood vessels.
- Assist the client to identify strategies to cope with the loss of vision and make referrals to community agencies.

Dehydration

- Dehydration is a state in which the body's fluid intake is not sufficient to meet the body's fluid needs, resulting in fluid volume deficit.
- There are three types of dehydration.
  1. Isotonic dehydration, in which water and dissolved electrolytes are lost in equal proportions. It involves loss of isotonic fluids from the extracellular fluid (ECF) space, including both the plasma and interstitial spaces. Causes of isotonic dehydration include
     a. Hemorrhage
     b. Vomiting, diarrhea
     c. Profuse salivation
     d. Fistulas, abscesses
     e. Ileostomy, cecostomy
     f. Frequent enemas
     g. Profuse diaphoresis
     h. Burns
     i. Severe wounds
     j. Long-term nothing by mouth (NPO) status
     k. Diuretic therapy
     l. Gastrointestinal suction, nasogastric suction
  2. Hypertonic dehydration occurs when water loss from the extracellular fluid is greater than the electrolyte loss. Causes of hypertonic dehydration include
     a. Excessive sweating
     b. Hyperventilation
     c. Ketoacidosis
     d. Diarrhea
     e. Early stage renal failure
     f. Diabetes insipidus
     g. Excessive fluid replacement (hypertonic)
     h. Excessive sodium bicarbonate administration
     i. Tube feedings, dysphagia
     j. Impaired thirst
     k. Unconsciousness
     l. Fever

  m. Impaired motor function

  n. Systemic infection

3. Hypotonic dehydration, in which electrolyte loss is greater than water loss, involves excessive loss of sodium and potassium from extracellular fluid. Causes of hypotonic dehydration include

  a. Chronic illness

  b. Excessive fluid replacement (hypotonic)

  c. Chronic renal failure

  d. Chronic or severe malnutrition

COLLABORATIVE MANAGEMENT

Assessment

- Record client information.
  - **1.** Medical history
    - **a.** Age
    - **b.** Past medical history
    - **c.** Recent surgery
    - **d.** Medication history
  - **2.** Height and weight: A weight change of 1 pound (0.45 kg) corresponds to a fluid volume change of about 500 mL.
  - **3.** Change in degree of tightness of clothing, rings, and shoes: A sudden decrease in tightness may indicate dehydration; an increase may reflect edema.
  - **4.** Orthostatic hypotension: palpitations or light-headedness
  - **5.** Abnormal or excessive fluid loss
  - **6.** Urinary output
    - **a.** Frequency and amount of voidings
    - **b.** Usual fluid intake and intake during the previous 24 hours
    - **c.** Type of fluids ingested
  - **7.** Amount of strenuous physical activity
- Assessment findings include
  - **1.** Cardiovascular manifestations
    - **a.** Increased pulse rate
    - **b.** Thready pulse quality
    - **c.** Decreased blood pressure
    - **d.** Postural hypotension (orthostatic hypotension)
    - **e.** Flat neck and hand veins in dependent positions
    - **f.** Diminished peripheral pulses

2. Respiratory manifestations
   a. Increased respiratory rate
   b. Increased depth of respirations
3. Neuromuscular manifestations
   a. Decreased central nervous system activity (lethargy to coma)
   b. Fever
4. Renal manifestations
   a. Decreased urine output
   b. Increased specific gravity
5. Integumentary manifestations
   a. Dry, scaly skin
   b. Turgor poor, tenting present
   c. Mouth dry and fissured with pastelike coating
6. Gastrointestinal manifestations
   a. Decreased motility
   b. Diminished bowel sounds
   c. Constipation
7. Psychosocial manifestations
   a. Behavioral changes
   b. Anxiety, restlessness
   c. Lethargy, confusion
8. Laboratory values
   a. Increased blood urea nitrogen and creatinine levels
   b. Changes in hemoglobin and hematocrit (depend on type of dehydration)
   c. Increased urine specific gravity (except in hypotonic dehydration)
9. Additional manifestation of hypotonic dehydration: skeletal muscle weakness
10. Additional manifestations of hypertonic dehydration
    a. Hyperactive deep-tendon reflexes
    b. Increased sensation of thirst
    c. Pitting edema

 Considerations for Older Adults

- Skin turgor for an older adult is assessed over the sternum, forehead, or abdomen because these areas are the most reliable indicators.

Planning and Implementation

NDx: Deficient Fluid Volume

- Replace fluids orally; intravenous fluid replacement may be necessary for severe dehydration.
- The rate of replacement and type of fluids used depend on the degree and type of dehydration and the presence of pre-existing cardiac, pulmonary, or renal problems. Commonly used fluids include
  1. Isotonic fluids such as 0.9% saline, 5% dextrose in water (D_5W), or Ringer's lactate
  2. Hypotonic fluids such as 0.45% normal saline
  3. Hypertonic fluids such as 10% dextrose in water, 5% dextrose in 0.9% saline, 5% dextrose in 0.45% saline, or 5% dextrose in Ringer's lactate
- Monitor pulse rate and quality and urine output during rehydration.
- Provide drug therapy, such as antidiarrheal medications, antiemetics, antimicrobials, or antipyretics, as ordered, to ameliorate or correct the underlying cause of the dehydration.
- Monitor serum and urine electrolyte values.
- Monitor orthostatic blood pressure and change in cardiac rhythm.
- Weigh the client daily.
- Maintain accurate intake and output record.
- Monitor color, quantity, and specific gravity of urine.
- Promote oral intake; encourage family or significant others to assist client with feedings.
- Provide frequent oral care.

NDx: Decreased Cardiac Output

- Drug therapy to increase venous return or improve cardiac contractility is used only when a cardiac problem is present.
- Oxygen therapy may be administered by mask or nasal cannula.
- Treatment includes
  1. Monitoring the client's vital signs and level of consciousness
  2. Monitoring skin color and moisture and urine output every hour until fluid balance is restored

- Keep the lips clean and moist.
- Provide mouth care every 8 hours to reduce the thick, sticky coating on the tongue and mouth during dehydration.
- Brush the client's teeth several times a day.
- Rinse the client's mouth frequently with lukewarm saline or tap water.
- Teach the client to avoid mouthwashes and swabs that contain alcohol or glycerine because these products dry the oral mucosa further and may sting open areas of the mucosa.
- Rinse the client's mouth no more than two times per day with diluted hydrogen peroxide.
- Encourage fluids.

◆**COLLABORATIVE PROBLEM:** Potential for Dysrhythmia

- Treatment includes
  1. Monitoring electrolyte levels, especially hypercalcemia and hyperkalemia
     a. Hypercalcemia may be treated with etidronate (Didronel) and plicamycin (Mithracin).
     b. Hyperkalemia may be treated with 20 units of regular insulin in 100 mL of dextrose.
  2. Assessing the rate, rhythm, and quality of the apical pulse
  3. Assessing the client for fatigue, chest pain, and shortness of breath
  4. Placing the client on a cardiac monitor and monitoring for dysrhythmia

Community-Based Care

- Clients most likely to be discharged before the imbalance is completely corrected and who are susceptible to recurrent episodes are those with chronic problems such as renal disease, diabetes, cancer, adrenal insufficiency, or other endocrine disorder.
- Discharge planning: Review with the client and family for
  1. Prescribed diet, drug regimens, and manifestations of dehydration
     a. Instruct the client to take medications as prescribed and not to increase the use of diuretics.
  2. The importance of daily weight monitoring using the

same scale at the same time of day, recording weight in a daily log book
  3. How and where to assess skin turgor
  4. How to take a peripheral pulse
- Refer to home health care and other community agencies as needed.
- Focused assessment for the home care nurse includes
  1. Cardiovascular assessment
  2. Cognition and mental status
  3. Condition of skin and mucous membranes
  4. Neuromuscular status
  5. Intake and output, diet, and weight
- Review medications, including over-the-counter medications.
- Assess client's understanding of illness and compliance with treatment.

Diabetes Insipidus

OVERVIEW

- Diabetes insipidus (DI) is a disorder of water metabolism caused by a deficiency of antidiuretic hormone (ADH), resulting from either a decrease in ADH synthesis or an inability of the kidney to respond appropriately to ADH.
- DI is classified into four types.
  1. Nephrogenic: an inherited defect in which the renal tubules do not respond to the actions of ADH, which results in inadequate water absorption by the kidney
  2. Primary: results from a defect in the hypothalamus or pituitary gland resulting in lack of ADH production or release
  3. Secondary: results from tumors in the hypothalamic-pituitary region, head trauma, infectious processes, surgical procedures, or metastatic tumors, usually from the lung or breast
  4. Drug-related: caused by lithium (Eskalith, Lithobid, Carbolith) and demeclocycline (Declomycin), which can interfere with the renal response to ADH

COLLABORATIVE MANAGEMENT

Assessment

- Assessment findings include
    1. History of known etiologic factors, such as recent surgery, head trauma, or medication
    2. Excretion of large amounts of dilute urine (more than 4 L in 24 hours)
    3. Dehydration
    4. Increased or excessive thirst
    5. Low urine specific gravity (below 1.005) and urine osmolality (50 to 200 mOsm/kg)
    6. Indications of circulatory collapse, shock
    7. Neurologic changes such as irritability, lethargy, decreased cognition

Interventions

- Nursing interventions include
    1. Monitoring strict intake and output
    2. Measuring urine specific gravity at least once daily
    3. Weighing the client every day
    4. Encouraging the client to drink fluids equal to the amount of urinary output (If the client is unable to do so, provide intravenous fluids, as ordered.)
    5. Monitoring carefully for indications of dehydration: dry skin, poor skin turgor, and dry or cracked mucous membranes
    6. Monitoring for signs of circulatory collapse such as vital sign changes
- Drug therapy may include
    1. Desmopressin acetate (DDAVP), a synthetic form of vasopressin given intranasally in a metered spray; frequency of dosing depends on client response
    2. Aqueous vasopressin for short-term therapy or when the dosage must be changed frequently
- Client education includes
    1. Teaching about the side effects of nasal sprays, including ulceration of the mucous membranes, allergy, sensation of chest tightness, and inhalation of the spray into the lungs, which precipitates pulmonary problems

2. Teaching what to do if side effects occur or if an upper respiratory infection develops (Sustained-action vasopressin [vasopressin tannate in oil] is administered intramuscularly.)
3. Providing education on vasopressin preparations for the client who will be discharged
4. Encouraging the client with chronic DI to wear a medical alert bracelet or necklace at all times

Diabetes Mellitus

OVERVIEW

- Diabetes mellitus is a genetically and clinically heterogeneous group of chronic systemic disorders of various causes affecting the metabolism of carbohydrates, protein, and fat as a result of insulin deficiency.
- Diabetes mellitus is characterized by polyuria, polydipsia, polyphagia, and fasting hyperglycemia or blood glucose levels above defined limits.
- Insulin, an anabolic hormone made in the beta cells of the islets of Langerhans in the pancreas, plays a key role in allowing body cells to store and use carbohydrates, fat, and protein. Insulin also acts as a catalyst to stimulate enzymes and chemicals necessary for cell function and energy production.
- Diabetes is classified according to the cause and presentation of the disease.
  1. *Type 1 (insulin-dependent) diabetes* is an autoimmune disorder in which beta cells of the pancreas are destroyed. Type 1 diabetes
     a. Is abrupt in onset
     b. Requires insulin injections to prevent ketosis and sustain health
     c. Affects 10% to 15% of the diabetic population
     d. Occurs primarily in childhood or adolescence but can occur at any age
     e. Causes clients to be thin and underweight

f. May be caused by a virus that initiates autoimmune destruction of pancreatic beta cells, where insulin is produced

2. *Type 2 diabetes* is characterized by a reduction in the ability of most cells to respond to insulin (insulin resistance), poor control of liver glucose output, and decreased beta cell function. Type 2 diabetes

a. Is generally slow in onset

b. May require insulin or sulfonylurea therapy to correct hyperglycemia

c. Is usually ketosis-resistant, but ketosis can occur during severe stress or infection

d. Affects about 90% of the diabetic population

e. Is usually found in middle-aged and older adults but may occur in younger people

f. Results in obesity in 80% of those affected

g. Has unknown cause, but risk factors include family history of diabetes; obesity; age over 40 years; previously identified impaired glucose tolerance, hypertension, or significant hyperlipidemia; and a history of gestational diabetes or delivery of babies weighing more than 9 pounds (4.1 kg)

3. *Genetic defects of the beta cells,* formerly referred to as MODY (maturity-onset diabetes of the young), is characterized by impaired insulin secretion with little or no defects in insulin action and is inherited in an autosomal dominant pattern.

4. Secondary diabetes

a. May occur with specific disorders such as pancreatic disease, endocrine disorders, or genetic disorders associated with glucose intolerance

b. May be induced by a chemical agent or drug such as steroids (steroid-induced diabetes) (uncommon occurrence)

5. Gestational diabetes mellitus (GDM)

a. Carbohydrate intolerance is noted during pregnancy and is confirmed by an oral glucose tolerance test.

b. Clients are at high risk for diabetes after pregnancy.

c. Children of mothers with GDM are at risk for neonatal mortality, congenital malformation, and large body size; they also have an increased risk of obesity and impaired glucose tolerance in late adolescence and young adulthood.

- Acute complications of diabetes mellitus include
  1. Diabetic ketoacidosis (DKA)
     a. DKA occurs in people with type 1 diabetes and is most often precipitated by concurrent illness, especially infection.
     b. Laboratory diagnosis is based on serum glucose level equal to or greater than 300 mg/dL (16.7 mmol/L), arterial pH level less than 7.38, arterial bicarbonate level less than 15 mEq/L, serum sodium level less than 136 mEq/L, blood urea nitrogen greater than 20 mg/dL, creatinine greater than 1.5 mg/dL, and ketonemia.
     c. DKA is preceded by polyuria, polydipsia, and polyphagia.
     d. Clinical evidence of dehydration and acidosis includes decreased skin turgor, dry mucous membranes, hypotension, tachycardia, tachypnea, Kussmaul respirations, abdominal pain, nausea, and vomiting; central nervous system depression results in changes in consciousness varying from lethargy to coma.
  2. Hyperglycemic hyperosmolar nonketotic coma (HHNC)
     a. HHNC is a hyperosmolar state caused by hyperglycemia of any origin; it is differentiated from DKA by the absence of significant ketosis and by the presence of a plasma glucose level and osmolality that are higher than average.
     b. Laboratory findings include plasma glucose level above 800 mg/dL and serum osmolality of at least 350 mOsm.
     c. Severe dehydration and electrolyte losses occur, and renal impairment results from decreased renal blood flow.
     d. HHNC occurs almost predominantly in older adults and almost exclusively in clients with type 2 diabetes.
     e. Conditions such as silent myocardial infarction, sepsis, pancreatitis, and stroke and drugs such as glucocorticoids, diuretics, phenytoin sodium, propranolol, and calcium channel blockers may precipitate HHNC.
     f. Older adults are more at risk than younger persons because of age-related changes in thirst perception,

loss of taste buds, and poor urine-concentrating abilities that lead to dehydration.

3. Hypoglycemia
   a. Neurogenic symptoms, which result from autonomic nervous system discharge triggered by hypoglycemia, including hunger, diaphoresis, weakness, and nervousness, occur when there is an *abrupt* decrease in the blood glucose level.
   b. Neuroglycopenic symptoms, which result directly from brain glucose deprivation, including headache, confusion, slurred speech, behavioral changes, and coma, occur with a more *gradual* decline in blood glucose level.

Considerations for Older Adults

- Older adults with diabetes are at the greatest risk for dehydration and subsequent HHNC. The onset of HHNC is insidious, and older adults typically seek medical attention later and are sicker than younger clients.
- The classic signs and symptoms of hypoglycemia may not appear in elderly diabetic clients; changes in levels of consciousness may be slow and progress through confusion and bizarre behavior. Coma may come without warning.

- Chronic complications of diabetes can be divided into macrovascular (large vessel) and microvascular (small vessel) problems.
  1. Macrovascular complications include
     a. Coronary heart disease
     b. Peripheral vascular disease (often leading to amputation)
     c. Cerebrovascular disease
  2. Microvascular complications include
     a. Ocular complications (can lead to blindness): diabetic retinopathy, retinal detachment, macular degeneration, myopia, cataracts, and glaucoma
     b. Diabetic neuropathy (damage to peripheral and autonomic nerves)
     c. Diabetic nephropathy (renal failure)
     d. Male erectile dysfunction

||| Cultural Considerations

- Diabetes is a significant problem for African Americans, Native Americans/American Indians, and Mexican Americans.
- In all populations, prevalence of diabetes rises with age.
- There is a strong correlation between relative weight and the prevalence of type 2 diabetes.
- Minority group members have a higher risk for complications than whites, even after adjusting for differences in blood glucose control.

COLLABORATIVE MANAGEMENT

Assessment

- Record client information.
    1. Age
    2. Birth weight of children
    3. Weight change
    4. Occurrence of a recent illness or extreme stress
    5. Omission of insulin or oral medications if the client is a known diabetic
    6. Change in eating habits
    7. Change in exercise schedule or activity level
    8. Duration of polyuria, polydipsia, polyphagia, and loss of energy
    9. History of small skin injuries becoming infected more easily or taking a longer time to heal
    10. History of or concurrent cardiovascular disease such as dysrhythmias, heart failure, hypertension, or stroke
- Assessment findings include
    1. Elevated blood glucose level
        a. Serum glucose
        b. Oral glucose tolerance test
        c. Capillary blood glucose monitoring
        d. Glycosylated hemoglobin assays (HbA1c)
        e. Glycosylated serum proteins and albumin
    2. Positive results for urinary ketones; presence of albumin and glucose in the urine
    3. Abdominal pain, nausea, and vomiting (in DKA)
    4. Dehydration

Planning and Implementation

◆**NDx:** Risk for Injury Related to Hyperglycemia

NONSURGICAL MANAGEMENT

- Medication is indicated when a client with type 2 diabetes cannot achieve blood glucose control with dietary modification, regular exercise, and stress management.

    1. *Sulfonylureas:* These agents are appropriate only for clients with pancreatic beta cell function; hypoglycemia is the most serious complication; other side effects include hematologic reactions, allergic skin reactions, and gastrointestinal effects.

    2. *Meglitinides:* Repaglinide (Prandin) action and side effects are similar to sulfonylurea agents. Adverse effects include hypoglycemia, gastrointestinal disturbances, upper respiratory infections, arthralgia, back pain, and headache.

    3. *Biguanides:* Metformin (Glucophage), the only biguanide available in the United States, can cause lactic acidosis in clients with renal insufficiency.

    4. *Alpha-glucosidase inhibitors:* Medications such as acarbose (Precose) reduce postprandial hyperglycemia by slowing digestion and absorption of carbohydrate within the intestine. Side effects include abdominal discomfort related to undigested carbohydrate in the intestinal tract.

    5. *Thiazolidinedione antidiabetic agents:* These agents enhance insulin action, promoting glucose utilization in peripheral tissues. Liver function studies should be done at the start of therapy and at regular intervals while on therapy.

    6. *D-Phenylalanine:* Derivatives lower blood glucose by triggering insulin secretion via interaction with the ATP-sensitive potassium channel on pancreatic beta cells.

    7. *Combination agents:* These are combinations from two different classes of medications, such as Glucovance.

- Insulin therapy is necessary for type 1 diabetes and for moderate to severe type 2 diabetes.

    1. Insulin is available in rapid-, short-, intermediate-, and long-acting forms, which may be injected separately or mixed in the same syringe.

2. Teach the client that insulin type, injection techniques, site of injection, and individual response can all affect absorption, onset, degree, and duration of insulin activity and reinforce that changing insulin may affect blood glucose control.

3. Insulin regimens try to duplicate the normal release pattern of insulin from the pancreas, including single daily injections, two-dose protocol, three-dose protocol, four-dose protocol, combination therapy, and intensified insulin regimens.

4. Complications of insulin therapy include
   a. Hypoglycemia
   b. Hypertrophic lipodystrophy, a spongy swelling at or around injection sites
   c. Lipoatrophy, a loss of subcutaneous fat in areas of repeated injection that is treated by injection of human insulin at the edges of the atrophied area
   d. Lipohypertrophy, an increased swelling of fat that occurs at the site of repeated injections and is treated by rotating injection sites
   e. Dawn phenomenon, a fasting hyperglycemia thought to result from nocturnal release of growth hormone secretion that may cause blood glucose elevations around 5 to 6 AM and is treated by providing more insulin for the overnight period
   f. Somogyi phenomenon, a morning hyperglycemia resulting from effective counter-regulatory response to nighttime hypoglycemia, that is treated by ensuring adequate dietary intake at bedtime and evaluating insulin dose and exercise program

5. Insulin may be administered by
   a. Subcutaneous injection
   b. Continuous subcutaneous infusion of insulin administered by an externally worn pump containing a syringe and reservoir with rapid or short-acting insulin connected to the client by an infusion set
   c. Insulin pumps implanted into the peritoneal cavity where insulin can be absorbed in a more physiologic manner

D

     d. Injection devices, whereby the needle is replaced by an ultrathin liquid stream of insulin forced through the skin under high pressure

     e. New technologies, including nasal spray administered via nebulizer and transdermal delivery of insulin, which is being investigated

  6. Teach the client about storage, dose preparation, injection procedures, and complications associated with drug therapy.

  7. Instruct the client to always buy the same type of syringes and use the same gauge and needle length; short needles are not used for an obese client.

■ Teach the client how to perform self-monitoring of blood glucose.

  1. Accuracy of the results depends on the accuracy of the specific blood glucose meter, operator proficiency, and test strip quality.

  2. Results are influenced by the amount of blood on the strip, the calibration of the meter to the strip currently in use; environmental conditions of altitude, temperature, and moisture; and client-specific conditions of hematocrit, triglyceride level, and presence of hypotension.

  3. Teach the client how to clean the equipment and how to prevent infection.

■ Instruct the client *not* to use alternative site testing (forearm, upper arm, abdomen, thigh, and calf) in the following situations:

  1. When client is hypoglycemic or susceptible to hypoglycemia (at time of peak activity of basal insulin)

  2. After exercise

  3. During an illness

  4. When blood glucose levels are changing rapidly

  5. Before driving

■ Provide diet therapy.

  1. Collaborate with the client, physician, and dietitian to formulate an individualized meal plan for the client.

  2. Day-to-day consistency in the timing and amount of food eaten helps control blood glucose. Clients taking insulin need to eat at consistent times that are coordinated with the timed action of insulin.

3. Base meal plan on blood glucose monitoring results, total blood lipid levels, and glycosylated hemoglobin.
4. Dietary guidelines are based on individual needs of the client.

   a. Protein intake: 15% to 20% of total daily calories is appropriate for clients with normal kidney function. In clients with microalbuminuria, reduction of protein to 10% of calories may slow progression of kidney failure.
   b. Less than 10% should be from saturated fat and up to 10% should be from polyunsaturated fat.
   c. Foods high in trans-fatty acids are avoided or severely restricted.
   d. Remaining calories are from monounsaturated fat and carbohydrates.
   e. High-fiber diets improve carbohydrate metabolism and lower cholesterol levels. High-fiber foods are added to the client's diet gradually to prevent cramping, loose stools, and flatulence.
   f. Suggest artificial sweeteners such as saccharin, aspartame, sucralose, and acesulfame K instead of sugar to enhance dietary compliance.
   g. Fat replacers may increase carbohydrate content in foods.
5. Teach the client that alcohol should be taken in moderation only if diabetes is well controlled.
6. Explain and reinforce how to read food labels.
7. Reinforce dietary teaching such as how to follow the exchange system for meal planning and how to perform carbohydrate counting.
8. Support and reinforce information provided by the dietitian regarding how to make adjustments in nutritional intake during illness, planned exercises, and social occasions.

Considerations for Older Adults

- A realistic approach to diet therapy is essential for older diabetic clients.
- Attempts to change long-time eating habits may be difficult.

- Clients who live alone, do their own food preparation, and have physical limitations may have difficulty following the diet recommended by the American Diabetes Association.
- Socioeconomic factors may also affect a client's ability to prepare the proper foods.

■ Regular physical exercise is a recommended component of a comprehensive diabetes treatment plan.
1. Collaborate with the client and rehabilitation specialist to develop an exercise program.
2. Instruct the client to have a complete physical examination before starting an exercise program at home.
3. Instruct the client to wear proper footwear with good traction and cushioning and to examine the feet after exercise.
4. Discourage exercise in extreme heat or cold or during periods of poor glucose control.
5. Advise the client to stay hydrated.
6. Clients with type 1 diabetes should perform vigorous exercise only if blood glucose levels are 80 to 250 mg/dL and no ketones are present in the urine.
7. Teach the client about the risks and complications related to exercise such as prolonged alterations in blood glucose levels, vitreous hemorrhage, or retinal detachment in clients with proliferative retinopathy, and increased proteinuria and foot and joint injury in clients with peripheral neuropathy.

SURGICAL MANAGEMENT

■ Whole pancreas transplantation can be performed in one of three ways: transplant of the pancreas transplantation alone (PTA) in the preuremic client, pancreas transplantation after successful kidney transplantation (PAK), and simultaneous pancreas-kidney transplantation (SPK).
1. Immunosuppressive therapy is given to prevent rejection of the transplanted pancreas.
2. Complications include venous thrombosis, rejection, and infection.
■ Islet cell transplantation has been limited by the technical inability to obtain a sufficient number of islet cells.

◆COLLABORATIVE PROBLEM:
Risk for Delayed Surgical Recovery

- Surgery is a physical and emotional stressor, making the diabetic client more at risk for intraoperative and post-operative complications.
- Provide preoperative care.
  1. Discontinue medications
     a. Chlorpropamide (Diabinese) 36 hours before surgery
     b. Metformin (Glucophage) 48 hours before surgery
     c. All other oral agents on the day of surgery
  2. Restart oral agents only after renal function has been reevaluated and found to be normal.
  3. Start intravenous fluids to maintain hydration when the client is admitted.
  4. Monitor blood glucose results and administer insulin as ordered.
- Intraoperative IV administration of short-acting insulin in 5% to 10% glucose is recommended for all insulin-treated clients and for drug-treated or diet-treated clients who are undergoing general anesthesia and whose diabetes is poorly controlled.
- Provide postoperative care.
  1. Monitor vital signs, especially temperature; hypothermia may cause high blood glucose levels.
  2. Monitor fluid and electrolyte balance; clients with azotemia may have problems with fluid management.
  3. Continue glucose and insulin infusions until the client is stable and able to tolerate oral feedings.
  4. May need to administer short-acting insulin until the client's usual medication regimen can be restarted.
  5. Provide pain management, ideally with patient-controlled analgesia (PCA) pump.
  6. Monitor for postoperative complications, including
     a. Hyperkalemia or hypokalemia
     b. Hypoglycemia (may be asymptomatic if the client's condition is well controlled on beta blockers)
     c. Impaired wound healing or wound infection
     d. Myocardial infarction
     e. Renal dysfunction
     f. Uncontrolled blood glucose

COLLABORATIVE PROBLEM:
Potential for Injury Related to Disturbed Sensory Perception

- Nonhealing foot wounds cause more inpatient hospital days than any other complication of diabetes.
- Loss of pain, pressure, and temperature sensation in the foot increases the risk for injury and ulceration.
- Foot deformities common in diabetic neuropathy may lead to callus formation, ulceration, and increased area of pressure.
- Foot care education includes
    1. Teaching preventive foot care to the client; sensory neuropathy, ischemia, and infection are the leading causes of foot disease.
    2. Recommending that the client have shoes fitted by an experienced shoe fitter such as a certified podiatrist and instructing the client to change shoes at midday and in the evening and to wear socks or stockings with shoes.
    3. Instructing the client on how to care for wounds.
- Refer the client to a specialist for orthotic devices to eliminate pressure on infected or open wounds of the foot.
- Topical application of platelet-derived growth factors may be used to accelerate tissue healing for long-standing foot ulcers.
- Wound care for diabetic ulcers includes a moist wound environment, debridement of necrotic tissue, and offloading or elimination of pressure.

COLLABORATIVE PROBLEM: Potential for Injury Related to Disturbed Sensory Perception (Visual)

- Encourage all clients to have a baseline ophthalmic examination and yearly follow-up examinations.
- Advise the client to seek a retinal specialist if problems are present.
- Collaborate with the rehabilitation specialist to recommend strategies to improve the client's visual abilities; strategies include improving lighting, placing dark equipment against a white background, coding objects such as insulin vials with bright colors or felt tip markers, and using large-type books and newspapers.
- Various stages of diabetic retinopathy can be treated with laser therapy or vitrectomy.

NDx: Chronic Pain

- Provide drug therapy as follows:
  1. Anticonvulsants for pain secondary to diabetic neuropathy
  2. Tricyclic antidepressants, particularly amitriptyline (Elavil, Levate), and nortriptyline (Pamelor) as ordered, to alleviate peripheral neuropathic pain
  3. Capsaicin cream 0.075% (e.g., Zostrix) topically to relieve neuropathic pain
- Use other nondrug pain management techniques as appropriate.

NDx: Ineffective Tissue Perfusion: Renal

- Interventions include
  1. Stressing the importance of maintaining a normal blood glucose level, maintaining a blood pressure level below 130/85 mm Hg, and being screened annually for microalbuminuria
  2. Limiting protein to 0.8 g/kg of body weight per day if the client has overt nephropathy
  3. Teaching the client about the signs and symptoms of urinary tract infection
  4. Adjustment by the health care provider of the insulin dosage for clients undergoing dialysis
  5. Advising the client not to take any over-the-counter medications without checking with the health care provider

COLLABORATIVE PROBLEM: Potential for Hypoglycemia

- Monitor glucose levels before administering hypoglycemic agents, before meals, at bedtime, and when the client is symptomatic.
- Treat the client with mild hypoglycemia (hungry, irritable, shaky, weak, headache, fully conscious, blood glucose less than 60 mg/dL [3.4 mmol/L]) who is able to swallow with one of the following:
  1. 2 to 3 glucose tablets
  2. 4 oz of fruit drink
  3. 4 oz of regular soft drink
  4. 8 oz of skim milk
  5. 6 saltines or 3 graham crackers
  6. 6 to 10 hard candies, 4 cubes of sugar, or 2 tsp of sugar

- Blood glucose level should be tested after 15 minutes.
- Treat the client with moderate hypoglycemia (cold and clammy skin, pale rapid pulse, rapid shallow respirations, marked changes in mood, drowsiness, blood glucose less than 40 mg/dL [2.2 mmol/L]) with 15 to 30 g of rapidly absorbed carbohydrates and additional food such as low-fat milk or cheese after 10 to 15 minutes.
- Treat the client with severe hypoglycemia (unable to swallow, unconscious or convulsing, blood glucose usually less than 20 mg/dL [1.0 mmol/L]) with glucagon subcutaneously or intramuscularly and 50% dextrose intravenously.
- Teach the client to prevent the four common causes of hypoglycemia: excess exercise, excess insulin, alcohol use, and deficient food intake.
- Encourage the client to wear an identification (medical alert) bracelet.

◀COLLABORATIVE PROBLEM:
Potential for Diabetic Ketoacidosis

- Interventions include
  1. Monitoring for signs and symptoms of diabetic ketoacidosis (DKA)
  2. Checking the client's blood pressure, pulse, and respirations every 15 minutes until stable
  3. Recording urine output, temperature, and mental status every hour
  4. Assessing the client's level of consciousness, hydration status, fluid and electrolyte balance, and blood glucose levels every hour until stable; once stable, assessing every 4 hours
  5. Giving insulin bolus as indicated, followed by a continuous drip
  6. Monitoring the client for hypokalemia (symptoms are muscle weakness, abdominal distention or paralytic ileus, hypotension, and weak pulse); before administration of potassium, ensuring that the client's urinary output is at least 30 mL/hour
  7. Replacing both fluid volume and ongoing losses; monitoring for congestive heart failure and pulmonary edema if large volume of IV fluid is administered

8. Instructing the client on how to prevent future episodes of DKA by contacting the primary health care provider when the blood glucose is greater than 250 mg/dL, when ketonuria is present for more than 24 hours, when unable to take food or fluids, and when illness persists for more than 1 to 2 days

◀COLLABORATIVE PROBLEM: Potential for Hyperglycemic Hyperosmolar Nonketotic Syndrome (HHNS)

- Administer IV fluids and insulin as indicated and monitor and assess the client's response to therapy.
- Assess for signs of cerebral edema and immediately report change in level of consciousness; change in pupil size, shape, or reaction to light; or seizure activity to the physician.

Community-Based Care

- Discharge planning includes
  1. Ensuring that the client understands the significance, symptoms, causes, and treatment of hypoglycemia and hyperglycemia
  2. In collaboration with the dietitian, teaching the client basic survival skills associated with medication, diet, exercise, and complications
  3. Assisting the client to identify the items needed for the administration of insulin and for glucose monitoring
  4. Providing information about community resources, for example, diabetic education programs
  5. Teaching the client how to monitor blood sugar level
  6. Teaching the client how to administer medication and prevent hypoglycemia
  7. Helping the client adapt to diabetes, including teaching stress management techniques and identifying coping mechanisms
  8. Referring the client to the American Diabetes Association and its resources
  9. Referring the client to a diabetic educator for the necessary education

Dislocation and Subluxation

- *Dislocation* of a joint occurs when the articulating surfaces are no longer in proximity; a *subluxation* is a partial dislocation. Both commonly occur in the shoulder, hip, knee, and finger.
- These injuries are most often caused by trauma but can be congenital or pathologic, resulting from joint disease such as rheumatoid arthritis.
- Pain, immobility, alteration in the contour of the joint, and rotation and deviation in the length of the extremity are typical manifestations.
- The treatment is a closed manipulation, or reduction, of the joint while the client is anesthetized.
- After reduction, the joint is immobilized by a cast or immobilizer until healing occurs.
- Clients with recurrent dislocations may require surgical intervention with internal fixation.

Dissection, Aortic

OVERVIEW

- Aortic dissection, traditionally referred to as a *dissecting aneurysm,* may be caused by a sudden tear in the aortic intima, opening the way for blood to enter the aortic wall.
- Degeneration of the aortic media and hypertension are contributing factors.
- Aortic dissection is frequently associated with aging and connective tissue disorders such as Marfan syndrome.
- The three types of aortic dissection are
  Type I: an intimal tear originating in the ascending (proximal) aorta, with extension into the descending (distal) aorta
  Type II: originating in and limited to the ascending aorta
  Type III: arising within the descending thoracic aorta and often progressing distally

Assessment

- Assessment findings include
  1. Pain that is described as "tearing" or "stabbing" and is located in the anterior chest, back, neck, throat, jaw, or teeth
  2. Diaphoresis
  3. Nausea and vomiting
  4. Faintness and apprehension
  5. Elevated blood pressure
  6. Decreased or absent peripheral pulses
  7. Musical murmur, heard best along the right sternal border
  8. Neurologic deficits, such as altered level of consciousness, paraparesis, or stroke

Interventions

- The goals of emergency treatment include the elimination of pain, the reduction of blood pressure, and a decrease in the velocity of left ventricular ejection.
- Drug therapy includes
  1. Continuous intravenous sodium nitroprusside (Nipride) to lower blood pressure; if this is ineffective, nicardipine hydrochloride (Cardene) may be used
  2. Intravenous push propranolol (Inderal, Apo-Propranolol) to decrease left ventricular ejection
- Subsequent treatment is based on the location of the dissection; surgical excision and graft replacement may be necessary.

Diverticula, Esophageal

- Diverticula are sacs resulting from the herniation of esophageal mucosa and submucosa into surrounding tissue.
- Clients with esophageal diverticula are at risk for esophageal perforation.

- The most common form of diverticulum is *Zenker's diverticulum,* which is usually located near the hypopharynx and occurs most often in older adults.

COLLABORATIVE MANAGEMENT

Assessment

- Assessment findings include
  1. Dysphagia
  2. Regurgitation
  3. Feelings of fullness or pressure
  4. Halitosis
  5. Nocturnal cough

Interventions

- Diet therapy and positioning are the primary interventions for controlling symptoms related to diverticula.
- Nursing interventions include
  1. Collaborating with the dietitian to determine the size and frequency of meals and the texture and consistency that can best be tolerated by the client
  2. Elevating the head of the bed for sleep
  3. Teaching the client to avoid the recumbent position and vigorous exercising for at least 2 hours after eating
  4. Teaching the client to avoid restrictive clothing and frequent stooping or bending
- Surgical management is aimed at excision of the diverticula.
- Postoperative care is as follows.
  1. Maintain the client on nothing by mouth (NPO) status for several days to promote healing.
  2. Do not irrigate the nasogastric tube used for decompression unless specifically ordered by the physician.
  3. Maintain hydration and nutrition status through intravenous fluids and tube feedings until oral intake is permitted.
  4. Manage the client's postoperative pain.
  5. Monitor for bleeding and perforation.
  6. Teach the client to observe for complications at home.
  7. Teach the client measures to take to prevent reflux (elevating head of bed, avoiding recumbent position).

Diverticular Disease

OVERVIEW

- Diverticular disease includes diverticulosis and diverticulitis.
  1. *Diverticulosis* is the presence of many abnormal pouchlike herniations in the wall of the intestine; these outpouchings, known as diverticula, are caused by significantly high pressures in the lumen of the intestines. They can occur in any part of the intestine but are most common in the sigmoid colon.
  2. *Diverticulitis*, or inflammation of one or more diverticula, results when the diverticulum retains undigested food, which compromises the blood supply to that area and facilitates bacterial invasion of the diverticular sac, which may then perforate. A perforated diverticulum can progress to intra-abdominal perforation with generalized peritonitis.

COLLABORATIVE MANAGEMENT

Assessment

- Clients with diverticulosis are usually asymptomatic.
- Assess for clinical manifestations of diverticulitis.
  1. Intermittent then steady left lower quadrant abdominal pain, which increases with coughing, straining, or lifting, and which may be intermittent
  2. Generalized abdominal pain (peritonitis)
  3. Temperature elevation with tachycardia
  4. Nausea and vomiting
  5. Abdominal distention and tenderness
  6. Palpable, tender abdominal or rectal mass
  7. Blood in the stool (microscopic to larger amounts)
  8. Elevated white blood cell (WBC) count
  9. Presence of diverticula on barium enema or upper gastrointestinal tract series (diverticulosis)
  10. Hypotension and dehydration occurs if massive bleeding occurs
  11. Signs of septic shock occur if peritonitis has occurred

Interventions

- Drug therapy
  1. Oral broad-spectrum antibiotics such as metronidazole (Flagyl) plus trimethoprim/sulfamethoxazole (Bactrim, Septra) or ciprofloxacin (Cipro)
  2. Intravenous antibiotics such as cefoxitin plus metronidazole for severe diverticulitis
  3. Anticholinergics to reduce intestinal hypermotility
  4. Pain medication with non-opioid drugs for mild cases and opioids such as meperidine hydrochloride (Demerol) or morphine sulfate for severe cases
- Laxatives are not given because they increase intestinal motility.
- Rest
  1. Recommend bedrest during the acute phase of the disease.
  2. Teach the client to refrain from lifting, straining, coughing, or bending to avoid increased intra-abdominal pressure.
- Diet therapy
  1. Provide clear liquids during the acute phase of the disease.
  2. Instruct the client that he or she will be restricted to nothing by mouth (NPO) status when experiencing severe symptoms and will receive intravenous fluids. A nasogastric tube is inserted for severe nausea, vomiting, or abdominal distention.
  3. Introduce a fiber-containing diet gradually when the inflammation is resolved.

SURGICAL MANAGEMENT

- Clients with diverticulitis need surgery if one of the following occurs.
  1. Rupture of the diverticulum with subsequent peritonitis
  2. Pelvic abscess
  3. Bowel obstruction
  4. Fistula
  5. Persistent fever or pain after 4 days of medical treatment
  6. Uncontrolled bleeding
- Surgical management includes a colon resection with an end-to-end anastomosis or temporary or permanent colostomy.

- Preoperative care includes
  1. Reinforcing physician teaching about the possible need for a temporary or permanent colostomy
  2. Teaching the importance of or provide bowel preparation consisting of enemas and laxatives (for the client who is *not* in the acute stage of diverticulitis)
  3. Administering intravenous fluids, antibiotics, and anti-inflammatory agents, if prescribed
  4. Maintaining NPO status with a nasogastric tube in place for clients having emergency surgery
- Postoperative care includes
  1. Maintaining drainage system at the abdominal incision site
  2. If a colostomy was created, monitoring colostomy stoma for color and integrity
  3. Maintaining the nasogastric tube for several days until peristalsis returns
  4. Introducing clear liquids slowly, and gradually advancing the diet as tolerated
  5. Providing the client with an opportunity to express feelings about the colostomy
  6. Providing additional postoperative care as described in Surgical Management under Cancer, Colorectal
  7. Providing written postoperative instructions on
     a. Inspection of the incision for redness, tenderness, swelling, and drainage
     b. Dressing change procedures, if necessary
     c. Avoidance of activities that increase intra-abdominal pressure, including straining at stool, bending, lifting heavy objects, and wearing restrictive clothing
     d. Pain management, including prescriptions
- Teach the client and family
  1. To follow dietary considerations for diverticulosis, which include
     a. Eating a diet high in cellulose and hemicellulose, which are found in wheat bran, whole grain breads, and cereals
     b. Eating fruits and vegetables with high-fiber content (unless *diverticulitis* occurs)
     c. If the recommended fiber requirements cannot be tolerated, taking a bulk-forming laxative to increase fecal size and consistency

    d. Encouraging fluids to prevent bloating that may accompany a high-fiber diet

    e. Avoiding foods that contain indigestible roughage or seeds

    f. Avoiding alcohol, which has an irritant effect on the bowel

    g. Not exceeding 30% of the total daily caloric intake in dietary fat

    h. Avoiding all fiber when the symptoms of diverticulitis are present

2. Signs and symptoms of diverticular disease, including fever, abdominal pain, and bloody stools

3. To avoid enemas and laxatives other than bulk-forming laxatives such as psyllium hydrophilic mucilloid (Metamucil)

Dysrhythmias, Cardiac

OVERVIEW

- Cardiac dysrhythmias are abnormal rhythms of the heart's electrical system, caused by disturbances of cardiac electrical impulse formation, conduction, or both.
- Many diseases (congenital heart disease, myocardial infarction), electrolyte imbalance, changes in oxygenation and drug toxicity can cause dysrhythmias.
- *Tachydysrhythmias* are heart rates greater than 100 beats/min.
  1. Signs and symptoms include palpitations, chest discomfort; pressure or pain from myocardial ischemia or infarction; restlessness; anxiety; pale, cool skin; and syncope from hypotension.
  2. They may cause heart failure as indicated by dyspnea, orthopnea, pulmonary crackles, distended neck veins, fatigue, and weakness.
- *Bradydysrhythmias* are characterized by a heart rate less than 60 beats/min.
  1. The client may tolerate a low heart rate if blood pressure is adequate.

2. Symptomatic bradydysrhythmias lead to myocardial ischemia or infarction, dysrhythmias, hypotension, and heart failure.

- *Premature complexes* are early complexes that occur when a cardiac cell or group of cells other than the sinoatrial (SA) node becomes irritable and fires an impulse before the next sinus impulse is generated.

    1. Bigeminy: when normal complexes and premature complexes occur alternately in a repetitive two-beat pattern, with a pause occurring after each premature complex so that complexes occur in pairs
    2. Trigeminy: a repetitive three-beat pattern, usually occurring as two sequential normal complexes followed by a premature complex and a pause, with the same pattern repeating itself in triplets
    3. Quadrigeminy: a repetitive four-beat pattern, usually occurring as three sequential normal complexes followed by a premature complex and a pause, with the same pattern repeating itself in a four-beat pattern

- Escape complexes and rhythms may occur when the SA node fails to discharge or is blocked or when a sinus impulse fails to depolarize the ventricles. The client may feel lightheaded, dizzy, or faint during the pause.
- Dysrhythmias are classified according to their site of origin.
- Sinus dysrhythmias include

    1. Sinus tachycardia occurs when the SA node discharge exceeds 100 beats/min. Treatment is based on identifying the underlying cause (e.g., angina, fever, hypovolemia, pain); beta-adrenergic blocking agents may be prescribed.
    2. *Sinus bradycardia,* a decreased rate of SA node discharge of less than 60 beats/min. If the client is symptomatic, treatment includes atropine, a pacemaker, and avoidance of parasympathetic stimulations such as prolonged suctioning.

- Atrial dysrhythmias include

    1. Premature atrial complex (PAC), which occurs when atrial tissue becomes irritable. This ectopic focus fires an impulse before the next sinus impulse is due, thus usurping the sinus pacemaker.
        a. No intervention is generally needed except to treat the cause, such as heart failure or valvular disease.

    b. Medications such as type 1A antidysrhythmics or other drugs may be prescribed.

  2. Supraventricular tachycardia (SVT), which involves the rapid stimulation of atrial tissue at a rate of 100 to 280 beats/min with a mean of 170 beats/min

    a. No intervention is generally needed except to treat the cause.

    b. Sustained SVT may need to be treated with radio-frequency catheter ablation.

    c. Oxygen therapy, antidysrhythmic drugs, or synchronized cardioversion may also be needed.

  3. *Atrial flutter,* a rapid arterial depolarization occurring at a rate of 250 to 350 times/min

    a. Drug treatment includes ibutilide (Covert), amiodarone (Cordarone), and diltiazem (Cardizem).

    b. Synchronized cardioversion is done if the client is hemodynamically compromised.

    c. Rapid atrial overdrive pacing or radiofrequency catheter ablation may be needed if none of the mentioned treatments are successful.

  4. Atrial fibrillation (AF), which consists of rapid impulses from many atrial foci at a rate of 350 to 600 times/min

    a. Treatment is the same as for atrial flutter.

    b. Anticoagulants may be given to clients considered to be at high risk for emboli.

- *Junctional dysrhythmias* may occur when the nodal cells in the atrioventricular (AV) junctional area generate an impulse when the SA node is excessively slow or may occur as irritable rhythms.

- Ventricular dysrhythmias include

  1. Idioventricular rhythm (ventricular escape rhythm), which occurs when the ventricular nodal cells pace the ventricles

    a. This rhythm is characterized by hypotension, shock, cardiac arrest, and no palpable pulses.

    b. Immediate resuscitation measures are required.

  2. *Premature ventricular complexes (PVCs),* which result from increased irritability of the ventricular cells. PVCs are early ventricular complexes followed by a pause and often occur in repetitive rhythms.

a. The client may be asymptomatic or may experience palpitations, chest discomfort, or diminished or absent peripheral pulses.

b. If there is no underlying heart disease, PVCs are not treated other than by eliminating any contributing cause.

c. Significant myocardial ischemia or infarction: significant PVCs are treated with oxygen and amiodarone (Cordarone); other drugs are prescribed if an MI occurs.

3. *Ventricular tachycardia (VT)*, or "V tach," which occurs with repetitive firing of an irritable ventricular ectopic focus, usually at a rate of 140 to 180 beats/min

a. Symptoms depend on ventricular rate; the client may be hemodynamically compromised and in cardiac arrest.

b. Sustained VT is treated with oxygen, amiodarone, lidocaine; or magnesium sulfate.

c. Unstable VT is treated with emergency cardioversion followed by oxygen and antidysrhythmic therapy.

d. With pulseless VT, immediately begin cardiopulmonary resuscitation (CPR) and defibrillate as soon as possible. If the client remains pulseless, continue CPR and other resuscitative measures.

e. Once the client has been successfully converted, attention is given to treating the reversible causes of VT.

4. Ventricular fibrillation (VF), sometimes called "V-fib," which is the result of electrical chaos in the ventricles

a. The client feels faint, immediately loses consciousness, and becomes pulseless and apneic, with seizure activity and absent blood pressure. Within minutes, the pupils are fixed and dilated and death occurs unless there is prompt restoration of an organized rhythm.

b. Immediate defibrillation is performed and Advanced Cardiac Life Support (ACLS) algorithm is followed.

5. Ventricular asystole, the complete absence of any ventricular rhythm. The client is in full cardiac arrest and is treated with CPR and by following the ACLS algorithm.

■ *Atrioventricular (AV) conduction blocks* exist when supraventricular impulses are excessively delayed or totally blocked in the AV node or intraventricular conduction system.

1. First-degree AV block: All sinus impulses eventually reach the ventricles; conduction is slowed.
   a. The client generally has no symptoms and no treatment is needed.
   b. If due to drug therapy, the offending drug is withheld and the health care provider notified.
   c. If associated with symptomatic bradycardia, oxygen is administered.
2. Second-degree AV block type I (AV Wenckebach or Mobitz type I): Each successive sinus impulse takes a little longer to conduct through the AV node, until one impulse is completely blocked and fails to depolarize the ventricles. The symptomatic client is treated with oxygen and atropine; a pacemaker may be needed.
3. Second-degree AV block type II (Mobitz type II): The block is actually infranodal, occurring below the His bundle, and involves a constant block in one of the bundle branches; impulse fails to reach ventricle.
   a. Symptoms depend on the frequency of the dropped rate.
   b. If client is symptomatic, he or she is treated with prophylactic pacing to avert the threat of sudden third-degree heart block.
   c. A permanent pacemaker may be required.
4. Third-degree heart block (complete heart block): None of the sinus impulses conducts to the ventricles.
   a. Clinical manifestations depend on the overall ventricular rate and cardiac output and may have hemodynamic consequences such as light-headedness, confusion, syncope, seizures, hypotension, or cardiac arrest.
   b. Oxygen and atropine are given to the client who is symptomatic; prophylactic pacing may be initiated.
5. Bundle branch block: A conduction delay or block occurs within one of the two main bundle branches below the bifurcation of the His bundle.
   a. There are no clinical manifestations and no specific interventions.
   b. Provide the client with sufficient rest and ensure adequate ventilation and oxygenation.

COLLABORATIVE MANAGEMENT

◄NDx: Decreased Cardiac Output and Ineffective Tissue Perfusion

Interventions

■ The major interventions are to assess for complications and monitor the client for response to treatment.

1. Monitor the client's electrocardiograph and assess for signs and symptoms of dysrhythmias.
2. Assess apical and radial pulses for a full minute for any irregularity.
3. Management includes
   a. Drug therapy
   b. Vagal maneuvers such as carotid sinus massage and Valsalva maneuvers
   c. Cardioversion
   d. Temporary or permanent pacing
   e. CPR or ACLS
   f. Defibrillation
   g. Radiofrequency catheter ablation
   h. Aneurysmectomy
   i. Coronary artery bypass grafting
   j. Insertion of an implantable cardioverter/defibrillator (ICD)

Community-Based Care

■ A case manager or care coordinator identifies the need for health care resources needed at home and coordinates access to the services.
■ Discharge planning and health care resources
   1. Provide information on lifestyle modifications including activity restrictions.
   2. Teach the client and family the name, dosage, schedule, and side effects of medications.
   3. Teach and observe the client and family taking a pulse.
   4. Stress the importance of reporting chest discomfort, shortness of breath, and change in heart rhythm and rate to the health care provider.
   5. Encourage the client to follow diet instructions and post emergency telephone numbers.

6. Instruct the client to keep all appointments with their health care provider.
7. Encourage family members to learn CPR.
8. Refer to American Heart Association or the provincial affiliate of the Heart and Stroke Foundation in Canada and other community agencies.

■ Give the following special instructions to a client with a pacemaker/ICD device:
1. Give instructions on how to care for the pacemaker and/or ICD and how it functions (if appropriate), and the importance of reporting any fever or any redness, swelling, or drainage at the pacemaker/ICD insertion site.
2. Keep your ICD identification card in your wallet and consider wearing a medical alert bracelet.
3. Do not wear tight clothing or belts that could cause irritation over the site.
4. Keep handheld cellular phones at least 6 inches away from the generator, with the handset on the ear opposite the side of the generator.
5. Avoid sources of strong electromagnet fields such as large electrical generators and radio or television transmitters and radar.
6. If you feel symptoms when you are near any device, move 5 to 10 feet away from it and check your pulse.
7. Notify all health care providers, including your dentist, that you have a pacemaker/ICD device.
8. Notify airport security personnel before passing through a metal detector (screening device) that you have an pacemaker/ICD and show them your identification card.
9. Magnetic resonance imagining is contraindicated.

■ Give the following special instructions to a client with a pacemaker:
1. Take your pulse for 1 minute at the same time each day and record the rate in your pacemaker diary.
2. Take your pulse any time you feel symptoms of possible pacemaker failure and report your heart rate and symptoms to your health care provider.
3. Know the rate at which your pacemaker is set and know the rate changes to report to your physician.
4. Know the indications of battery failure and report these findings to your health care provider.

5. Check your pulse and report any of the following symptoms to your health care provider: difficulty breathing, dizziness, fainting, chest pain, weight gain, and prolonged hiccupping.

6. Do not operate electrical appliances directly over your pacemaker site because they may cause it to malfunction. Be sure electrical appliances are properly grounded.

7. Do not lean over electrical or gasoline engines or motors.

- Give the following special instructions to a client with an ICD.
  1. Sit or lie down immediately if you feel dizzy, faint, or light-headed.
  2. Avoid activities that involve rough contact with the ICD implantation site.
  3. Avoid sources of strong electromagnet fields such as large electrical generators and radio or television transmitters because they may inhibit tachydysrhythmia detection and therapy or may cause inadvertent antitachycardial pacing or shocks. If beeping tones are heard coming from the device, move away from the electromagnetic field immediately before the inactivation sequence is completed and notify the health care provider.
  4. Report symptoms such as fainting, nausea, weakness, blackout, and rapid pulse to your health care provider.
  5. Know how to perform cough CPR as instructed.
  6. Notify your health care provider if your ICD device discharges.
  7. Avoid strenuous activities that may cause your heart rate to meet or exceed the rate cutoff of your ICD device because this causes the device to discharge inappropriately.

Dystrophy, Muscular

- Five types of muscular dystrophy are seen in adults.
  1. Duchenne
     a. Sex-linked recessive variety exclusive to males
     b. Manifested by symmetric pelvic and shoulder girdle weakness, waddling gait, cardiac involvement, and possible mental retardation

    c. Death from respiratory or cardiac failure usually occurring between ages 10 and 30

2. Becker

    a. Sex-linked recessive variety exclusive to males

    b. Manifested by wasting of pelvic and shoulder muscles and normal cardiac and mental function; slowly progressive; inability to walk seen 25 years after onset

    c. Normal life span

3. Limb-girdle

    a. Usually autosomal dominant and found in either sex

    b. Manifested by upper extremity and neck muscle weakness and lower extremity and hip muscle weakness; severe disability within 10 to 20 years

    c. Life span shortened by 10 to 20 years

4. Facioscapulohumeral or Landouzy-Dejerine

    a. Autosomal dominant and found in either sex

    b. Manifested by facial and shoulder girdle muscle involvement

    c. Normal life span

5. Myotonic

    a. Autosomal dominant and found in either sex

    b. Manifested by muscle atrophy with multiple organ involvement (heart, lungs, smooth muscles, and endocrine system)

    c. Gradual progression if onset in adulthood

- Management and nursing care is supportive (see also Rehabilitation in Part I).
- An experimental treatment called myoblast transfer therapy (MTT) is supported by the Food and Drug Administration. It involves injections of healthy muscle cells (myoblasts) taken from a donor and multiplied in a laboratory. The cells are then given to the client with MD where, theoretically, they fuse with each other and the recipient's unhealthy muscle cells.

Ectasia, Ductal

- Ductal ectasia is a benign breast problem in women approaching mensopause, caused by dilation and thickening of collecting ducts in the subareolar area.
- The ducts become distended and filled with cellular debris, which initiates an inflammatory response.
- Clinical signs are a hard, tender mass with irregular borders; greenish-brown nipple discharge; enlarged axillary nodes; redness; and edema over the mass.
- Microscopic examination of nipple discharge is performed for atypical or malignant cells.
- The affected area may be excised.
- Interventions include alleviating anxiety associated with the threat of breast cancer and supporting the client during diagnostic and treatment procedures.

Embolism, Pulmonary

OVERVIEW

- Pulmonary embolism (PE) is a collection of particulate matter (solids, liquids, or gaseous substances) that enters venous circulation and lodges in the pulmonary artery.
- Physiologic responses include platelet accumulation, triggering the release of potent vasoconstrictors and causing widespread pulmonary vasoconstriction, which impairs ventilation and perfusion.
- Clients susceptible to pulmonary embolism are those with risk factors for deep venous thrombosis (DVT), including prolonged immobilization, central venous catheters, surgery, obesity, pregnancy, estrogen therapy, heart failure, advanced age, and a history of thromboembolism.

COLLABORATIVE MANAGEMENT

Assessment

- Assessment findings include
  1. Sudden onset of dyspnea
  2. Pleuritic chest pain
  3. Apprehension, restlessness
  4. Feeling of impending doom
  5. Dry cough
  6. Hemoptysis
  7. Tachypnea
  8. Crackles
  9. Tachycardia
  10. Pleural friction rub
  11. Low-grade fever
  12. Distended neck veins
  13. Cyanosis
  14. S_3 or S_4 heart sound
  15. Low arterial carbon dioxide partial pressure (PCO_2) value
  16. Syncope
  17. Petechiae over chest and axillae
  18. Diaphoresis

Interventions

- Interventions include the following:
  1. Administer oxygen via nasal cannula or mask. Intubation and mechanical ventilation are used in cases of severe hypoxemia.
  2. Check vital signs, pulse oximetry, lung sounds, and cardiac and respiratory status every hour.
  3. Document increasing dysrhythmias, distended neck veins, and pedal or sacral edema.
  4. Give anticoagulation or fibrinolytic therapy.
     a. Give intravenous heparin (bolus followed by continuous infusion) during the acute phase; give warfarin (Coumadin) orally when the heparin drip is discontinued.
     b. Thrombolytics may be used to break up an existing clot if the PE is massive or the client is hemodynamically unstable. Monitor for an allergic response or anaphylaxis if urokinase is administered.

    c. Monitor partial thromboplastin time before therapy is started, every 4 hours when therapy begins, and then daily.

    d. Frequently assess the client for bleeding and protect from situations that could lead to bleeding.

5. Surgical interventions include embolectomy and/or the insertion of an inferior vena caval filter.

6. Prevent decreased cardiac output.

    a. Intravenous fluids restore plasma volume and prevent shock.

    b. Positive inotropic agents are used to improve cardiac output.

    c. Vasodilators decrease pulmonary pressure if it is impeding cardiac contractility.

7. Monitor laboratory values daily.

8. Acknowledge the client's anxiety and speak calmly and clearly.

9. Assure the client that appropriate measures are being taken.

10. Conduct discharge planning.

    a. Teach the client and family about bleeding precautions, activities to reduce the risk for DVT and recurrence of PE, signs and symptoms of complications, medications, and the importance of follow-up care.

    b. Refer to home care or anticoagulant clinic for follow up of anticoagulant treatment.

Empyema, Pulmonary

OVERVIEW

- Pulmonary empyema is a collection of pus in the pleural space; the fluid is thick, opaque, and foul smelling.
- The most common cause is pulmonary infection, infected pleural effusion, or lung abscess, which spreads across the pleura or obstructs lymph nodes and causes a retrograde flood of infected lymph into the pleural space.

COLLABORATIVE MANAGEMENT

- Client history includes recent febrile illnesses (including pneumonia), chest pain, dyspnea, cough, and trauma.
- Physical assessment includes diminished chest wall movement, decreased breath sounds, decreased or absent fremitus, a flat percussion note, abnormal breath sounds, fever, chills, weight loss, and night sweats.
- Chest x-ray examination and examination of the pleural fluid by thoracentesis are usually performed to help make the diagnosis.
- Therapy is based on emptying the empyema cavity, re-expanding the lung, and controlling the infection.
- Chest tubes are placed in the lower parts of the empyema sac to promote drainage and lung expansion, and antibiotics are given.
- An open thoracotomy and removal of portion of the pleura may be needed for thick pus and marked pleural thickening.

Encephalitis

- Encephalitis, an inflammation of the brain parenchyma (brain tissue) and often the meninges, is most often caused by viral agents such as
  1. Arboviruses transmitted through the bite of an infected tick or mosquito
  2. Enteroviruses associated with mumps and chickenpox
  3. Herpes simplex virus type I, which is the most common nonepidemic type
- Amebas such as *Naegleria* and *Acanthamoeba*, found in warm freshwater, may also be involved.

COLLABORATIVE MANAGEMENT

Assessment

- Assessment findings include
  1. Fever
  2. Nausea and vomiting

3. Stiff neck
4. Change in level of consciousness and mental status
5. Motor dysfunction
6. Focal neurologic deficits
7. Symptoms of increased intracranial pressure
8. Ocular palsies
9. Facial weakness
10. Abnormal cerebrospinal fluid analysis
11. Elevated white blood cell (WBC) count

Interventions

- The treatment for encephalitis is similar to that for meningitis.
    1. Maintain a patent airway to prevent development of pneumonia and atelectasis.
    2. Encourage and assist the client to turn, cough, and deep breathe every 2 hours; suction if respiratory status is compromised.
    3. Monitor vital signs and neurologic signs.
    4. Elevate the head of the bed 30 to 45 degrees.
    5. Administer acyclovir (Zovirax) for herpes encephalitis; no specific drug therapy is available for infection by arboviruses or enteroviruses.
- If there are permanent neurologic disabilities, the client is discharged to a rehabilitation setting or a long-term care facility.

Endocarditis, Infective

OVERVIEW

- Infective endocarditis (previously called bacterial endocarditis) refers to a microbial infection (virus, bacteria, fungi) involving the endocardium.
- Infective endocarditis occurs primarily in clients who are intravenous (IV) drug abusers, have had cardiac valve replacements, have experienced systemic infection, or have structural cardia defects.
- Portals of entry for infecting organisms include
    1. Oral cavity, especially if dental procedures have been performed

2. Skin rashes, lesions, or abscesses
3. Infections (cutaneous, genitourinary or gastrointestinal, systemic)
4. Surgical or invasive procedures, including IV line placement

COLLABORATIVE MANAGEMENT

Assessment

- Assessment findings include
  1. Signs of infection, including high fever, chills, malaise, night sweats, and fatigue
     a. Older adults may remain afebrile.
  2. Heart murmurs, usually regurgitant in nature
  3. Right-sided heart failure, evidenced by
     a. Peripheral edema
     b. Weight gain
     c. Anorexia
  4. Left-sided heart failure, evidenced by
     a. Fatigue
     b. Shortness of breath
     c. Crackles
  5. Evidence of arterial embolization in the form of fragments of vegetation, which may travel to the spleen, kidneys, gastrointestinal tract, brain, pulmonary circulation, or extremities
  6. Manifestations of embolic complications include
     a. Splenic infarction: sudden abdominal pain and radiation to the left shoulder
     b. Renal infarction: flank pain that radiates to the groin and is accompanied by hematuria or pyuria
     c. Mesenteric emboli: diffuse abdominal pain, often after eating and abdominal distention
     d. Brain emboli: confusion, reduced concentration and aphasia or dysphagia
     e. Pulmonary infarction: pleuritic chest pain, dyspnea, and cough
  7. Petechiae of the neck, shoulders, wrists, ankles, mucous membranes, or conjunctivae
  8. Splinter hemorrhages, or black longitudinal lines or small red streaks in the nail bed

9. Osler's nodes (reddish tender lesions with a white center on the pads of the fingers, hands, and toes)
10. Janeway's lesion (nontender hemorrhagic lesion found on the fingers, toes, nose, and earlobes)
11. Positive blood culture
12. Low hemoglobin level and hematocrit
13. Abnormal transesophageal echocardiography

Interventions

- Interventions include
  1. Administering IV antimicrobial therapy
  2. Monitoring the client's tolerance to activity
  3. Consistently using aseptic techniques to protect the client from contact with potentially infective organisms
  4. Monitoring for signs of embolization, including rapid pulse, dyspnea, new heart murmurs, and signs of heart failure
- Surgical intervention includes removal of the infected valve, repair or removal of congenital shunts, repair of injured valves and chordae tendineae, and draining abscesses in the heart or elsewhere.
- Preoperative and postoperative care for the client having surgery involving the valves is similar to that described for clients undergoing a coronary artery bypass grafting or valve replacement.

Community-Based Care

- Teach the client and family
  1. Information on the cause of the disease and its course, medication regimens, signs and symptoms of infection, and practices to prevent future infections
  2. How to administer IV antibiotic and care for the IV site; ensure that all supplies are available to the client discharged to home
  3. The importance of good personal and oral hygiene such as using a soft toothbrush, brushing the teeth twice a day, and rinsing the mouth with water after brushing
  4. To avoid the use of irrigation devices and dental floss
  5. The need to inform health care providers and dentists of the history of endocarditis so that prophylactic antibiotics are given before treatment

Endometriosis

OVERVIEW

- Endometriosis is a benign problem of endometrial tissue implantation outside the uterine cavity typically appearing on the ovaries and the cul-de-sac and less commonly on other pelvic organs and structures.
- The tissue responds to hormonal stimulation and goes through the same cyclic changes.
- Bleeding occurs at the site of implantation, and the blood is trapped in the tissues, causing scarring and adhesions.

COLLABORATIVE MANAGEMENT

Assessment

- Record client information
    1. Menstrual history
    2. Sexual history
    3. Characteristics of bleeding
    4. Lower abdominal pain occurring before the menstrual flow (the most common symptom)
    5. Rectal pressure
    6. Dyspareunia (painful intercourse)
    7. Painful defecation
    8. Sacral backache
    9. Hypermenorrhea
    10. Infertility

Interventions

- Drug therapy includes
    1. Mild analgesics or nonsteroidal anti-inflammatory drugs (NSAIDs) for pain relief
    2. Hormonal therapy
        a. Pseudopregnancy induced with oral contraceptives and progesterone ingestion
        b. Pseudomenopause or ovarian suppression induced by using danazol (Danocrine, Cyclomen), an anti-gonadotropin testosterone derivative

    c. Gonadotropin-releasing hormone (GnRH) agonists to produce a reversible medical oophorectomy
- Other therapy includes
  1. Applying a heating pad to the abdomen or sacrum
  2. Teaching relaxation techniques, yoga, or biofeedback
- Surgical management by removing endometrial implants and adhesions with carbon dioxide laser or hysterectomy may be required.

Epididymitis

- Epididymitis is an inflammation of the epididymis, which may result from an infection or noninfectious source such as trauma.
- Bacterial infection is the most common cause
- It may be a complication of a sexually transmitted disease.
- Less frequently, it may be a complication of long-term indwelling catheters, prostatic surgery, and, occasionally, cystoscopic examination.
- *Chlamydia trachomatis* is the major cause of epididymitis in men under 35 years of age.

COLLABORATIVE MANAGEMENT

- Assessment findings include
  1. Pain along the inguinal canal and the vas deferens, leading to pain and swelling in the scrotum and groin.
  2. Epididymis is swollen and painful
  3. Pyuria
  4. Bacteriuria
  5. Fever and chills
- Treatment interventions include
  1. Bedrest with scrotal elevation
  2. Wearing a scrotal support when ambulating
  3. Antibiotics
  4. Sexual partner treatment if chlamydial or gonorrheal in origin

5. Comfort measures, including ice packs, sitz baths, and analgesics
   6. Advising the client to avoid lifting, straining, or sexual activity until the infection is under control
- An orchiectomy may be required if an abscess forms.
- Epididymectomy (removal of epididymis from testicle) may be done if condition is recurrent or chronically painful.

Erectile Dysfunction

- Erectile dysfunction (ED) is the inability to achieve or maintain an erection firm enough for sexual intercourse.
- *Organic* ED is characterized by a gradual deterioration of function. The man first notices diminishing firmness and a decrease in frequency of erections. Causes include
   1. Inflammation of the prostate, urethra, or seminal vesicles
   2. Surgical procedures including prostatectomy
   3. Lumbosacral injuries
   4. Vascular disease, including hypertension
   5. Chronic neurologic conditions, such as Parkinson disease or multiple sclerosis
   6. Endocrine disorders, such as diabetes mellitus or thyroid disorders
   7. Smoking or alcohol consumption
   8. Medications such as antihypertensives and psychotropic agents may cause ED.
   9. Poor overall health that prevents sexual intercourse
- If the client has episodes of ED, it usually has a *functional* (psychologic) cause. The client has normal nocturnal and morning erections. Symptoms appear suddenly and are preceded by a period of high stress.

COLLABORATIVE MANAGEMENT

- Assess sexual, medical, and social history; determine if there is a medical cause.
- Nonsurgical management includes
   1. Psychosocial intervention

2. Change or adjustment in medication
3. Control of underlying disease
4. Mechanical devices or pharmacologic injection to increase blood flow to the penis
5. Viagra, a drug that increases blood flow; Viagra should not be given to clients with cardiac disease, especially those clients taking nitrates

Fatigue Syndrome, Chronic (CFS)

- Also know as chronic fatigue and immune dysfunction syndrome (CFIDS), manifested by severe fatigue for 6 months or longer, usually following flu-like symptoms.
- Four or more of the following criteria must be met:
  1. Sore throat
  2. Substantial impairment in short-term memory or concentration
  3. Tender lymph nodes
  4. Muscle pain
  5. Multiple joint pain with redness or swelling
  6. Headaches of a new type, patter, or severity
  7. Unrefreshing sleep
  8. Post-exertional malaise lasting more than 24 hours
- Treatment
  1. Supportive, focusing on alleviation or reduction of symptoms
  2. Drug therapy, including nonsteroidal anti-inflammatory drugs or low-dose antidepressants
  3. Teaching the client to follow good health practices such as obtaining adequate sleep, proper nutrition, regular exercise, stress management, and energy conservation
  4. Complementary and alternative therapies such as acupuncture, tai chi, massage, and herbal supplements
- Refer the client to the National Chronic Fatigue Syndrome and Fibromyalgia Association, American Association for Chronic Fatigue Syndrome, and the Chronic Fatigue and Immune Dysfunction Syndrome Association of America.

Fibroadenoma, Breast

- Breast fibroadenoma is the most common breast lump that occurs during the teenage years, although it may occur into the 30s.
- A fibroadenoma is a solid, benign mass of connective tissue unattached to the surrounding breast tissue.
- The lump is characteristically firm, hard but not cystic, easily movable, and clearly delineated from surrounding tissue; it is usually located in the upper outer quadrant of the breast.
- A needle aspiration is performed to establish whether the lump is cystic or solid.
- Solid lumps are usually excised on an outpatient basis by local anesthesia.

Fibroma, Ovarian

- Ovarian fibromas are the most common benign, solid ovarian neoplasms.
- Fibromas appear as pearly white tumors of connective tissue origin with low malignancy potential.
- Fibromas range from small nodules to masses weighing more than 50 pounds; the average size is 6 cm.
- Fibromas tend to have a unilateral occurrence and on examination have a slightly irregular contour and are mobile.
- Fibromas larger than 6 cm may be associated with ascites and may cause feelings of pelvic pressure or abdominal enlargement.
- Fibromas often occur after menopause.
- Management is surgical removal of the tumor. Oophorectomy (removal of an ovary) may be performed; if both ovaries are removed, instruct the client to expect decreased vaginal lubrication, hot flashes, and atrophy of the vaginal epithelium, which may be treated with estrogen therapy.

Fibromyalgia Syndrome

- Fibromyalgia is manifested by pain and tenderness at specific sites in the back of the neck, upper chest, trunk, low back, and extremities.
- The tender points (trigger points) can be palpated to elicit pain in a predictable, reproducible pattern.
- Other symptoms include
  1. Mild to severe fatigue
  2. Sleep disturbances
  3. Numbness or tingling in the extremities
  4. Sensitivity to noxious odors, loud noises and bright lights
  5. Headache and jaw pain
  6. Gastrointestinal: abdominal pain, diarrhea, constipation, heartburn
  7. Genitourinary: dysuria, urinary frequency, urgency, and pelvic pain
  8. Cardiovascular: dyspnea, chest pain, dysrhythmias
  9. Visual: blurred vision, dry eyes
- Interventions include
  1. Antidepressive agents to promote sleep and reduce pain or muscle spasms
  2. Selective serotonin reuptake inhibitors for depression
  3. Nonsteroidal anti-inflammatory drugs
  4. Physical therapy
  5. Regular exercise, which includes stretching, strengthening, and low impact aerobic exercise
  6. Complementary and alternative therapies such as tai chi, acupuncture, hypnosis, and stress management
- Refer to the National Chronic Fatigue Syndrome and Fibromyalgia Association for additional information.

Fissure, Anal

- An anal fissure is a superficial erosion of the anal canal.
- *Acute* anal fissures are superficial and heal spontaneously with conservative treatment.
- *Chronic* fissures recur and often warrant surgery.
- Pain during and after defecation is the most common symptom, but bleeding may also occur.
- Other symptoms associated with chronic fissures are pruritus, urinary frequency or retention, dysuria, and dyspareunia.
- Diagnosis is made by physical examination.
- Nonsurgical interventions include local, symptomatic relief measures such as warm sitz baths, analgesics, and bulk-forming agents.
- Topical anti-inflammatories or opiate suppositories are helpful if spasms are severe.
- Surgical excision of the fissure may be necessary if the fissures do not respond to medical management.

Fistula, Anal

- An anal fistula, or *fistula in ano,* is an abnormal tract leading from the anal canal to the perianal skin.
- Most anal fistulas result from anorectal abscesses, but they can be associated with tuberculosis, Crohn's disease, or cancer.
- Symptoms include pruritus, purulent discharge, and tenderness or pain aggravated by bowel movements.
- Because fistulas do not heal spontaneously, surgery (fistulotomy) is necessary.
- Pain relief measures, such as sitz baths, analgesics, and stool softeners, are used to reduce tissue trauma and discomfort.

Flail Chest

OVERVIEW

- Flail chest (paradoxical respiration) is the inward movement of the thorax during inspiration with outward movement during expiration, usually involving one side of the chest.
- Blunt chest trauma results in hemothorax and rib fractures, causing a loose segment of the chest wall to become paradoxical to the expansion and contraction of the rest of the chest wall.
- Gas exchange, the ability to cough, and secretion removal are impaired.

COLLABORATIVE MANAGEMENT

- The client is assessed for paradoxical chest movement, dyspnea, cyanosis, tachycardia, hypotension, pain, and anxiety.
- Interventions include
  1. Humidified oxygen
  2. Pain management
  3. Promotion of lung expansions through deep breathing and positioning
  4. Coughing and tracheal aspiration
  5. Psychosocial support
  6. Intubation with mechanical ventilation with positive end-expiratory pressure (PEEP) for severe flail chest associated with respiratory failure and shock
- Monitor the client's
  1. Arterial blood gases
  2. Vital capacity
  3. Vital signs
  4. Fluid and electrolyte balance
  5. Central venous pressure

Food Poisoning

- Food poisoning is caused by ingestion of infectious organisms in food.
- There are three common types of food poisoning.
  1. Staphylococcal food poisoning
     a. *Staphylococcus* grows in meats and dairy products and can be transmitted by human carriers.
     b. Symptoms of staphylococcal infection include abrupt onset of vomiting, diarrhea, and abdominal cramping, usually 2 to 4 hours after the ingestion of contaminated food.
     c. The diagnosis is made when stool culture yields 100,000 enterotoxin-producing staphylococci.
     d. Treatment includes oral or intravenous (IV) fluids if fluid volume is grossly depleted.
  2. *Escherichia coli* infection
     a. Increasingly, *E. coli* is associated with food poisoning.
     b. Symptoms include vomiting, diarrhea, abdominal cramping, and fever.
     c. Treatment includes intravenous (IV) fluids and antibiotic therapy.
  3. Botulism
     a. Botulism is a severe, life-threatening food poisoning associated with a high mortality rate; it is most commonly acquired from improperly processed canned foods.
     b. The incubation period is 18 to 36 hours and the illness may be mild or severe.
     c. *Clostridium botulinum* enters the bloodstream from the intestines and causes symptoms of diplopia, dysphagia, dysphonia, respiratory muscle paralysis, nausea, vomiting, and diarrhea or constipation.
     d. The diagnosis is made by history and stool culture revealing *C. botulinum;* the serum may be positive for toxins.
     e. Treatment of botulism includes trivalent botulism antitoxin (ABE), stomach lavage, IV fluids, and

tracheostomy with mechanical ventilation if respiratory paralysis occurs.

    f. To prevent botulism, discard cans of food that are punctured, swollen, or have defective seals.

- *Salmonellosis* is a bacterial infection that is classified as either a food poisoning or gastroenteritis.
  1. Incubation is 8 to 48 hours after ingestion of contaminated food or drink.
  2. Fever, nausea, vomiting, cramping abdominal pain, and severe diarrhea, which may be bloody, last 3 to 5 days.
  3. Diagnosis is made by stool culture.
  4. Treatment is based on symptoms.
  5. Salmonellosis can be transmitted by the "five F's": flies, fingers, food, feces, and fomites; therefore strict handwashing is essential to avoid transmission.

Fracture, Nasal

- A nasal fracture often results from injuries received during falls and sports activities, motor vehicle accidents, or physical assaults.
- Bone or cartilage displacement can cause airway obstruction and cosmetic deformity.
- Assessment findings include deviation of the nose to one side, malaligned bridge, crepitus, and midface bruising, bleeding, and pain.
- Treatment includes
  1. Simple, closed reduction with local anesthesia (the treatment of choice)
  2. Rhinoplasty, or surgical reconstruction, for severe fractures
  3. Nasoseptoplasty to straighten a deviated septum to improve airflow and sinus drainage
- Postoperative assessment includes
  1. Check the nasal packing and change the "moustache" dressing or drip pad as needed.
  2. Check for edema, bleeding.

3. Check vital signs every 4 hours.
4. Assess for increased swallowing, which may indicate posterior nasal bleeding.
5. Place the client in a semi-Fowler's position.
6. Apply cool compresses to the nose, eyes, and face.
7. Encourage the client to drink at least 2500 mL/day.
- The client is instructed to
  1. Avoid the Valsalva maneuver.
  2. Use laxatives or stool softeners.
  3. Avoid aspirin and nonsteroidal anti-inflammatory drugs (NSAIDs).
  4. Take the full antibiotic prescription.
  5. Recommend that the client use a humidifier at home to prevent excessive drying of the mucosa.

Fractures

OVERVIEW

- A fracture is a break or disruption in the continuity of a bone.
- Fractures can be classified as complete or incomplete.
  1. Complete fracture: The break is across the entire width of the bone such that the bone is divided into two distinct sections.
  2. Incomplete fracture: The fracture does not divide the bone into two distinct sections.
- Fractures can also be grouped according to the extent of the soft tissue damage accompanying the fracture.
  1. Open or compound fracture: The skin surface over the broken bone is disrupted, causing an external wound; compound fractures are graded to define the extent of the injury.
     a. Grade I is the least severe injury; skin damage is minimal.
     b. Grade II, an open fracture, is accompanied by skin and muscle contusions.
     c. Grade III is the most severe injury. There is damage to skin, muscle, nerve tissue, and blood vessels; the

wound is more than 6 to 8 cm (2.4 to 3.2 inches) in diameter.

  2. Closed or simple fracture: The break does not extend through the skin.

■ Fractures can also be classified based on cause.

  1. Pathologic (spontaneous) fracture: The break occurs after minimal trauma to a bone that has been weakened by disease.

  2. Fatigue or stress fracture: The break results from excessive strain and stress on bone.

  3. Compression fractures are produced by a loading force applied to the long axis of cancellous bone.

■ Complications of fractures include

  1. Acute compartment syndrome (ACS): ACS is a serious condition in which increased pressure within one or more compartments causes compromise of circulation to the area; the most common sites are the lower leg and the dorsal and volar compartments of the forearm. Infection, motor weakness, contracture, and myoglobinuric renal failure can result; fasciotomy is the surgical treatment.

  2. Shock: Hypovolemic shock can occur as a result of hemorrhage from severed arteries.

  3. Fat embolism syndrome (FES): FES is a serious complication in which fat globules are released from the yellow bone marrow into the bloodstream. The emboli migrate to the pulmonary capillary bed, causing confusion (low arterial oxygen), dyspnea, tachycardia, fever, and petechiae.

  4. Thromboembolitic complications: Deep venous thrombosis (DVT) is the most common complication of lower extremity surgery or trauma and the most commonly fatal complication of musculoskeletal surgery.

  5. Infection: Osteomyelitis (bone infection) is most commonly seen in open fractures.

  6. Ischemic necrosis sometimes referred to as aseptic or avascular necrosis (AVN) is bone death resulting from disruption of blood supply.

  7. Delayed union, nonunion, and malunion: *Delayed union* is a fracture that has not healed within 6 months of the time of injury; *nonunion* fractures never completely heal; *malunion* is incorrect healing of a fracture.

COLLABORATIVE MANAGEMENT

Assessment

- Record client information.
  1. Events leading to the fracture and immediate postinjury care
  2. The client's medical history
  3. Current medications, including substance (recreational drug) and alcohol use
  4. Nutritional history and recreational history
  5. Occupation
- Assessment findings include
  1. Trauma to other body systems (priority assessment)
  2. Change in bone alignment
  3. Shortening or change in bone shape
  4. Neurovascular changes
     - a. Skin color
     - b. Skin temperature
     - c. Movement (if pain is elicited, stop immediately)
     - d. Sensation
     - e. Pulses distal to injury
     - f. Pain: location, nature, frequency
  5. Changes in skin integrity, such as ecchymosis, subcutaneous emphysema, or swelling
  6. Capillary refill (if an extremity is involved)
  7. Hemorrhage (open fracture)
  8. Muscle spasm
  9. Respiratory compromise
- Special assessment considerations are as follows:
  1. Fractures of the shoulder and upper arm are assessed with the client in the sitting or standing position so that shoulder drooping or abnormal positioning can be seen.
  2. More distal areas of the arm are assessed with the client supine so that the extremity can be elevated to reduce swelling.
  3. The client is in the supine position when fractures of the lower extremity and pelvis are suspected.
  4. Some fractures can cause internal organ damage, resulting in hemorrhage.
  5. With a pelvic fracture, assess vital signs, skin color,

and level of consciousness for indications of possible hypovolemic shock.

- Psychosocial assessment of the client depends on the extent of the injury and other complications.
- Stresses that result from prolonged hospitalization may affect relationships between the client and his or her family, body image, sexuality, and financial resources.

Emergency Care

- A fracture may be accompanied by multiple injuries to vital organs. First, assess the client for respiratory distress, bleeding, and head injury. Lifesaving care is provided before treatment for the fracture.
  1. Control bleeding.
  2. Prevent shock.
  3. Check vital signs.
  4. Place the client in a supine position.
  5. Keep the client warm with coverings.
- Complete a neurovascular assessment.
  1. Inspect the fracture site for intactness of skin, swelling, and deformity.
  2. Palpate the area lightly to determine temperature, decreased sensation, and blanching.
  3. Assess distal pulses.
  4. Assess motor function.
- Immobilize the area to prevent further damage, reduce pain, and increase circulation; perform another neurovascular assessment.
- If the skin is broken, loosely apply a clean (preferably sterile) cloth to prevent further contamination of the wound.
- Fracture management in the emergency department, physician's office, or clinic begins with reduction and immobilization.
  1. *Closed reduction* involves manipulating the bone ends so that they realign while applying a manual pull, or traction, on the bone.
  2. *Bandages* and *splints* are used to immobilize areas such as the scapula and clavicle.
  3. *Casts* are used to hold bone fragments in place after reduction; they allow early mobility, correct and prevent deformity, and reduce pain.

- Cast materials include
  1. Plaster of Paris
     a. Requires application of a well-fitted stockinette and web padding before the application of wet plaster rolls.
     b. The cast takes 24 to 72 hours to dry.
     c. The client is warned that heat will be felt immediately after the cast is applied.
     d. To facilitate drying, the cast is not covered, and the client is turned every 1 to 2 hours.
     e. The nurse handles the cast with the palms of the hands to prevent indentations and resulting areas of pressure on skin.
  2. Fiberglass is lighter weight and takes less time to dry than plaster of Paris.
  3. Polyester-cotton knit is lighter weight and takes less time to dry than plaster of Paris.
- Types of casts include
  1. Arm cast
     a. When the client is in bed, the arm is elevated above the heart to reduce swelling; the hand should be higher than the elbow.
     b. When the client is out of bed, the arm is supported by a sling placed around the neck; the sling should distribute the weight over a large area of the shoulders and trunk, not just the neck.
  2. Leg cast
     a. Leg cast permits mobility and requires the client to use ambulatory aids.
     b. A cast shoe, sandal, or boot that attaches to the foot, or a rubber walking pad attached to the sole of the cast assists in ambulation (if weight bearing is allowed) and helps prevent falls or damage to the cast.
     c. Elevate the leg on pillows when the client is in bed to reduce swelling.
  3. Cast brace
     a. This device enables the client to bend unaffected joints while the fracture is healing; the fracture must show signs of healing and minimal tissue edema before the cast is applied.
     b. As healing continues, the cast may be replaced by a leg immobilizer or soft brace.

4. Body and spica casts
   a. A body cast encircles the body, whereas a spica cast encircles a portion of the trunk and one or two extremities.
   b. The client is at risk for skin breakdown, pneumonia or atelectasis, joint contracture, and constipation.
   c. *Cast syndrome* (superior mesenteric artery syndrome) results in partial or complete upper intestinal obstruction manifested by abdominal distention, epigastric pain, nausea, and vomiting.
      (1) Placing a window in the abdominal portion of the cast or bivalving may be sufficient to relieve pressure on the duodenum.

■ Cast care
   1. Handle a wet plaster cast with the palms of hands to prevent indentations and resultant areas of pressure on the skin.
   2. To prevent skin irritation from rough and crumbling edges, "petal" or finish the cast by placing tape over the rough edges if the underlying stockinette does not cover the edges of the cast.
   3. The health care provider may cut a window in the cast so that a wound, if present, can be observed and cared for.
   4. Ensure that the cast is not too tight by inserting a finger between the cast and the skin; if it is too tight, the health care provider may cut it to relieve pressure.
   5. The health care provider may bivalve the cast, cutting it lengthwise into two equal pieces. Either half can be removed for inspection or provision of care; the two pieces are reunited by an elastic bandage wrap.
   6. Encase a long leg or body cast in a protective covering around the perineum to prevent contamination by urine or feces; make a fracture bedpan available.
   7. Frequently monitor the client's neurovascular status.
   8. Inspect the cast daily for drainage, cracking, crumbling, alignment, and fit once it is dry.
      a. Circle, date, and monitor for change areas of drainage on the cast; it is not unusual for bloody drainage to seep through the cast from an open fracture site.
      b. Immediately report to the physician a sudden increase in the amount of drainage or a change in the integrity of the cast.

    c. Clean a soiled cast with mild detergent and a damp cloth.

  9. Do not use lotion or powder on skin around the cast.

10. Teach the client not to place foreign objects beneath the cast.

11. Smell the cast for foul odor and palpate for hot areas every shift.

12. Have a cast cutter available at all times.

13. Observe for and report complications from casting.
    a. Infection
    b. Circulation impairment
    c. Peripheral nerve damage
    d. Pressure necrosis
    e. Contracture of joint
    f. Degenerative arthritis
    g. Muscle atrophy
    h. Thromboembolism

- Traction is the application of a pulling force to a part of the body to provide reduction, alignment, and rest; it may also decrease muscle spasm and prevent or correct deformity.

  1. Traction types include
    a. *Running:* The pulling force is in one direction and the client's body acts as countertraction; moving the bed or body can alter the countertraction force.
    b. *Balanced suspension:* Countertraction is provided in such a way that the pulling force of the traction is not altered; commonly used to treat fractures of the femur.
    c. *Skin (Buck's traction):* A Velcro boot, belt, or halter is secured around a body part to decrease painful muscle spasms; weight is limited to 5 to 10 pounds.
    d. *Skeletal:* Pins, wires, tongs (Crutchfield), or screws are surgically inserted directly into bone, which allows the use of a longer traction time and heavier weights, usually from 15 to 30 pounds (6.8 to 13.6 kg). It aids in bone realignment.
    e. *Plaster traction:* A combination of skeletal traction and a plaster cast is used.
    f. *Brace devices:* Braces exert a pull to correct alignment deformities.

2. Care for the client in traction includes
   a. Maintaining correct balance between traction pull and countertraction force
   b. Not removing weights without a physician's order
   c. Allowing the weights to hang freely at all times
   d. Inspecting ropes, knots, and pulleys every 8 hours for loosening, fraying, and positioning
   e. Checking the weight for consistency with the physician's order every 8 hours; if not correct, notifying the physician
   f. Noting that if the client complains of severe pain from muscle spasms, the weights may be too heavy or the client may need realignment
   g. Inspecting the skin every 8 hours for signs of irritation and inflammation, especially at points of entry for wires, screws, or pins, and observing for drainage, color, odor, and severe redness
   h. Performing pin care as required by hospital policy
   i. Performing a neurovascular assessment at least every 8 hours, or more often if clinically indicated

Considerations for Older Adults

* Older adults are at risk for problems caused by skin or skeletal traction because of inadequate circulation and sensation.
* Traction of any type is not ideal treatment because it necessitates prolonged immobilization and serious complications such as pneumonia, and pulmonary emboli can result.

SURGICAL MANAGEMENT

■ *Open reduction with internal fixation (ORIF)* permits early mobilization. Open reduction allows direct visualization of the fracture site and internal fixation uses metal pins, rods, plates, and prosthesis to immobilize the fracture during healing.

■ *External fixation* involves fracture reduction and the insertion of pins into the bone through small percutaneous incisions. The pins are held in place by a large, external metal frame to prevent bone movement.

1. External fixation allows for early ambulation and exercise while relieving pain.

2. The device maintains alignment in closed fractures that will not maintain position in a cast and stabilizes comminuted fractures that require bone grafting.
3. In open fractures, the device permits easy access to the wound and promotes healing.
4. Pin tract infection that can lead to osteomyelitis is a potential complication.
5. The Ilizarov fixator promotes rotation, angulation, shortening, lengthening, and widening of bone for congenital anomalies, joint contractures, bone segmental defects, and deformities from malunion or nonunion fractures.

- Provide routine preoperative and postoperative care, as well as
    1. Monitor neurovascular status at least every hour for the first 24 hours after injury, every 2 hours for the next 12 to 24 hours, and every 4 hours for the next few days.
    2. Monitor the complete blood count for signs of anemia resulting from blood loss.
    3. Observe for and report complications such as infection.
- Electrical bone stimulation, ultrasound fracture treatment, and bone grafting are methods for treating nonunion or failure of the bone to heal.

◀NDx: Acute Pain

- Musculoskeletal pain is one of the most severe types of pain; the client may have pain for a prolonged time, making pain management difficult.
- To manage pain
    1. Administer opioid analgesics, anti-inflammatory drugs, and muscle relaxants, as ordered.
    2. Observe for effectiveness of drug therapy (an early sign of acute compartment syndrome is the sudden inability of pain medication to relieve pain).
    3. Use temporary pain relief measures such as ice, heat, massage, distraction, imagery, music therapy, and relaxation techniques.

◀NDx: Risk for Infection

- Interventions include
    1. Using strict aseptic technique for dressing changes and wound irrigations

2. Monitoring for signs of infection such as swelling, drainage, and fever
   3. Administering antibiotics to clients with open fractures to prevent infection

◆NDx: Impaired Physical Mobility

- Prevent and assess for complications of immobility.
- Collaborate with the physical therapist to promote client mobility.

F

PROMOTIONS OF MOBILITY

- *Crutches* require strong upper extremities, balance, and coordination.
   1. To prevent pressure on the axillary nerve, there should be the distance of two or three finger widths between the axilla and the top of the crutch when the crutch tip is at least 6 inches diagonally in front of the foot.
   2. The crutch is adjusted so that the elbow is flexed no more than 30 degrees.
   3. The most common gait for crutch walking is the three-point gait, which allows no weight bearing on the affected leg.
- A *walker* is most often used by the elderly client who needs additional support for balance.
- A *cane* is used if minimal support is needed.
   1. The cane is placed on the unaffected side.
   2. The cane should create no more than 30 degrees of flexion of the elbow.
   3. The top of the cane should be parallel to the greater trochanter of the femur.

◆NDx: Imbalanced Nutrition: Less than Body Requirements

- Focus on meeting the client's nutritional needs.
   1. Assess the client's food likes and dislikes.
   2. Collaborate with the dietitian to plan meals that are both appealing and nutritional (high protein, high calorie).
   3. Administer supplements of vitamins B and C, as prescribed.
   4. Encourage the client to increase dietary intake of milk and milk products to prevent hypocalcemia.
   5. Encourage the client to consume foods high in iron to prevent anemia; an iron supplement may be ordered.

- Discharge planning includes
  1. Identifying structural barriers to mobility in the home before discharge.
  2. Collaborating with the case manager to identify the need for a home care nurse or care aide, or a physical or occupational therapist; ensuring that needed support services and supplies are available at time of discharge
  3. Providing verbal and written instructions for the care of casts, splints, braces, or external fixator
  4. Providing verbal and written instructions on wound care, as needed
  5. Teaching the client and family how to recognize complications such as infection, as well as when and where to contact professional health care if complications arise
  6. Referring the client for assistance with financial issues, understanding the long-term nature of the recovery period, job counseling, and so forth, depending on the nature and severity of the fracture
  7. Emphasizing the importance of follow-up visits with the health care provider and other therapists
- Teach the client how to care for the extremity after cast removal. Instruct the client to
  1. Remove scaly, dead skin carefully by soaking, not scrubbing.
  2. Move the extremity carefully and expect discomfort, weakness, and decreased range of motion.
  3. Exercise slowly as instructed.
  4. Wear support stockings or elastic bandages to prevent swelling (for lower extremity).

Fractures of Specific Sites

- *Clavicular: Self-healing.* A splint or bandage is used for immobilization.
- *Scapular*: Immobilized with a sling and swathe or shoulder immobilizer until healing occurs. Serious internal trauma

can occur, including pneumothorax, pulmonary contusions, and fractured ribs.

- *Humeral shaft:* Corrected by closed reduction and the application of a hanging arm cast or splint. An impacted injury is treated conservatively with a sling. A displaced fracture may require open reduction with internal fixation (ORIF) with pins or a prosthetic device.

- *Olecranon:* Treated by closed reduction and application of a cast. Healing may take 2 months, and several additional months may be needed before full use of the elbow returns. For displaced fractures, ORIF is performed, and a splint is worn.

- *Radius and ulna:* Treated with closed reduction and casting. If displaced, ORIF with intramedullary rods or plates and screws is performed.

- *Wrist and hand:* Treated with closed reduction and casting. Metacarpal fractures are immobilized for 3 to 4 weeks; phalangeal fractures are immobilized in finger splints for 10 to 14 days.

- *Hip:* Classified as *intracapsular* (within the joint capsule) or *extracapsular* (outside the joint capsule). Treatment of choice is surgical repair (usually ORIF) to allow the client to get out of bed. Bucks traction may be applied before surgery.

Considerations for Older Adults with a Hip Fracture

- Hip fractures occur most often in older women with osteoporosis.
- As many as one third of older clients die within 1 year of injury from medical complications caused by the fracture or by immobility that occurs after the fracture.
- Approximately 50% of older clients cannot return home or live independently after a hip fracture.

- *Femur:* Seldom immobilized by casting. Skeletal traction followed by a cast brace or hip spica cast is used. ORIF may be needed.

- *Patella:* Repaired with closed reduction and casting or internal fixation with screws.

- *Tibia and fibula:* Treated with closed reduction with casting for 8 to 10 weeks; internal fixation and long leg cast for

4 to 6 weeks; or external fixation when the fracture causes extensive skin and soft tissue damage.

- *Ankle*: Generally spiral, transverse, or oblique breaks that are difficult to treat and present problems in healing. Treatment consists of a combination of closed and open techniques, depending on the severity and extent of the fracture.
- *Foot or phalanges:* Very painful fractures that are treated with either open or closed techniques.
- *Ribs and sternum:* Major complication is puncture of the lungs, heart, or arteries by bone fragments or ends. Treat pain so that adequate ventilation is maintained.
- *Pelvis:* The second most common cause of death from trauma after head injuries. The pelvis is vascular and close to major organs and blood vessels. When a non–weight-bearing part of the pelvis is fractured, treatment involves bedrest. A weight-bearing fracture may require the use of a pelvic sling, skeletal traction, double hip spica cast, or external fixator.
- Compression fractures of the spine associated with osteoporosis are treated with bedrest, analgesics, and physical therapy. Surgical treatment involves vertebroplasty and kyphoplasty in which bone cement is injected directly into the fracture site to provide immediate pain relief; kyphoplasty is the additional step of using an inflated balloon to restore height to the vertebrae.

Frostbite

- Frostbite is a cold injury of the skin; severity depends on temperature, duration of exposure, and tissue hypoxia at exposure.
- Cell death is due to microvascular vasoconstriction, with subsequent interference of blood flow and stasis.
- Continued exposure to cold causes vascular necrosis and gangrene.
- Increased risk factors include age, immobility, alcohol use, vascular disease, and psychiatric disorders.

- Treatment includes rapid and continuous rewarming of the tissue in a warm bath for 15 to 20 minutes or until skin flushing occurs; thawing can be painful.
- Slow thawing or interrupted periods of warmth are avoided because they can contribute to increased cellular damage.
- After thawing, the tissue is exposed so that tissue changes can be monitored.
- Frostbite blisters are left intact.
- Over time, the degree of actual tissue destruction is evident, and local care to eschar is indicated.
- Long-term complications of cold injury include thickened nail plates, depigmentation, scarring, and amputation.

Gastritis

OVERVIEW

- Gastritis is defined as the inflammation of the gastric mucosa.
- Mucosal injury occurs and is worsened by histamine release and vagal nerve stimulation.
- Hydrochloric acid diffuses into the mucosa and injures small vessels, resulting in edema, hemorrhage, and erosion of the gastric lining.
- Gastritis can be classified as acute or chronic.
    1. *Acute* gastritis, the inflammation of gastric mucosa or submucosa, may result from the onset of infection *(Helicobacter pylori, Escherichia coli)* after exposure to local irritants such as alcohol or aspirin, nonsteroidal anti-inflammatory drugs (NSAIDs), bacterial endotoxins, or ingestion of corrosive substances, or from the lack of stimulation of normal gastric secretions. It occurs in varying degrees of mucosal necrosis and inflammation, with complete regeneration and healing usually occurring within a few days and complete recovery with no residual damage usually ensuing.
    2. *Chronic* gastritis is a diffuse chronic inflammatory process involving the mucosal lining of the stomach that

usually heals without scarring but can progress to hemorrhage and ulcer formation. It may be caused by chronic local irritation from alcohol, drugs, smoking, radiation, infectious agents (e.g., *H. pylori*), and environmental agents. Of clients with gastric ulcers, 50% have associated chronic gastritis.

- The three subtypes of chronic gastritis are
    1. *Type A,* associated with the presence of antibodies to parietal cells. An autoimmune pathogenesis has been proposed. Type A accompanies pernicious anemia.
    2. *Type B,* generally caused by *H. pylori* infection.
    3. *Atrophic gastritis,* found most often in older adults after exposure to toxic substances in the workplace or *H. pylori* infection, or it can be related to autoimmune factors.

COLLABORATIVE MANAGEMENT

Assessment

- Acute gastritis: assess for
    1. Abdominal tenderness and bloating
    2. Anorexia, cramping, nausea and vomiting
    3. Hematemesis, melena
    4. In stress-induced gastritis, possible symptoms of intravascular volume depletion and shock
    5. Aspirin-related gastritis may result in dyspepsia
- Chronic gastritis: assess for
    1. Vague complaints or periodic epigastric distress, which may be relieved by food
    2. Anorexia
    3. Pain that worsens with intake of food, especially spicy or fatty food
    4. Weight loss

Interventions

- Acute gastritis is treated symptomatically and supportively. If the client experienced a gastrointestinal bleed with severe hemorrhage, a blood transfusion may be needed. Fluid replacement is indicated for severe fluid loss.
- Treatment of chronic gastritis varies with the cause.
- Drug therapy includes
    1. H_2 antagonists to block gastric acid secretions

2. Antacids are used as buffering agents
3. Proton pump inhibitors
4. Vitamin B_{12}, as ordered, for clients with pernicious anemia
5. Bismuth subsalicylates or a proton pump inhibitor, metronidazole (Flagyl, Novonidazole), tetracycline, or ampicillin (Amcill, Ampicin), if *H. pylori* is present
6. Instructing the client to avoid using drugs associated with gastric irritation, including steroids, aspirin, chemotherapeutic agents, and NSAIDs
- Diet therapy includes
  1. Instructing the client to avoid foods and spices that contribute to distress, including tea, coffee, cola, chocolate, mustard, paprika, cloves, pepper, and Tabasco sauce
  2. Instructing the client to avoid consuming large, heavy meals
  3. Providing a soft, bland diet
- Teach client ways to reduce stress.
  1. Teach techniques to reduce discomfort, such as progressive relaxation, cutaneous stimulation, guided imagery, and distraction.
  2. Advise the client to stop smoking, if appropriate, and to avoid alcohol and caffeine.
- Surgery is indicated when conservative measures have failed to control bleeding (see Surgical Management under Peptic Ulcer Disease).

Gastroenteritis

OVERVIEW

- Gastroenteritis is an increase in the frequency and water content of stools and/or vomiting as a result of inflammation of the mucous membranes of the stomach and intestines, primarily affecting the small bowel.
- The disease may be viral or bacterial in origin, causing an inflammatory response in one of three ways.
  1. Release of enterotoxin, causing local inflammation and diarrhea

2. Penetration of the organism into the intestine, causing cellular destruction, necrosis, and ulceration (diarrhea occurs with white blood cells or red blood cells)
3. Attachment of the organism to the mucosal epithelium, destroying cells of the intestinal villi with resultant malabsorption

- *Viral* gastroenteritis can be classified as either epidemic viral gastroenteritis or rotavirus gastroenteritis (incubation about 48 hours and affecting infants and young children).
  1. Norwalk virus is spread by the oral-fecal route and is a common cause of waterborne epidemics of gastroenteritis.
- *Bacterial* gastroenteritis can be divided into three general types.
  1. *Campylobacter* enteritis
  2. *Escherichia coli* diarrhea
  3. Shigellosis

COLLABORATIVE MANAGEMENT

Assessment

- The client's history can provide information related to the potential cause.
  1. Onset of diarrhea with accompanying abdominal cramping or pain
  2. Nausea and vomiting
  3. Bloody, mucous, or watery, foul-smelling stool
  4. Fever; temperature may be normal or elevated from 101° to 103° F (38.2° to 39.2° C)
  5. Dehydration exhibited by poor skin turgor, dry mucous membranes, orthostatic blood pressure changes, hypotension, and oliguria
  6. Viral symptoms such as myalgia, headache, or malaise
  7. Positive result of a stool culture

Interventions

- Provide fluid replacement therapy as ordered.
  1. Administer oral rehydration therapy with commercially prepared products such as Resol.
  2. Administer hypotonic intravenous fluids for severe dehydration; add potassium if the client is hypokalemic.

3. Check vital signs and orthostatic blood pressure as clinically indicated.
4. Check weight daily.
5. Maintain strict intake and output.
6. Depending on the type of gastroenteritis, notify the local health department.
- Provide diet therapy.
  1. Advise the client to take small volumes of clear liquids with electrolytes.
  2. Advise the client not to drink water because it does not contain any electrolytes to replace those lost.
  3. Slowly progress diet to include saltine crackers and toast and jelly; when this is tolerated, bland foods (e.g., nonfat soup, custard, yogurt, cottage cheese, baked or mashed potatoes, and cooked vegetables) may be added, then progress to the client's regular diet.
  4. Advise the client to avoid caffeine.
- Provide drug therapy as ordered.
  1. Drugs that suppress intestinal motility suppressants such as antiemetics or anticholinergics for bacterial or viral gastroenteritis are *not* routinely given.
  2. Antibiotics may be given if gastroenteritis is due to bacterial infection.
  3. Anti-infective agents, such as trimethoprim/sulfamethoxazole (Septra, Bactrim), are given if shigellosis is present.
  4. Antiperistaltic agents may be given.
  5. Diarrhea that continues for 10 days is probably not due to gastroenteritis and an investigation for other causes is done.
- Provide skin care.
  1. Teach the client to avoid toilet paper and harsh soaps and to gently clean the area with warm water and absorbent cotton, followed by thorough drying with absorbent cotton.
  2. Cream, oil, or gel can be applied to a damp, warm washcloth to remove excrement adhering to excoriated skin.
  3. Hydrocortisone cream or protective barrier cream should be applied to the skin between stools; witch hazel compresses (e.g., Tucks) and sitz baths can relieve discomfort.

- Teach the client the following health practices.
  1. Replace lost fluids.
  2. Follow the recommended diet.
  3. Wash hands after each bowel movement to minimize the risk of disease transmission.
  4. Do not share eating utensils, glasses, and dishes and to maintain strict personal hygiene.
  5. Maintain clean bathroom facilities.
  6. Inform the health care provider if symptoms persist beyond 3 days.
  7. Adhere to these precautions for up to 7 weeks after the illness or up to several months if *Shigella* was the causative organism.
  8. Follow written instructions for medication, if ordered, including dosage, schedule of administration, and side effects.

Gastroesophageal Reflux Disease

- Gastroesophageal reflux disease (GERD) occurs as the result of the backward flow (reflux) of gastrointestinal (GI) contents into the esophagus, exposing the esophageal mucosa to the irritating effects of gastric or duodenal contents, resulting in inflammatory changes of the esophageal mucosa.
- The degree of inflammation is related to the acid concentration of the refluxed material, the number of reflux episodes, and the length of time that the esophagus is exposed to the irritant.

COLLABORATIVE MANAGEMENT

Assessment
- Record client information.
  1. Pain location
  2. Dyspepsia (also called heartburn or pyrosis), the primary symptom, described as a substernal or retrosternal burning sensation that tends to move up and down the chest in

a wavelike fashion; severe heartburn may radiate to the neck or jaw or may be felt in the back

3. Pain aggravated by bending over, straining, or lying in a recumbent position
4. Pain occurring after each meal and persisting for 20 minutes to 2 hours
5. Regurgitation not associated with belching or nausea; warm fluid traveling up the throat, resulting in a sour or bitter taste in the mouth
6. Water brash (reflex salivary hypersecretion)
7. Dysphagia (difficulty swallowing) or odynophagia (painful swallowing)
8. Chest pain from esophageal spasm
9. Chronic cough that occurs mostly at night
10. Belching and a feeling of flatulence or bloating after eating
11. Results of 24-hour pH monitoring, esophageal manometry (motility testing), and scintigraphy (measure of reflux of radioisotope)

Interventions

NONSURGICAL MANAGEMENT

- Explore the client's meal plan and food preferences, and in collaboration with the dietitian meet with the client and family to plan diet modifications to reduce GERD symptoms. Teach the client to
  1. Avoid fatty foods, coffee, tea, cola, chocolate, spicy foods, acidic foods, and alcohol because they reduce esophageal sphincter (LES) pressure or cause local irritation.
  2. Eat four to six small meals a day.
  3. Avoid having snacks in the evening or eating 3 hours before bedtime.
  4. Eat slowly and chew food thoroughly to facilitate digestion and prevent eructation (belching).
  5. Limit or eliminate alcohol and tobacco.
  6. Remain upright after meals for 1 to 2 hours.

Client Education

- Teach risk factors that can exacerbate the disease.
- Stress the importance of ongoing monitoring.

- Encourage lifestyle changes.
    1. If the client is obese, collaborate with the dietitian and meet with the client and family to examine approaches to weight reduction.
    2. Explore the possibility and means of smoking cessation and make appropriate referrals.
    3. Instruct the client to elevate the head of the bed by 6 inches to prevent nighttime reflux.
    4. Instruct the client to sleep in the left lateral decubitus (side-lying) position.
    5. Encourage the client to avoid wearing tight-fitting clothing and working in a bent-over or stooped position.
- Drug therapy includes
    1. Antacids for acid-neutralizing effects
    2. Histamine receptor antagonist to reduce gastric acid production, provide symptom improvement, and support healing of the inflamed esophageal tissue
    3. Proton pumps are the *main* treatment for GERD by providing effective, long-acting inhibition of gastric acid secretion
    4. Prokinetic drugs to accelerate gastric emptying and improve LES pressure and esophageal peristalsis
- Identify whether the client is on any medications that may lower LES pressure and cause reflux such as oral contraceptives, anticholinergic agents, beta-adrenergic agonists, nitrates, and calcium channel blockers.

SURGICAL MANAGEMENT

- Noninvasive endoscopic procedures include
    1. The Stretta procedure involves the application of radio-frequency energy near the gastroesophageal junction, which inhibits the activity of the vagus nerve thus reducing discomfort for the client.
    2. In the Enteryx procedure, a soft, spongy permanent implant is injected into the LES muscle to tighten the LES and prevent reflux.
    3. The Bard EndoCinch Suturing System (BESS) involves suturing near the LES.
- The major surgical procedure for clients who have not responded to aggressive medical management is the *laparoscopic Nissen fundoplication.*

- Synthetic *Angelchik prosthesis* placement is an alternative surgical procedure. A laparotomy is performed, and a C-shaped silicone prosthesis filled with gel is tied around the distal esophagus, anchoring the LES in the abdomen and reinforcing sphincter pressure.

Glaucoma

OVERVIEW

- Glaucoma is a group of ocular diseases that result in increased ocular pressure.
- Left untreated, glaucoma can result in blindness.
- In most common forms of glaucoma, vision is lost gradually and painlessly, without the person's awareness.
- Types of glaucoma include
    1. *Primary,* in which the structures that are involved in circulation or reabsorption of the aqueous humor undergo direct pathologic change
        a. Primary open-angle glaucoma (POAG) develops slowly, usually without symptoms.
        b. Angle closure, also known as closed angle, narrow angle, or acute angle, has a sudden onset and is treated as an emergency.
    2. *Secondary,* which results from ocular diseases that cause a narrowed angle or an increased volume of fluid within the eye

COLLABORATIVE MANAGEMENT

Assessment

- Assessment findings include
    1. Increased intraocular pressure
    2. Diminished accommodation
- Assessment findings for *late* manifestations of glaucoma include
    1. Visual field losses
    2. Decreased visual acuity not correctable with glasses
    3. Appearance of halos around lights

4. Headache or eye pain (pain is sudden and excruciating in acute glaucoma)
5. Increased cupping and atrophy of the optic disc
6. Pale optic disc
7. Anxiety and fear
8. Increased tonometry reading

Interventions

NONSURGICAL MANAGEMENT

- Drug therapy includes
    1. Miotics to constrict the pupil and contract the ciliary muscle, which may cause vision to be blurred for 1 to 2 hours after use and adaptation to dark environments difficult
    2. When used as eye drops, beta blockers inhibit formation of aqueous humor, which include timolol (Timoptic, Apo-Timoptic), and levobunolol (Betagan)
    3. Carbonic anhydrase inhibitors to reduce production of aqueous humor; side effects include numbness and tingling of the hands and feet, nausea, and malaise
    4. Systemic osmotic agents given to clients with acute glaucoma to reduce ocular pressure

SURGICAL MANAGEMENT

- *Laser trabeculoplasty* is performed under local anesthesia for open-angle glaucoma to produce scars in the trabecular meshwork, causing the meshwork to tighten and thus increase the outflow of aqueous humor.
- For angle-closure glaucoma, the laser is used to create a hole in the periphery of the iris, which allows aqueous humor to flow from the posterior chamber to the anterior chamber and then into the trabecular meshwork.
- A postoperative ocular steroid ointment may be prescribed following laser surgery.
- The most serious complication of laser surgery is choroidal hemorrhage indicated by acute pain deep in the eye, decreased vision, and vital sign changes.
- Other surgical procedures may be performed if the glaucoma fails to respond to pharmacologic or laser management.

Glomerulonephritis, Acute

OVERVIEW

- Acute glomerulonephritis, or acute nephritic syndrome, is an inflammatory process of the glomeruli initiated by activation of immunologic responses as a result of infection.
- *Infectious* causes include
  1. Group A beta-hemolytic *Streptococcus*
  2. Staphylococcal or pneumococcal bacteremia
  3. Syphilis
  4. Visceral abscesses
  5. Infective endocarditis
  6. Hepatitis B
  7. Infectious mononucleosis
  8. Measles
  9. Mumps
  10. Cytomegaloviral infections
  11. Parasitic, fungal, or viral infections
- *Secondary* causes related to systemic disease include
  1. Systemic lupus erythematosus
  2. Systemic necrotizing vasculitis
  3. Thrombocytopenia purpura
  4. Diabetic glomerulopathy
  5. Henoch-Schönlein purpura
  6. Goodpasture's syndrome
  7. Wegener's granulomatosis
  8. Polyarteritis nodosa
  9. Hemolytic-uremic syndrome

COLLABORATIVE MANAGEMENT

Assessment

- Record client information.
  1. History of recent infections, particularly skin and upper respiratory infections
  2. Recent travel
  3. Activities with exposure to viruses, bacteria, fungi, or parasites

4. Recent illnesses
5. Recent surgeries or invasive procedures
6. Known systemic diseases

- Assessment findings include
  1. Skin lesions or incisions
  2. Edema of the face, eyelids, hands, and peripheral tissue
  3. Fluid overload and circulatory congestion
  4. Difficulty breathing, nocturnal or exertional dyspnea or orthopnea
  5. Crackles in lung fields
  6. S_3 heart sound (gallop rhythm)
  7. Neck vein distention
  8. Changes in patterns of urination
  9. Smoky, reddish-brown, or cola-colored urine
  10. Dysuria
  11. Decreased urine output
  12. Mild to moderate hypertension
  13. Changes in weight
  14. Fatigue and malaise
  15. Anorexia, nausea, or vomiting
  16. Red blood cells and protein in the urine
- A percutaneous needle biopsy may define the pathologic condition, assist in determining prognosis, and help outline treatment.

Interventions

- Appropriate anti-infective agents such as penicillin, erythromycin, or azithromycin are given to treat infection.
- To prevent infection spread, the health care provider may order anti-infective drugs for persons in immediate close contact with the client.
- Sodium and water restriction, along with diuretics, may be needed for the client with hypertension, circulatory congestions, and edema.
  1. Antihypertensives are given to treat hypertension.
  2. The usual fluid allowance is equal to the 24-hour urinary output, plus 500 to 600 mL for insensible fluid loss.
- Potassium and protein intake may be restricted to prevent hyperkalemia and additional uremic manifestations of the elevated blood urea nitrogen (BUN) level.

- Plasmapheresis may also be attempted.
- Energy management includes
  1. Encouraging and promoting a restful environment
  2. Teaching and demonstrating energy conservation techniques
  3. Encouraging the client to practice relaxation techniques
- Health teaching includes
  1. Reviewing prescribed medication instructions, including purpose, timing, frequency, duration, and side effects
  2. Ensure that the client and family understand dietary and fluid modifications
  3. Advising the client to measure weight and blood pressure daily and to notify the health care provider of any sudden changes
  4. Advising the client to exercise each day, as tolerated
  5. Teaching the importance of rest
  6. Instructing the client about peritoneal or vascular access care if short-term dialysis is required to control excess fluid volume or uremic symptoms

Glomerulonephritis, Chronic

OVERVIEW

- Chronic glomerulonephritis, or chronic nephritic syndrome, is the diagnostic name given to known and unknown causes of renal deterioration or renal failure that develop over 20 to 30 years.
- The exact cause is unknown. Changes are believed to be due to the effects of hypertension, intermittent or recurrent infections and inflammation, and poor blood flow to the kidneys.
- Kidney tissue atrophies, and the functional mass of nephrons decreases, which alters glomerular filtration.
- Glomerular injury results in proteinuria because of increased permeability of the glomerular basement membrane.
- The process eventually results in end-stage renal disease (ESRD) and uremia, requiring dialysis or transplantation.

COLLABORATIVE MANAGEMENT

Assessment

- Record client history.
    1. Health problems, including systemic disease
    2. Renal or urologic problems
    3. Childhood infectious diseases, such as with *Streptococcus*
    4. Recent exposure to infections
    5. Overall assessment of health status
    6. Changes in urinary status, including frequency of voiding and changes in urine color, clarity, and odor
    7. Changes in activity tolerance
    8. Presence of edema
    9. Changes in mental concentration or memory
    10. Proteinuria
    11. Decreased creatinine clearance
    12. Serum electrolyte changes
- Perform a physical assessment.
    1. Inspect the skin for yellow color, ecchymosis, and rashes.
    2. Inspect for evidence of edema in tissues.
    3. Measure blood pressure and weight.
    4. Auscultate the heart for an S_3 sound.
    5. Auscultate the lungs for the presence of rales or crackles.
    6. Observe the rate and depth of breathing pattern.
    7. Inspect neck veins for engorgement.
    8. Inspect and analyze urine.
    9. Assess for uremic symptoms such as slurred speech, ataxia, tremors or asterixis (flapping tremor of the fingers or the inability to maintain a fixed posture with the arms extended and wrists hyperextended).

Interventions

- Management of chronic glomerulonephritis is similar to conservative management for ESRD.
- Treatment consists of dietary modification, fluid intake sufficient to prevent reduced blood flow volume to the kidneys, and medication therapy to temporarily control the symptoms of uremia.
- Eventually the client requires dialysis or transplantation.

Glomerulonephritis, Rapidly Progressive

- Rapidly progressive glomerulonephritis, a type of acute nephritis, develops over several weeks or months and causes a significant loss of renal function.
- Manifestations include fluid volume excess, hypertension, oliguria, electrolyte imbalance. and uremic symptoms.
- Renal deterioration often progresses to end-stage renal disease.

Gonorrhea

- Gonorrhea is a sexually transmitted disease (STD) caused by *Neisseria gonorrhoeae*, a gram-negative diplococcus.
- The disease is transmitted by direct sexual contact and through an infected birth canal to the neonate.
- Initial symptoms occur 3 to 10 days after sexual contact with an infected person, or the client may be asymptomatic.

COLLABORATIVE MANAGEMENT

Assessment

- Assessment findings include
  1. Male
     a. Dysuria
     b. Penile discharge that is either profuse yellowish-green fluid or clear, scant fluid
     c. Anal itching and irritation
     d. Rectal bleeding
     e. Painful defecation
     f. Pharyngitis
  2. Female
     a. Change in vaginal discharge
     b. Urinary frequency

    c. Dysuria
    d. Anal itching and irritation
    e. Rectal bleeding
    f. Painful defecation
    g. Pharyngitis
- In males, the urethra is the site most commonly affected, but gonorrhea can spread to the prostate, seminal vesicles, and epididymis.
- In females, the cervix and urethra are the most common sites, but upward spread can cause pelvic inflammatory disease, endometritis, salpingitis, and pelvic peritonitis.
- Also assesses for
  1. Sexual history
     a. Types and frequency of sexual activity
     b. Number of sexual contacts
     c. History of STDs
     d. Potential sites of infection
     e. Sexual preference
  2. Gram stain smears for gram-negative diplococci (culture provides a definitive diagnosis)

Interventions

- Antibiotics that may be given include ceftriaxone (Rocephin), ciprofloxacin (Cipro), or ofloxacin (Floxin), plus azithromycin (Zithromax), or doxycycline (Monodox, Novodoxyclin).
- Quinolones (ciprofloxacin, ofloxacin) are not recommended in areas with high quinolone resistance (Hawaii, California, Asia, and Pacific rim); treat with intramuscular ceftriaxone.
- The client should be tested and treated for *Chlamydia* infection that is frequently seen in clients with gonorrhea.
- Inform the client that sexual partners need to be treated.
- Teach the client about
  1. Transmission and treatment
  2. Prevention of reinfection
  3. Avoidance of sexual activity until the infection is cured
  4. Use of condoms if sexually active
  5. The need to report the disease
- Encourage the client to express feelings about having the disease.
- Provide privacy for teaching and maintain the confidentiality of medical record.

Gout

G

OVERVIEW

- Gout is a systemic disease in which urate crystals deposit in joints and other body tissues, causing inflammation.
- Two major types of gout are
  1. *Primary* gout, which results from one of several inborn errors of purine metabolism. Uric acid production exceeds the kidney's excretion capability, and sodium urate deposits in synovium and other tissues, resulting in inflammation. It is inherited as an X-linked trait.
  2. *Secondary* gout, which involves excessive uric acid in the blood caused by another disease.
- Four phases of the disease process are
  1. *Asymptomatic hyperuricemia,* in which there are no symptoms but serum uric acid is elevated
  2. *Acute* gout, which is characterized by excruciating pain and inflammation of one or more small joints, especially the great toe
  3. *Intercritical* or *intercurrent* gout, which is asymptomatic, with no abnormalities found on examination (between acute attacks)
  4. *Chronic* gout, in which repeated episodes of acute gout result in the deposit of urate crystals under the skin and within major organs, especially the renal system

COLLABORATIVE MANAGEMENT

Assessment

- Assessment findings include
  1. A family history of the disease
  2. Joint inflammation
  3. Excruciating pain in the involved joints
  4. Tophi: hard, fairly large irregular-shaped deposits in the skin that may break open, with a yellow, gritty substance discharged (seen in chronic gout)
  5. Renal calculi or dysfunction

Interventions

- Drug therapy includes
  1. For *acute* gout only, colchicine (Colsalide, Novocolchicine) and nonsteroidal anti-inflammatory drugs (NSAIDs) until the inflammation subsides, usually for 4 to 7 days
  2. For *chronic* gout, allopurinol (Zyloprim, Alloprin) or probenecid (Benemid), or combination drugs that contain probenecid and colchicine (ColBenemid) with serum uric acid levels monitored to determine the effectiveness of the drug
- Dietary restrictions are controversial but may include a strict low-purine diet with avoidance of organ meats, shellfish, and oily fish with bones.
- Excessive alcohol intake and fad "starvation" diets can cause a gout attack.
- Instruct the client to avoid
  1. Aspirin in any form
  2. Diuretics
  3. Excessive physical or emotional stress
- Teach the client to
  1. Force fluids
  2. Increase urinary pH by eating alkaline ash foods such as citrus fruits and juices, milk, and other dairy products

Guillain-Barré Syndrome

OVERVIEW

- Guillain-Barré syndrome (GBS) is an acute autoimmune disorder characterized by varying degrees of motor weakness and paralysis.
- Three stages make up the acute course and include the
  1. *Initial* period, which begins with the onset of the first definitive symptoms and ends when no further deterioration is noted (usually 1 to 3 weeks)
  2. *Plateau* period, which is a time of little change and lasts several days to 2 weeks
  3. *Recovery* period, which is thought to coincide with remyelination and axonal regeneration and lasts 4 to 6 months

- Chronic inflammatory demyelinating polyneuropathy (CIDP) is an unusual type of GBS that progresses over a longer period; complete recovery rarely occurs.
- The cause of GBS remains obscure, although most evidence implicates a cell-mediated immunologic reaction.
- The client often relates a history of acute illness, trauma, surgery, or immunization 1 to 8 weeks before the onset of neurologic signs and symptoms.
- Three types of GBS are ascending, descending, and Miller-Fisher variant.

  1. *Ascending,* the most common clinical pattern, occurs with weakness and paresthesia beginning in the lower extremities and progressing upward to include the trunk and arms or affecting the cranial nerves and sometimes with respiratory compromise. *Pure motor* GBS is identical to the ascending variant, except sensory signs and symptoms are absent.
  2. In *descending* type, there is weakness of the face or bulbar muscles of the jaw; the sternocleidomastoid muscles; and muscles of the tongue, pharynx, and larynx, progressing downward to involve the limbs. Respiratory compromise can occur quickly.
  3. The *Miller-Fisher variant* consists of a triad of ophthalmoplegia, areflexia, and severe ataxia, with normal motor strength and intact sensory function.

||| Cultural Considerations

- GBS has worldwide distribution and affects people of all races and ages.
- The highest rates have been noted in people 45 years of age and older.
- The incidence is higher in whites than in blacks.

COLLABORATIVE MANAGEMENT

Assessment

- Record past medical and surgical history, including
  1. Occurrence of antecedent illness 1 to 8 weeks before the onset of GBS
  2. Description of symptoms (in chronological order)

- Assessment findings include
  1. Paresthesia (numbness or tingling)
  2. Pain, resembling that of a charley horse
  3. Cranial nerve dysfunction
     a. Facial weakness
     b. Dysphagia
     c. Diplopia
  4. Difficulty walking
  5. Muscle weakness or flaccid paralysis without muscle wasting in an ascending, distal to proximal progression
  6. Respiratory compromise or failure
     a. Dyspnea
     b. Decreased breath sound
     c. Decreased tidal volume or vital capacity
  7. Bowel and bladder incontinence
  8. Autonomic dysfunction evidenced by
     a. Labile blood pressure
     b. Cardiac dysrhythmias
     c. Tachycardia
  9. Decreased or absent deep tendon reflexes
  10. Ability to cope with illness
  11. Anxiety, fear, and panic
  12. Anger and depression

Planning and Implementation

◆**NDx:** Ineffective Breathing Pattern; Ineffective Airway Clearance; Impaired Gas Exchange

- Perform a respiratory assessment
  1. Assess every 4 hours; auscultate breath sounds.
  2. Observe for dyspnea, air hunger, adventitious breath sounds, cyanosis, and confusion.
  3. Measure vital capacity every 2 to 4 hours.
  4. Obtains arterial blood gases as indicated by the client's clinical status.
  5. Remove secretions by encouraging coughing or suctioning; monitor the color, consistency, and amount of secretions obtained.
  6. Administer humidified air or oxygen as appropriate.
  7. Administer ultrasonic nebulizer treatments as appropriate.

8. Keep equipment for intubation and a ventilator available.
9. Perform chest physiotherapy; encourage the client to cough and deep breathe.

- Monitor the client for dysrhythmias
- Monitor vital signs.
- Maintain strict intake and output and monitor for urinary retention.
- Immunoglobulin therapy may be used.
  1. Monitor for side effects such as chills, mild fever, myalgia, headache, anaphylaxis, aseptic meningitis, retinal necrosis, and acute renal failure.
- Plasmapheresis may be used to remove the circulating antibodies thought to be responsible for the disease. Plasma is selectively separated from whole blood; blood cells are returned to the client without the plasma.
  1. Provide information and reassurance to the client.
  2. Weigh the client before and after treatment.
  3. Administer proper care to the shunt by maintaining patency of the shunt, checking for bruits every 2 to 4 hours, and observing the puncture site for bleeding or ecchymosis.
  4. Monitor vital signs.
  5. Keep double bulldog clamps at the bedside.
- Complications of plasmapheresis include hypovolemia, hypokalemia, hypocalcemia, temporary circumoral and distal extremity paresthesia, muscle twitching, nausea, and vomiting.

◆NDx: Acute Pain

- Assess the severity and nature of the client's pain, which is typically worse at night.
- Pain is best treated with opiates, which can be administered via a patient-controlled analgesia (PCA) pump or continuous intravenous drip. Document the client's response to pain medication.
- Other interventions include frequent positioning, massage, ice, heat, relaxation techniques, guided imagery, and distractions.

- The health care team collaborates with the client to develop interventions to prevent complications of immobility and address deficits in self-care.
  1. Assess motor function every 2 to 4 hours.
  2. Assist client with ambulation, transfers from bed to chair, position changes, and maintenance of proper body alignment.
  3. Conduct range-of-motion (ROM) exercises every 2 to 4 hours while client is awake.
  4. Monitor the client's response to or tolerance of activity.
  5. Provide adequate rest periods between activities and therapy session.
  6. Collaborate with the dietitian to develop a nutrition plan; assist with meals as needed.
- Complications of immobility include atelectasis, pneumonia, pressure ulcers, deep vein thrombosis, and pulmonary emboli.
  1. Take actions to prevent or manage these complications such as turning the client and encouraging coughing and deep breathing.
  2. If complications develop, notify the health care provider.

◄NDx: Impaired Verbal Communication

- Interventions include
  1. Assisting the client to develop a communication system in collaboration with the speech-language pathologist.
  2. Developing a communication board that lists common requests.

◄NDx: Powerlessness

- Collaborative interventions include
  1. Encouraging the client to verbalize feelings concerning the illness and its effects
  2. Providing information regarding the disease process
  3. Encouraging the client to participate in his or her care and to make as many choices as possible
  4. Providing encouragement and positive reinforcement
  5. Identifying factors that increase coping abilities through asking the client and family to describe situations that they have successfully coped with in the past

6. Keeping necessary items (call light, radio, or television control) within the client's reach
7. Using the client's own personal items, when feasible

Community-Based Care

- Discharge planning includes
  1. Providing a detailed plan of care at the time of discharge for clients to be transferred to a long-term care or rehabilitation facility (rehabilitation may be lengthy)
  2. Assessing the client and family's knowledge and understanding of the disease
  3. Providing oral and written information on
     a. Techniques to facilitate mobility
     b. Prevention of skin breakdown
     c. ROM exercises
     d. Positioning techniques
  4. Ensuring that client and family members understand how to use assistive devices safely and properly
  5. Referring the client to local or community agencies for assistance in the home setting
  6. Ensuring that adaptive equipment is available
  7. Referring the client to the Guillain-Barré Foundation for information about local resources and educational materials

Gynecomastia

- Gynecomastia is a benign condition of breast enlargement, usually bilateral, in males.
- The condition is caused by proliferation of the glandular tissue, including mammary ducts and ductal stroma.
- Etiologic factors include drugs, aging, and obesity; underlying diseases causing estrogen excess such as malnutrition, liver disease, or hyperthyroidism; and androgen deficiency states such as aging or chronic renal failure.
- The client with gynecomastia is evaluated for breast cancer.

Headache, Cluster

OVERVIEW

- Cluster headaches manifest as unilateral, oculotemporal, or oculofrontal pain described as excruciating, boring, and nonthrobbing.
- They occur every 8 to 12 (and up to 24) hours daily at the same time for a period of 6 to 8 weeks (hence the term *cluster*), followed by a period of remission for 9 months to a year.
- Cluster headaches occur more often in adult men between 20 and 50 years of age than in women.
- The headache, which lasts for approximately 10 to 45 minutes, is accompanied by ipsilateral (same side) tearing of the eye, rhinorrhea or congestion, ptosis, miosis, bradycardia, flushing or pallor of the skin, increased intraocular pressure, and increased skin temperature.

COLLABORATIVE MANAGEMENT

Interventions

- The same types of drugs used to treat migraine headache are used to treat cluster headaches.
- In addition to drugs, 100% oxygen via mask at 5 L/min with the client in a sitting position may be administered for no longer than 15 minutes and is discontinued when the headache is relieved. Oxygen reduces cerebral blood flow and inhibits the activity of the carotid bodies.
- Other interventions include
  1. Instructing the client to wear sunglasses and sit away from windows while the headache is occurring
  2. Helping the client identify precipitating factors such as bursts of anger, excessive physical activity, and excitement
  3. Teaching the client the importance of a consistent sleep-wake cycle

Headache, Migraine

OVERVIEW

- A migraine headache is an episodic disorder manifested by unilateral, frontotemporal, throbbing pain in the head, which is often worse behind one eye or ear.
- This type of headache is often accompanied by a sensitive scalp, anorexia, photophobia, and nausea with or without vomiting.
- Three categories of migraine headache are migraine *with* aura ("classic migraine"), migraine *without* aura, and atypical migraines.

COLLABORATIVE MANAGEMENT

Interventions

- Collaborate with the client to determine factors, if any, that may trigger the development of a headache (e.g., the consumption of monosodium glutamate [MSG], aged cheese, caffeine, chocolate, nitrates, and red wine). Many clients are sensitive to odors from tobacco products, paint or gasoline fumes, perfumes, or aftershave lotion.
- For preventive therapy, the client may take
  1. Nonsteroidal anti-inflammatory drugs (NSAIDs)
  2. Beta blockers such as propranolol (Inderal, Apo-Propranolol) and timolol (Blocadren, Apo-Timol)
  3. Calcium channel blockers
  4. Tricyclic or selective serotonin reuptake inhibitor antidepressants, antiepileptics, or riboflavin (vitamin B_2)
- Drugs used to treat pain after the headache starts include
  1. Ergotamine derivatives such as dihydroergotamine (DHE). DHE should not be given within 24 hours of a triptan preparation.
  2. NSAIDs, acetaminophen (Tylenol, Abenol)
  3. Triptans such as sumatriptan (Imitrex)
     a. Triptans are contraindicated in clients with actual or suspected ischemic heart disease, hypertension, or peripheral vascular disease and in pregnant women.

4. Isometheptene combinations
5. Antiemetics
6. Complementary and alternative therapies that may be used include yoga, meditation, biofeedback, relaxation techniques, acupuncture, and various herbals.

Headache, Tension

OVERVIEW

- Tension headaches are characterized by neck and shoulder muscle tenderness and bilateral pain at the base of the skull and in the forehead.
- Nausea, vomiting, photophobia, phonophobia, and aggravation of the headache with activity may occur.
- Treatment includes non-opioid analgesics, NSAIDs, and muscle relaxants.

Hearing Loss

OVERVIEW

- Hearing loss, one of the most common physical handicaps in North America, is generally thought of as conductive, sensorineural, or a combination of the two.
  1. *Conductive* hearing loss occurs when sound waves are blocked from coming to the inner ear nerve fibers because of external ear or middle ear disorders such as an inflammatory process or an obstruction.
  2. *Sensorineural* hearing loss is caused by a pathologic process of the inner ear or of the sensory fibers that lead to the cerebral cortex (VIII cranial nerve); common causes are prolonged exposure to loud noise, ototoxic drugs, aging (presbycusis), metabolic and circulatory disorders, and bacterial or viral infections.
  3. *Mixed conductive-sensorineural* hearing loss is a combination of the two.

- The etiology of hearing loss determines the degree to which the hearing loss can be corrected and the amount of normal hearing that will return.

Considerations for Older Adults

- It is estimated that 30% to 35% of adults 65 to 75 years of age have some degree of hearing loss, and as much as 50% of the adult population older than 85 years of age has some degree of hearing loss.

COLLABORATIVE MANAGEMENT

Assessment

- Assess for
  1. Pain
  2. Feeling of fullness or congestion
  3. Dizziness or vertigo
  4. Tinnitus
  5. Difficulty understanding conversations, especially in a noisy room
  6. Difficulty hearing sounds; needing to strain to hear
  7. Frequency of asking people to repeat statements
  8. Failure to respond when not looking in the direction of the sound
  9. High volume of television or radio
  10. Avoidance of large groups
  11. Abnormality of the tympanic membrane or ear canal
  12. Abnormally soft or loud voice
  13. Abnormal Rinne test
     a. Air conduction greater than bone conduction in *conductive* hearing loss
     b. Bone conduction greater than air conduction in *sensorineural* hearing loss
  14. Abnormal Weber test
     a. Lateralization to the affected ear in *conductive* hearing loss
     b. Lateralization to the unaffected ear in *sensorineural* hearing loss
  15. Poor hearing in a loud environment; high-frequency soft-discriminating consonants are lost first, especially sounds such as *s, sh, f, th,* and *ch.*
  16. Social isolation

Planning and Implementation

◆**NDx:** Disturbed Sensory Perception (Auditory)

NONSURGICAL MANAGEMENT

- Interventions include the following:
    1. Use the written word if the client is able to see, read, and write.
    2. Use pictures of familiar phrases and objects.
    3. Eliminate distracting noises when talking to the client.
    4. Ensure that there is adequate lighting in the room, when appropriate, especially if the client can read lips.
    5. Do not shout.
    6. Keep hands and other objects away from the mouth when talking to the client.
    7. Position self close to and in front of the client and speak slowly and clearly.
    8. Use lower tones when communicating with a client with a high-frequency hearing loss.
    9. Validate with the client the understanding of statements made by asking the client to repeat what was said.
    10. Administer antibiotics, analgesics, antihistamines, and antiemetics, as ordered, to treat the underlying cause of the hearing loss.
    11. Prevent sudden movements of the client or the client's bed.
    12. Recommend the use of devices such as telephone amplifiers, flashing lights activated by the ringing telephone or doorbell, and a specially trained dog to help the client be aware of sound.
- Cochlear implant is a new and experimental method to treat a sensorineural hearing loss.
- Hearing with a hearing aid can be much different from normal hearing.
    1. Encourage the client to start using the aid slowly to develop an appreciation for the device.
    2. Remind the client that background noises will be amplified as well.
    3. Remind the client to remove the hearing aid when he or she is fatigued.

SURGICAL MANAGEMENT

- The type of surgery performed depends on the cause of the hearing loss.
- *Tympanoplasty* involves reconstruction of the middle ear.
  1. Type I tympanoplasty is also known as a myringoplasty.
  2. Higher grades of tympanoplasties require more extensive reconstruction.
  3. Preoperative care includes
     a. Administering antibiotic drops and irrigating the ear
     b. Instructing the client to avoid people with upper respiratory infections, to get adequate rest, and to maintain nutrition and hydration
     c. Teaching the importance of deep breathing post-operatively (forceful coughing is avoided)
  4. Postoperative care includes
     a. Providing routine postoperative care
     b. Keeping the client flat with the operative ear up for at least 12 hours postoperatively
     c. Monitoring ear canal packing and dressing for drainage and changing dressing when needed using sterile technique
     d. Administering prophylactic antibiotics
     e. Using communication techniques for the hearing impaired until the packing is removed
     f. Instructing the client in postoperative care and activity restrictions
        (1) Avoid straining when having a bowel movement.
        (2) Do not drink through a straw for 2 to 3 weeks.
        (3) Avoid air travel for 2 to 3 weeks.
        (4) Avoid coughing excessively for 2 to 3 weeks.
        (5) Stay away from people with colds.
        (6) Blow the nose gently, one side at a time with mouth open.
        (7) Avoid getting the head wet, washing hair, and showering for the first week after surgery.
        (8) Keep the affected ear dry for 6 weeks by placing a cotton ball coated with petroleum jelly in it; change the cotton ball daily.
        (9) Avoid rapid head movements, bouncing, and bending over for 3 weeks.

(10) Change the dressing on the ear every day or as directed by the physician.

(11) Report excessive drainage from the ear immediately to the physician.

■ A *partial stapedectomy* or *complete stapedectomy* with a prosthesis is most effective for clients with otosclerosis.

1. Preoperative care includes
   a. Assessing for signs and symptoms of external ear infection
   b. Reviewing the expectations from surgery, including an initial increase in hearing loss
   c. Reinforcing with the client that complications such as permanent deafness, prolonged vertigo, infection, and facial nerve damage are possible

2. Postoperative care includes
   a. Providing routine postoperative care
   b. Reminding the client that hearing is temporarily worse after surgery as a result of ear packing and tissue swelling
   c. Administering antibiotics and analgesics
   d. Observing for surgical damage to cranial nerves VII, VIII, and X, including facial weakness, changes in tactile sensation, and changes in taste sensation
   e. Administering antivertiginous drugs such as meclizine hydrochloride (Antivert, Bonamine) and antiemetic drugs such as droperidol (Inapsine) for vertigo, nausea, and vomiting
   f. Assisting the client with ambulation during the first 1 to 2 days after surgery because vertigo is a common complaint
   g. Teaching the client the precautions listed previously under postoperative care for the client having a tympanoplasty

◆**NDx:** Anxiety

■ Nursing interventions include
1. Using special techniques for communicating with the hearing-impaired client (see Nonsurgical Management under the nursing diagnosis Disturbed Sensory Perception)
2. Suggesting that the client obtain closed-captioned programming for the television and an amplifier for the telephone

3. Reminding the client to wear a hearing aid, if appropriate
4. Recommending formal lip reading and sign language classes
5. Helping the client identify support systems and resources to make social contact satisfying

Community-Based Care

- To prevent postoperative complications, instruct the client as follows:
  1. Do not use small objects such as cotton-tipped applicators, matches, toothpicks, or hairpins to clean your external ear canal.
  2. Wash your external ear and canal daily in the shower or while washing your hair.
  3. Blow your nose gently.
  4. Do not occlude one nostril while blowing your nose.
  5. Sneeze with your mouth open.
  6. Wear sound protection around loud or continuous noises.
  7. Avoid activities with high risk for head or ear trauma such as wrestling, motorcycle riding, and skateboarding.
  8. Keep the volume on head receivers at the lowest setting that allows you to hear.
  9. Frequently clean objects that come into contact with your ear (e.g., telephone receiver, headphones).
  10. Avoid environmental conditions with rapid changes in air pressure.
- Discharge planning includes
  1. Assisting the client and family in identifying potential hazards at home to prevent falls associated with vertigo
  2. Providing verbal and written instructions about how to take medications and when to return for follow-up care
  3. Referring the client to the American Speech-Language-Hearing Association, the National Association of Hearing and Speech Agencies, and Self-Help for Hard-of-Hearing People (Shhh)
  4. Referring the client to a home health agency as needed

Heart Failure

OVERVIEW

- *Heart failure* (HF), also called *pump failure,* is the inadequacy of the heart to pump blood throughout the body.
- Heart failure causes insufficient perfusion of body tissue with vital nutrients and oxygen.
- Basic cardiac physiologic mechanisms such as stroke volume, heart rate, cardiac output, and contractility are altered in heart failure.
- Compensatory mechanisms to maintain normal cardiac function are
  1. Increased sympathetic nervous system response, causing increased heart rate, improved stroke volume (Starling's "law of the heart" states that increased myocardial stretch results in more forceful contraction, increasing stroke volume and cardiac output), and arterial vasoconstriction (which also increases afterload)
  2. Sodium and water retention (caused by activation of the renin-angiotensin-aldosterone mechanism when blood flow to the kidney decreases)
  3. Myocardial hypertrophy, which provides more muscle mass, resulting in more effective cardiac contractility, and further increasing cardiac output
- Compensatory mechanisms may eventually cause harmful effects on pump function, contributing to increased myocardial oxygen consumption, causing the signs and symptoms of heart failure.
- The major *types* of heart failure are
  1. Left heart failure, which is further subdivided into systolic heart failure and diastolic heart failure
  2. Right heart failure
  3. High-output failure
- *Left Heart Failure*
  1. Systolic heart failure (systolic ventricular dysfunction)
     a. Systolic failure results when the heart is unable to contract forcefully enough during systole to eject adequate amounts of blood into the circulation, resulting in diminished tissue perfusion.

    b. Preload increases with decreased contractility and afterload increases as a result of increased peripheral resistance.

    c. The ejection fraction drops from a normal of 50% to 70% to below 40%.

    d. Tissue perfusion diminishes and blood accumulates in the pulmonary vessels.

2. Diastolic heart failure (diastolic ventricular function)

    a. Diastolic failure occurs when the left ventricle is unable to relax adequately during diastole, which prevents the ventricle from filling with sufficient blood to ensure an adequate cardiac output.

    b. Ejection fraction may remain near normal.

■ *Right heart (ventricular) failure* occurs when the right ventricle is unable to empty completely.

    1. Increased volume and pressure develop in the systemic veins, and systemic venous congestion develops with peripheral edema.

    2. Right HF in the absence of left failure is most often the result of pulmonary problems.

    3. Acute respiratory distress syndrome may also occur.

    4. *High-output failure* can occur when cardiac output remains normal or above normal and is caused by increased metabolic needs or hyperkinetic conditions such as septicemia, anemia, and hyperthyroidism.

    5. Heart failure may also be categorized by its effect on the client's functional status or staging the disease, which is centered on its risk, evolution, and progression.

    6. Compensatory mechanism operating to improve cardiac output when it is insufficient to meet the demands of the body are

        a. Sympathetic nervous system stimulation

        b. Renin-angiotensin system (RAS) activation

        c. Other neurohumoral responses

        d. Myocardial hypertrophy

Considerations for Older Adults

♦ Heart failure is caused by systemic hypertension in 75% of the cases.

♦ Long-term nonsteroidal anti-inflammatory drugs and thiazolidinediones used for diabetic clients can cause fluid and sodium retention leading to hypertension and subsequently heart failure.

♦ Prevalence of HF increases with age.

COLLABORATIVE MANAGEMENT

Assessment

■ Record client information and assess for
1. Medical history
   a. Hypertension
   b. Angina
   c. Myocardial infarction
   d. Rheumatic heart disease
   e. Valvular disorders
   f. Endocarditis
   g. Pericarditis
2. Perception of breathing pattern
3. Fluid volume status; urinary pattern
4. Response to activity
5. LV failure complaints and assessment
   a. Change in ability to perform activities of daily living (ADLs)
   b. Unusual fatigue or weakness
   c. Feelings of heaviness in arms and legs
   d. Mental status changes, confusion, dizziness
   e. Nocturnal cough; frothy, pink-tinged sputum
   f. Dyspnea; orthopnea, breathlessness
   g. Crackles and wheezes
   h. Orthostatic (postural) hypotension
   i. S_3 or S_4 heart sounds
   j. Increased heart size (assess by palpating the precordium)
   k. Tachycardia
   l. Oliguria
6. RV failure complaints and assessment
   a. Peripheral edema
   b. Weight gain
   c. Gastrointestinal problems such as nausea and anorexia
   d. Diuresis at night
   e. Tight-fitting shoes

f. Indentations from shoes or socks developing on swollen feet
   g. Inability to wear ring because of swollen fingers
   h. Jugular venous distention
   i. Enlarged liver and spleen
   j. Dependent edema (legs and sacrum)
7. Nutritional history
8. Possible kidney function study abnormalities such as elevated blood urea nitrogen (BUN) levels
9. Abnormal arterial blood gas (low arterial oxygen)
10. Enlarged heart on x-ray
11. Dysrhythmias, ventricular hypertrophy, or myocardial ischemia on electrocardiogram (ECG)
12. Elevated pulmonary artery and pulmonary artery wedge pressures in LV failure

Planning and Implementation

◆**NDx:** Impaired Gas Exchange

- Interventions include
   1. Monitoring respiratory rate, rhythm, and character every 1 to 4 hours and auscultating breath sounds
   2. Titrating the amount of supplemental oxygen delivered to maintain oxygen saturation at 92% or greater
   3. Placing the client experiencing respiratory difficulty in high Fowler's position with pillows under each arm to maximize chest expansion and improve oxygenation
   4. Encouraging the client to cough and deep breathe every 2 hours while awake

◆**NDx:** Decreased Cardiac Output

NONSURGICAL MANAGEMENT

- Drug therapy to reduce afterload includes
   1. Angiotensin-converting enzyme (ACE) inhibitors, a group of arterial vasodilators given to prevent conversion of angiotensin I to angiotensin II, resulting in arterial resistance, arterial dilation, and increased stroke volume. ACE inhibitors block aldosterone, which prevents sodium and water retention, thus decreasing fluid overload.
      a. These drugs may cause a rapid drop in blood pressure (BP), especially in clients with a systolic BP less than

100, those who are older than 75 years of age, those who have a serum sodium level less than 136 mEq/L, or those who are volume depleted.

   b. Monitor serum potassium level for hyperkalemia and serum creatinine level for renal dysfunction and the client for development of a cough.

2. Many health care providers maintain the client's systolic BP at 90 to 110 mm Hg. Monitor the client for orthostatic hypotension, confusion, poor peripheral perfusion, and reduced urine output.

- Human B-type natriuretic peptides (hBNP) such as Nesiritide (Natrecor) lowers pulmonary capillary wedge pressure and improves glomerular filtration. This drug may cause dysrhythmias.

- To reduce preload in clients in heart failure who have congestion with total body sodium and water overload, take the following actions:

   1. Collaborate with the dietitian and client to select foods that meet a sodium-restricted diet and to understand the importance of eliminating table salt and salt used in cooking.

   2. Limit the clients with excessive aldosterone secretion who experience thirst to 2 L/day of fluids, including IV fluids.

   3. Weigh the client every morning before breakfast using the same scale; this is the most reliable indicator of fluid gain or loss. (1 kg of weight gain or loss equals 1 L of fluid retained or lost).

   4. Monitor and record intake and output.

- When diet and fluid restrictions are not effective, diuretics are most effective for treating fluid volume overload.

   1. Older clients receiving loop diuretics, especially those with type 2 diabetes mellitus, are susceptible to dehydration.

   2. Thiazide diuretics may be used in older clients with mild volume overload to avoid the excessive diuresis and dehydration that may occur with loop diuretics.

- Monitor for and prevent potassium deficiency from diuretic therapy. If the client's potassium is below 4.0 mEq/L,

   1. A potassium-sparing diuretic may be added to the regimen.

   2. Increase client's intake of potassium-rich foods.

   3. A potassium supplement may be prescribed.

- Recognize that clients with renal problems may develop *hyperkalemia*. Renal problems are indicated by a creatinine level greater than 1.8.
- Venous vasodilators are prescribed for the client in heart failure with persistent dyspnea.
  1. Venous vasodilators are used to return venous vasculature to a more normal capacity, decrease the volume of blood returning to the heart, and improve left ventricular function.
  2. Monitor blood pressure when the medication is first given or the dosage increased.
- Medications are prescribed for clients in heart failure with sinus rhythm and atrial fibrillation.
  1. Digoxin (Lanoxin) increases contractility, reduces heart rate, slows conduction through the arteriovenous node, and inhibits sympathetic activity while enhancing parasympathetic activity; older clients, particularly those who are hypokalemic, are susceptible to digoxin toxicity.
  2. Beta blockers may be started after the client has been on an ACE inhibitor and a diuretic and has been stabilized for 2 weeks.
     a. The first dose is low and the client is monitored for bradycardia, hypotension, and weight gain; the dose is gradually adjusted upward.
     b. Benefits of therapy accrue over time and are not immediate.
- For clients with *diastolic* heart failure, drug therapy has not been as effective. Calcium channel blockers, ACE inhibitors, and beta blockers have been used with varying degrees of success.
- Other options to treat heart failure include
  1. Continuous positive airway pressure (CPAP) improves sleep apnea and cardiac output and ejection fraction.
  2. Cardiac resynchronization therapy (CRT) uses a permanent pacemaker alone or in combination with an implantable cardioverter-defibrillator to provide biventricular pacing.
  3. Investigative gene therapy, which replaces damaged genes with normal or modified genes by a series of injections of growth factor into the left ventricle

- Heart transplantation is the ultimate choice for end-stage heart failure.
- Procedures to improve cardiac output in clients who are not candidates for heart transplant or are awaiting transplant include
  1. Left ventricular assist device (LVAD)
  2. Right ventricular assist device (RVAD)
- Newer surgical therapies to reshape the left ventricle in clients with heart failure include
  1. Partial left ventriculectomy
  2. Endoventricular circular patch
  3. Acorn cardiac support device
  4. Myosplint

◆NDx: Activity Intolerance

- The purpose of interdisciplinary interventions is to regulate energy to prevent fatigue and optimize function.
  1. Provide periods of uninterrupted rest.
  2. Assess the client's response to increased activity. Before and after check for changes in BP and pulse (increase in BP of more than 20 mm Hg or increase in pulse rate of more than 20 beats/min from baseline) and oxygen saturation.
  3. Assess for increased fatigue, dyspnea, or chest pain when activity increases.

◆NDx: Potential for Pulmonary Edema

- Interventions include
  1. Assessing the client with heart failure for acute *pulmonary edema*. Clinical manifestations include extreme anxiety; tachycardia; air hunger; moist cough productive of frothy, blood-tinged sputum; and cold, clammy, cyanotic skin, crackles in lung bases, disorientation, and confusion.
  2. Administering rapid-acting diuretics, as prescribed
  3. Providing oxygen and maintaining the client in a high Fowler's position
  4. Administering morphine sulfate intravenously, 1 to 2 mg at a time, to reduce venous return (preload), decrease anxiety, and reduce the work of breathing
  5. Administering other drugs such as bronchodilators and vasodilators

6. Monitoring vital signs closely including pulse oximetry
7. Monitoring intake and output; catheterizing if prescribed
8. Monitoring the client carefully to determine the necessity of intubation and mechanical ventilation

Community-Based Care

- Collaborate with the case manager or social worker to assess the client's needs for health care resources (home care nurse, etc.) and social support (family and friends to help with care if needed), and facilitate appropriate placement.
- Discharge preparation includes
    1. Encouraging the client to stay as active as possible and developing a regular exercise program
        a. Begin walking 200 to 400 feet/day 3 times per week, then gradually increase the frequency and duration.
        b. If the client experiences chest pain or pronounced dyspnea while exercising, or experiences fatigue the next day, he or she is probably advancing the activity too quickly and should slow down.
    2. Instructing the client to watch for and report to the physician
        a. Weight gain of more than 3 pounds in 1 week or 1 to 2 pounds overnight
        b. Decrease in exercise tolerance lasting 2 to 3 days
        c. Cold symptoms (cough) lasting more than 3 to 5 days
        d. Frequent urination at night
        e. Development of dyspnea or angina at rest, or worsening angina
        f. Increased swelling in the feet, ankles, and hands
    3. Providing oral and written instructions concerning medications. If discharged on digoxin, teaching the client and caregiver how to take and record the pulse rate
    4. Instructing the client to weigh him- or herself each day in the morning
    5. Reviewing the signs and symptoms of hypokalemia for clients on diuretics and providing information on foods high in potassium
    6. Recommending that the client restrict dietary sodium, providing written instructions on low-salt diets, and identifying food flavorings to use as a substitute for salt, such as lemon, garlic, and herbs

7. Discussing the importance of advance directives with the client or family. If resuscitation is desired, the family should know how to activate the Emergency Medical System and how to provide CPR until an ambulance arrives. If CPR is not desired, the client and family should be given resources on what to do and how to respond.
8. Referring the client to the American Heart Association for information and support groups

Hemophilia

OVERVIEW

- Hemophilia comprises two hereditary bleeding disorders resulting from deficiencies of specific clotting factors that impair the hemostatic response and the capacity to form a stable fibrin clot.
  1. *Hemophilia A* (classic hemophilia) is a deficiency of factor VIII and accounts for 80% of all cases.
  2. *Hemophilia B* (Christmas disease) is a deficiency of factor IX and accounts for 20% of all cases.
- Hemophilia is an X-linked recessive trait; female carriers risk transmitting the gene for hemophilia to half of their daughters (who are then carriers) and to half of their sons (who will have overt hemophilia).
- Abnormal bleeding occurs, which may be mild, moderate, or severe, depending on the degree of factor deficiency in response to any trauma.

COLLABORATIVE MANAGEMENT

- Assess for
  1. Excessive hemorrhage from minor cuts, bruises, or abrasions
  2. Joint and muscle hemorrhages (degenerative)
  3. Tendency to bruise easily
  4. Prolonged and potentially fatal postoperative hemorrhage
  5. Prolonged partial thromboplastin time, normal bleeding time, and normal prothrombin time

- The bleeding problems of hemophilia A are managed by either regularly scheduled intravenous infusions of factor VIII cryoprecipitate or intermittent infusions as needed.

Hemorrhoids

OVERVIEW

- Hemorrhoids are unnaturally swollen or distended veins in the anorectal region that are common and not significant unless they cause pain or bleeding.
- Increased intra-abdominal pressure causes elevated systemic and portal venous pressure, which is transmitted to the anorectal veins.
- *Internal* hemorrhoids cannot be seen on inspection of the perianal area and lie above the anal sphincter.
- *External* hemorrhoids can be seen on inspection and lie below the anal sphincter.
- *Prolapsed* hemorrhoids can become thrombosed or inflamed, or they can bleed.
- Common causes of repeated increased abdominal pressure are straining at stool, pregnancy, and portal hypertension.

COLLABORATIVE MANAGEMENT

Assessment

- Common symptoms are bleeding, which is characteristically bright red and found on toilet tissue or outside the stool; pain associated with thrombosis; itching; and mucous discharge.
- Diagnosis is made by inspection, digital examination, and proctoscopy, if needed.

Interventions

- Conservative treatment, which is aimed at reducing symptoms, includes
  1. Application of cold packs to the anorectal area followed by tepid sitz baths

2. Witch hazel soaks and topical anesthetics such as lidocaine (Xylocaine)
3. Over-the-counter remedies such as Nupercainal ointment used temporarily; prolonged use can mask worsening symptoms and delay diagnosis of a severe disorder
4. High-fiber diet and fluids to promote regular bowel movements without straining
5. Stool softeners
6. Teaching the client to cleanse the anal area with moistened cleaning tissues and to gently dab the area rather than wipe

SURGICAL MANAGEMENT

- Surgical methods, including ultrasound, sclerotherapy, circular stapling, or hemorrhoidectomy, are indicated for recurring symptoms.
- Instruct the client with hemorrhoids to
  1. Adhere to a high-fiber, high-fluid diet to promote regular bowel patterns.
  2. Use local treatments for symptom relief.
- Postoperative care includes
  1. Monitor for bleeding and pain.
  2. Apply moist heat (e.g., sitz baths) three to four times a day after the first 12 hours postoperatively.
  3. Administer stool softeners such as docusate sodium (Colace).
  4. Administer opioid analgesia postoperatively and before the first defecation.

Hemothorax

- Hemothorax is blood loss into the thoracic cavity and is a common result of blunt chest trauma or penetrating injuries.
  1. *Simple hemothorax* is a blood loss of less than 1500 mL
  2. *Massive hemothorax* is a blood loss of more than 1500 mL
- The bleeding is caused by injuries to the lung parenchyma and is associated with rib and sternal fractures.

- Massive intrathoracic bleeding stems from injury to the heart, great vessels, or major systemic arteries.
- Physical assessment findings depend on the size of the hemothorax.
  1. Asymptomatic for small hemothorax
  2. Respiratory distress for large hemothorax with diminished breath sounds and a dull percussion note on the affected side
- Interventions, aimed at removing blood in the pleural space to normalize pulmonary function and prevent infection, include anterior and posterolateral chest tube insertion.
- An open thoracotomy may be considered if there is an initial evacuation of 1500 to 2000 mL of blood or persistent bleeding of more than 200 mL/hr over 3 hours.
- Nursing interventions include all of the following:
  1. Monitor the client's vital signs.
  2. Monitor for increased blood loss.
  3. Measure intake and output.
  4. Assess the client's response to chest tubes.
  5. Administer intravenous fluids and blood, as ordered. Autotransfusion of blood lost through chest drainage may be considered.

Hepatitis

OVERVIEW

- Hepatitis is the widespread inflammation of liver cells, resulting in enlargement of the liver and congestion with inflammatory cells.
- Viral hepatitis is the most prevalent type and is caused by one of five common viruses.
  1. **Hepatitis A virus (HAV)**
     a. HAV is spread by the fecal-oral route, by the oral ingestion of fecal contaminants, or by oral-anal sexual activity. It is characterized by a mild course and often goes unrecognized. HAV is the most common type of viral hepatitis.

b. Sources of infection include contaminated water, shellfish caught in contaminated water, and food contaminated by food handlers infected with the HAV.

c. The incubation period is usually between 15 and 50 days, with an average of 4 weeks.

2. **Hepatitis B virus (HBV)**

a. Formerly known as serum hepatitis, HBV is transmitted via the skin and mucous membrane route by contamination with blood and serous fluids.

b. Lower concentrations of HBV are also found in semen, vaginal fluid, and saliva.

c. HBV is also spread via sexual contact, shared needles, accidental needlesticks or injuries from sharp instruments, blood transfusion, hemodialysis, acupuncture, tattooing, ear/body piercing, and mother-fetal route.

d. The clinical course is varied, with an insidious onset and mild symptoms (anorexia, nausea, vomiting, fever, fatigue, dark urine with light stool).

e. The incubation period is generally between 25 and 180 days.

f. Chronic liver disease develops in approximately 1% to 10% of adult clients with acute HBV infection.

3. **Hepatitis C virus (HCV)**

a. The causative virus is an enveloped, single-strand RNA virus that is transmitted by exposure of the skin and mucous membrane to blood and plasma.

b. HCV is spread by contaminated items such as illicit intravenous (IV) drug needles, blood, blood products or organ transplants received before 1992, needle stick injury with HCV-contaminated blood, tattoo, and intranasal cocaine use.

c. It is not transmitted by casual contact or intimate household contacts. However, those infected should not share razors, toothbrushes, or pierced earrings because there may be microscopic blood on these items.

d. The incubation period is 21 to 140 days, with an average incubation period of 7 weeks.

e. Chronic liver disease occurs in 85% of those infected and is the leading indicator for liver transplantation.

4. **Delta hepatitis (hepatitis D virus or HDV)**
    a. Hepatitis D virus is caused by a defective RNA virus that needs the helper function of HBV. HDV co-infects with HBV and needs its presence for viral replications.
    b. Incubation period is 14 to 56 days.
    c. HDV is transmitted primarily by parenteral routes.
5. **Hepatitis E virus (HEV)**
    a. HEV was originally identified by its association with epidemics of hepatitis in the Indian subcontinent and has since been found in epidemics in Asia, Africa, Mexico, the Middle East, and Central and South America.
    b. In the United States and Canada, HEV has occurred in people who have visited these endemic areas.
    c. HEV is transmitted by the oral-fecal route and resembles HAV. Incubation period is 15 to 64 days.
- Toxic and drug-induced hepatitis result from exposure to hepatotoxins such as industrial toxins, alcohol, or medication. Treatment is supportive.
- Hepatitis may occur as a secondary infection during the course of other viral infections such as cytomegalovirus, Epstein-Barr virus, herpes simplex virus, and varicella zoster virus.
- Fulminant hepatitis is a failure of the liver cells to regenerate, with progression of the necrotic process that is often fatal.
- Liver inflammation persisting longer than 6 months is considered chronic hepatitis.

COLLABORATIVE MANAGEMENT

Assessment
- Record client information.
    1. Known exposure to hepatitis
    2. Recent blood transfusions or blood transfusion before 1992
    3. History of hemodialysis
    4. Sexual preferences
    5. Injectable drug use
    6. Recent ear or body piercing
    7. Recent tattooing
    8. Living accommodations, including crowded facilities

9. Health care employment history
  10. Recent travel to foreign countries
  11. Recent ingestion of shellfish or contaminated water
- Assessment finding for viral hepatitis include
   1. Weakness and fatigue
   2. Loss of appetite
   3. Abdominal pain
   4. Myalgias (muscle pain)
   5. Arthralgia (joint pain)
   6. Diarrhea/constipation
   7. Irritability
   8. Malaise
   9. Nausea and vomiting
  10. Liver tenderness in the right upper quadrant
  11. Jaundice of the skin, mucous membranes, and sclera
  12. Dark urine
  13. Clay-colored stools
  14. Rashes, pruritus
  15. Fever
  16. Elevated serum liver enzymes
  17. Elevated total bilirubin (serum and urine)
  18. Serologic markers for hepatitis A, B, C, or D
- The clinical manifestations of toxic and drug-induced hepatitis depend on the causative agent.
- Clients may be angry about being sick and being fatigued; may feel guilty about having exposed others to the disease; may be embarrassed by the isolation and hygiene precautions that are necessary; and may be worried about the loss of wages, cost of hospitalization, and general financial issues.
- Family members may be afraid of contracting the disease and therefore distance themselves from the client.

Interventions

- Promote rest.
   1. Maintain physical rest alternating with periods of activity to promote liver cell regeneration by reducing the liver's metabolic needs.

2. Individualize the client's plan of care and change it to reflect the severity of symptoms, fatigue, and results of liver function tests and enzyme determinations.
3. Promote emotional and psychological rest.

- Provide diet therapy. A special diet is not needed, but diet should be high in carbohydrates and calories with moderate amounts of fat and protein.
  1. Determine food preferences.
  2. Provide small, frequent meals.
  3. Provide high-calorie snacks as needed.
- Drug therapy includes
  1. Supplemental vitamins
  2. Antiemetics, such as trimethobenzamide hydrochloride (Tigan, Tegamide) or dimenhydrinate (Dramamine, Travamine), as ordered, to relieve nausea
  3. Drugs for HBV and HCV include antiviral medications and immunomodulators
  4. Drugs for HBV include lamivudine (Epivir-HBV) and adefovir dipivoxil (Hepsera), which are oral antiviral drugs and interferon.
  5. Drugs for HCV include subcutaneous interferon and oral ribavirin.
- Liver transplantation may be performed for clients with chronic hepatitis.

Community-Based Care

- Provide health teaching on
  1. Modes of transmission of hepatitis
  2. Observation of measures to prevent infection transmission
  3. Avoiding alcohol and checking with the health care provider before taking any over-the-counter medication or any vitamin, supplement, or herbal preparation
  4. Determination of activity tolerance and rest
  5. Eating small, frequent meals of high-carbohydrate and low-fat foods
  6. Avoiding sexual activity until HBV surface antigen (HBsAg) testing results are negative

Hernia

- A hernia is a weakness in the abdominal muscle wall through which a segment of bowel or other abdominal structure protrudes. It results from a defect in the integrity of the muscular wall and increased intra-abdominal pressure.
- Common types of hernias are
  1. *Indirect inguinal* hernia, a sac formed from the peritoneum that contains a portion of the intestine or omentum; in males, indirect hernias can become large and descend into the scrotum
  2. *Direct inguinal* hernia, which passes through a weak point in the abdominal wall
  3. *Femoral* hernia, which occurs through the femoral ring as a plug of fat in the femoral canal that enlarges and pulls the peritoneum and the bladder into the sac
  4. *Umbilical* hernia, which is congenital (infancy) or acquired as a result of increased intra-abdominal pressure, most often in obese persons
  5. *Incisional* (ventral) hernia, which occurs at the site of a previous surgical incision as a result of inadequate healing, postoperative wound infection, inadequate nutrition, or obesity
- A *reducible* hernia allows the contents of the hernial sac to be reduced or placed back into the abdominal cavity.
- An *irreducible,* or incarcerated, hernia cannot be reduced or placed back into the abdominal cavity. It requires immediate surgical evaluation.
- A *strangulated* hernia results when the blood supply to the herniated segment of the bowel is cut off by pressure from the hernial ring, causing ischemia and obstruction of the bowel loop; this can lead to bowel necrosis and perforation.

Considerations for Older Adults

- The older adult with a strangulated hernia may not complain of pain but usually has nausea and vomiting.
- Direct inguinal hernias occur more often in older adults than in younger persons.

COLLABORATIVE MANAGEMENT

Assessment

- Assess for hernia presence when the client is lying down and again when the client is standing; if it is reducible, it may disappear when the client is lying flat.
- Listen for bowel sounds (absence may indicate obstruction) and palpate the hernia and its location.

Interventions

NONSURGICAL MANAGEMENT

- A truss (a pad with firm support) may be used for older or debilitated clients who are poor surgical risks.

SURGICAL MANAGEMENT

- *Herniorrhaphy,* the surgical treatment of choice, involves replacing the contents of the hernial sac into the abdominal cavity and closing the opening.
- *Hernioplasty* may be required to reinforce the weakened muscular wall with a mesh patch.
- Postoperative instructions include
  1. Avoid coughing.
  2. Deep breathe and turn frequently to promote lung expansion.
  3. For indirect inguinal hernia repair, wear a scrotal support and apply an ice bag to the scrotum to prevent swelling.
- Nursing care includes
  1. For indirect inguinal hernia repair, elevating the scrotum with a soft pillow
  2. Encouraging early ambulation unless contraindicated
  3. Using techniques to stimulate voiding, such as assisting the male client to stand
  4. Ensuring an intake of at least 1500 to 2500 mL of fluids per day
  5. Catheterizing the client every 6 to 8 hours if he or she is unable to void

Community-Based Care

- Teach the client
  1. How to care for the incision

2. To limit activity, including avoiding lifting and straining, for 2 weeks after surgery.
3. To report symptoms such as fever and chills, wound drainage, redness or separation of the incision, and increasing incisional pain to the health care provider.

Hernia, Hiatal

OVERVIEW

- Hiatal hernias, also called diaphragmatic hernias, involve the protrusion of the stomach through the esophageal hiatus of the diaphragm into the thorax.
- There are two major types of hiatal hernia.
  1. *Sliding* hernia, which occurs when the esophagogastric junction and a portion of the fundus of the stomach slide upward through the esophageal hiatus into the thorax, with the hernia moving freely and sliding into and out of the thorax when there are changes in position or intra-abdominal pressure increases
  2. *Paraesophageal* or rolling hernia, which occurs when the gastroesophageal junction stays below the diaphragm but the fundus and portions of the greater curvature of the stomach roll through the esophageal hiatus and into the thorax beside the esophagus; risk for volvulus, obstruction, and strangulation are high

COLLABORATIVE MANAGEMENT

Assessment

- Assess for
  1. General appearance and nutritional status
  2. Heartburn
  3. Regurgitation (esophageal reflux)
  4. Pain
  5. Dysphagia
  6. Belching
  7. Symptoms of sliding hernia associated with reflux

8. Symptoms of rolling hernia include
   a. A feeling of fullness after eating
   b. A feeling of breathlessness or suffocation
9. Increased symptoms when in a recumbent position
- Barium swallow study with fluoroscopy is the most specific diagnostic test.

Interventions

NONSURGICAL MANAGEMENT

- Drug therapy includes the use of antacids and histamine receptor antagonists to control esophageal reflux and its symptoms.
- Teach the client to avoid fatty foods, coffee, tea, cola, chocolate, alcohol, spicy foods, and acidic foods such as orange juice.
- Encourage the client to eat four to six small meals per day.
- Teach the client to avoid nighttime snacking to ensure that the stomach is empty before bedtime.
- Encourage weight reduction because obesity increases intra-abdominal pressure.
- Elevate the head of the bed 6 inches to reduce the incidence of esophageal reflux.
- Instruct the client to avoid lying down several hours after eating, straining or excessively vigorous exercise, or wearing tight or constrictive clothing.

SURGICAL MANAGEMENT

- Elective surgery is indicated when the risk of complications such as aspiration are high and damage from chronic reflux is severe.
- Provide routine preoperative care. In addition
  1. If the surgery is not urgent, encourage the client who is overweight to lose weight and the client who smokes to significantly cut back on tobacco use before surgery.
  2. Inform the client that he or she will have a nasogastric tube (NG) after surgery.
  3. Determine whether the client will have a chest tube after surgery and include this information in preoperative teaching.

- Surgical approaches for sliding hernias involve reinforcement of the lower esophageal sphincter (LES) to restore sphincter competence and prevent reflux, through some degree of *fundoplication,* or the wrapping of a portion of the stomach fundus around the distal esophagus to anchor it and reinforce the LES.
- Provide postoperative care similar to that for any client with esophageal surgery.
  1. Assess for complications of surgery, such as temporary dysphagia after oral feeding begins, gas bloat syndrome, atelectasis or pneumonia, and obstruction of the NG tube.
  2. Provide adequate pain relief.
  3. Elevate the head of the bed at least 30 degrees.
  4. Teach the client to support the incisional area during coughing and deep breathing.
  5. Teach the client to use the incentive spirometer.
  6. Ensure correct placement and patency of the NG tube.
  7. Supervise the first oral feedings.
  8. Teach the client to avoid drinking carbonated beverages, eating gas-producing foods (especially high-fat foods), chewing gum, and drinking with a straw.
  9. Encourage frequent position changes and ambulation.

Community-Based Care

- Teach the client
  1. Activity restriction following hiatal hernia repair, including avoidance of straining and lifting and restrictions on stair climbing
  2. To inspect the surgical wound daily and report the incidence of swelling, redness, tenderness, or discharge to the physician
  3. The importance of reporting fever to the physician
  4. To avoid prolonged coughing episodes to prevent dehiscence of the fundoplication
  5. Smoking cessation
  6. Diet restrictions, including modifying the size and timing of meals, avoiding irritating foods and liquids, and reporting recurrence of reflux symptoms to the physician
  7. To avoid straining and prevent constipation while having a bowel movement; stool softeners or bulk laxatives may be needed

Herpes, Genital

- Genital herpes simplex is an acute, recurring, incurable viral disease.
- The two types of herpes simplex are
  Type 1 HSV, which causes most nongenital lesions, including cold sores
  Type 2 HSV, which causes most genital lesions
- The incubation period is 2 to 20 days, with an average of 1 week.

H

COLLABORATIVE MANAGEMENT

Assessment

- Assess for
  1. Tingling sensation on the skin
  2. Appearance of vesicles (blisters) in a characteristic cluster on the penis, scrotum, vulva, perineum, vagina, cervix, or perianal region
  3. Headache
  4. Fever
  5. Generalized malaise
  6. Painful urination
  7. Positive result of a culture
- After lesions heal, the virus remains in a dormant state in the nerve ganglia.
- Periodically, the virus may activate, and episodes of infection recur.
- Recurrent episodes are usually less severe and of shorter duration than the primary infection. Some clients have no symptoms; however, there is viral shedding and the client is infectious.
- Long-term complications of genital herpes include the risks of cervical cancer, neonatal transmission, and HIV infection.

Interventions

- Antiviral drugs are used to decrease the severity, promote healing, and decrease the frequency of recurrent outbreaks.

- Mild recurrent episodes do not benefit from treatment with antiviral drugs.
- Emphasize the risk of fetal infection; maternity care providers should know of this history to ensure appropriate care for the mother and infant.
- Teach the client to prevent infection by
  1. Encouraging genital hygiene and keeping the skin clean and dry
  2. Wearing gloves while applying ointments
  3. Avoiding sexual activity when lesions are present
  4. Using condoms during all sexual activity
- Help clients cope with the diagnosis
  1. Assess the client's response to the diagnosis of genital herpes
  2. Be sensitive and supportive during care
  3. Refer the client to support groups, such as HELP

Hodgkin's Lymphoma and Non-Hodgkin's Lymphoma

OVERVIEW

- *Hodgkin's lymphoma* is a cancer originating in a single lymph node or a single chain of nodes. The lymphoid tissues within the node undergo malignant transformation. These nodes contain a specific transformed cell type, the Reed-Sternberg cell, which is a characteristic marker of Hodgkin's lymphoma.
- *Non-Hodgkin's lymphoma* includes all lymphoid cancers that do not have the Reed-Sternberg cells and is treated with aggressive chemotherapy.
- The initially localized disease (both forms) first spreads in a predictable manner to nearby lymph tissues and eventually invades nonlymphoid tissues.
- Factors implicated as causes include viral infections and exposure to chemical agents.
- Common first assessment finding is a large but painless lymph node or nodes, usually in the neck, fever, malaise and night sweats.

COLLABORATIVE MANAGEMENT

- Treatment is based on staging procedures (biopsy of distant nodes, computed tomography [CT] of thorax and abdomen, complete blood count [CBC], liver function studies, and bilateral bone marrow biopsies), which determine the exact extent of the disease.
- Treatment includes extensive external radiation of involved lymph node regions for stages I and II without mediastinal node involvement; more extensive disease requires radiation coupled with combination chemotherapy.
- Nursing management focuses on the side effects of therapy, especially
  1. Infection
  2. Bleeding
  3. Anemia
  4. Nausea and vomiting
  5. Skin problems at the site of radiation
  6. Impaired hepatic function
  7. Permanent sterility in men receiving radiation in an inverted Y pattern to the abdominopelvic region along with specific chemotherapeutic agents (Men are given the option of sperm storage in a sperm bank before treatment begins.)

Huntington's Chorea

OVERVIEW

- Huntington's chorea is a hereditary disorder transmitted as an autosomal dominant trait at the time of conception.
- It is most prevalent in people of western European ancestry.
- The two main symptoms of the disease are progressive mental status changes leading to dementia and choreiform movements.
- Other clinical manifestations of Huntington's chorea include poor balance, hesitant or explosive speech, dysphagia, impaired respirations, and bowel and bladder incontinence. Mental status changes include decreased attention span, poor

judgment, memory loss, personality changes, and later, dementia.

COLLABORATIVE MANAGEMENT

- There is no known cure or treatment of the disease.
- The only way to prevent transmission of the gene is for those affected to refrain from having children.
- Genetic testing is an option for people at risk of Huntington's chorea to determine whether they have the gene on chromosome 4; however, results of the test are subject to error.
- Management of the disease is symptomatic.
- Nursing interventions are directed toward treating the following nursing diagnoses:
  1. Impaired physical mobility
  2. Imbalanced nutrition: less than body requirements
  3. Total urinary incontinence
  4. Total self-care deficit
  5. Disturbed body image and ineffective role performance
  6. Risk for injury
  7. Ineffective airway clearance, ineffective breathing pattern, and impaired gas exchange
- As the symptoms progress, the client's status deteriorates, and death occurs from complications of immobility, such as pneumonia or sepsis.

Hydrocele

OVERVIEW

- A hydrocele is a cystic mass, usually filled with straw-colored fluid, that forms around the testes.
- A hydrocele is the result of a disorder in the lymphatic drainage of the scrotum, causing a swelling of the tunica vaginalis, which surrounds the testes.

- A hydrocele may be aspirated via needle and syringe or surgically removed.
- Provide postoperative care.
  1. Inform the client that if an incision drain is present, there is usually some serosanguineous drainage for the first 24 to 48 hours after surgery.
  2. Teach the client the importance of wearing a scrotal support to keep the scrotal dressing in place and keep the scrotum elevated to prevent edema.
  3. Assess the client for pain and infection.
  4. Reassure the client that swelling will subside over several weeks.

Hydronephrosis, Hydroureter, and Urethral Stricture

OVERVIEW

- Several disorders are associated with obstruction of the outflow of urine.
- In *hydronephrosis,* the kidney becomes enlarged as urine accumulates in the renal pelvis and the calyces. Obstruction within the pelvis or ureteropelvic junction results in renal pelvic distention, and extensive damage to the vasculature and renal tubules can result.
- *Hydroureter* is the obstruction of the ureter at the point of the iliac vessel crossing or the ureterovesical entry. Dilation of the ureter occurs at the point proximal to the obstruction as urine accumulates.
- A *urethral stricture* is the most distal point of obstruction, with bladder distention occurring before hydroureter and hydronephrosis.
- *Urinary tract obstruction* results in direct pressure buildup on the tissue, causing structural damage.

- Within the nephron, the tubular filtrate pressure increases as drainage through the collecting system is impaired, resulting in decreased glomerular filtration and renal failure.
- Causes of hydronephrosis and hydroureter include tumors, stones, trauma, congenital structural defects, and retroperitoneal fibrosis; pregnancy may cause ureteral dilation.
- Urethral stricture occurs from chronic inflammation.

COLLABORATIVE MANAGEMENT

- Record client information.
  1. History of known renal or urologic disorders
  2. Childhood urinary tract problems
  3. Pattern of urination, including amount and frequency
  4. Description of urine, including color, clarity, and odor
  5. Report of symptoms, including flank or abdominal pain, chills, fever, and malaise
- Assess for
  1. Flank asymmetry and pain
  2. Abdominal tenderness or pain
  3. Bladder distention
  4. Urine leakage with abdominal pressure
  5. Bacteria or white blood cells in the urine if infection is present
  6. Enlarged ureter or kidney on x-ray film and intravenous pyelography
- Urinary retention and risk for infection are primary problems.
- Treatment measures are aimed at correcting the cause of obstruction.
- Failure to treat the cause of urinary obstruction may result in renal failure.

Hyperaldosteronism

OVERVIEW

- Hyperaldosteronism is defined as an increased secretion of aldosterone by the adrenal glands, resulting in mineralocorticoid excess.

- Primary hyperaldosteronism (Conn's syndrome), which results from excessive secretion of aldosterone from one or both adrenal glands, is usually caused by the presence of an adenoma.
- Secondary hyperaldosteronism, the continuous excessive secretion of aldosterone, is caused by high levels of angiotensin II that are stimulated by high plasma renin levels caused by renal hypoxemia and the use of thiazide diuretics.
- Hyperaldosteronism is manifested by hypernatremia, hypokalemia, metabolic alkalosis, hypertension, headache, fatigue, muscle weakness, and nocturia.

COLLABORATIVE MANAGEMENT

- *Adrenalectomy,* either unilateral or bilateral, is the surgery of choice in most cases.
- Provide preoperative care.
    1. Correct abnormal potassium levels by administering potassium supplements, if needed.
    2. Provide a low-sodium diet preoperatively as ordered; there are no restrictions postoperatively.
    3. Administer temporary glucocorticoid replacement if a unilateral adrenalectomy is performed or permanent replacement if a bilateral adrenalectomy is performed.
    4. Before surgery or if surgery is inadvisable, administer spironolactone (Aldactone, Sincomen), a potassium-sparing diuretic and aldosterone antagonist, to promote fluid balance.
    5. Instruct the client about side effects of spironolactone.
        a. Hyperkalemia (in the client with impaired renal function or excessive potassium intake)
        b. Hyponatremia (dry mouth, thirst, lethargy)
        c. Gynecomastia
        d. Diarrhea
        e. Urticaria, rash
        f. Inability to maintain an erection, hirsutism, and amenorrhea

Hypercalcemia

OVERVIEW

- Hypercalcemia is a serum calcium level exceeding 10.5 mg/dL or 2.75 mmol/L.
- Small increases in serum calcium can have severe effects on body function.
- Common causes of hypercalcemia include
  1. Increased absorption of calcium
     a. Excessive oral intake of calcium
     b. Excessive oral intake of vitamin D
  2. Decreased excretion of calcium
     a. Renal failure
     b. Use of thiazide diuretics
  3. Increased bone resorption of calcium
     a. Hyperparathyroidism
     b. Malignancy
        (1) Direct invasion (cancers of breast, lung, prostate, and osteoclastic bone and multiple myeloma)
        (2) Indirect resorption (liver cancer, small cell lung cancer, cancer of the adrenal gland)
     c. Hyperthyroidism
     d. Immobility
     e. Use of glucocorticoids
  4. Hemoconcentration
     a. Dehydration
     b. Use of lithium
     c. Adrenal insufficiency

COLLABORATIVE MANAGEMENT

Assessment

- Assess for
  1. Cardiovascular manifestations, the most serious and life-threatening changes
     a. Increased heart rate
     b. Increased blood pressure
     c. Bounding, full peripheral pulses

    d. Electrocardiogram (ECG) abnormalities (severe or prolonged hypercalcemia)

       (1) Shortened ST segment

       (2) Widened T wave

          (a) Assess for presence of Homans' sign

          (b) Potentiation of digoxin-associated toxicities

          (c) Decreased clotting time

          (d) Late-phase manifestations

       (3) Bradycardia

       (4) Cardiac arrest, sinus arrest

2. Neuromuscular manifestations

    a. Disorientation, lethargy, coma

    b. Profound muscle weakness

    c. Diminished or absent deep tendon reflexes

3. Gastrointestinal manifestations

    a. Decreased motility

    b. Hypoactive bowel sounds

    c. Anorexia, nausea

    d. Abdominal distention

    e. Constipation

4. Respiratory manifestations (ineffective respiratory movement related to profound skeletal muscle weakness)

5. Renal manifestations

    a. Increased urinary output

    b. Dehydration

    c. Formation of renal calculi

Interventions

- Provide drug therapy.

    1. Discontinue all intravenous (IV) infusions and oral medications containing calcium.

    2. Discontinue drugs containing calcium or vitamin D.

    3. Discontinue thiazide diuretics; furosemide (Lasix, Furoside ✦) may be administered to increase the excretion of calcium.

    4. May administer

       a. Intravenous normal saline because sodium increases excretion of calcium in the urine

       b. Calcium chelators or binders such as penicillamine (Cuprimine, Pendramine)

5. May administer drugs that inhibit calcium resorption from the bone
   a. Phosphorus
   b. Calcitonin (Calcimar)
   c. Bisphosphonates (Etidronate)
   d. Prostaglandin synthesis inhibitors (aspirin, nonsteroidal anti-inflammatory drugs [NSAIDs])

- Peritoneal dialysis, hemodialysis, and blood ultrafiltration may be used to treat the client with life-threatening hypercalcemia.
- Continuous cardiac monitoring may be ordered.
   1. Compare recent ECG tracings with the client's baseline tracings or tracings obtained when the client's serum calcium was normal.
   2. Examine the ECG for changes in T waves and the QT interval, as well as for changes in rate and rhythm.
- Other interventions include
   1. Monitor intake and output
   2. Monitor for fluid overload
   3. Encourage mobilization to prevent bone resorption

Hypercortisolism (Cushing's Syndrome)

OVERVIEW

- Hypersecretion by the adrenal cortex results in hypercortisolism, or Cushing's syndrome, hyperaldosteronism (excessive mineralocorticoid production), or excessive androgen production.
- Cushing's syndrome is a group of clinical problems caused by an excess or cortisol secreted by the adrenal cortex (endogenous) or given for another clinical disorder (exogenous or iatrogenic).

COLLABORATIVE MANAGEMENT

Assessment

- Record client information.
  1. Change in activity or sleep pattern
  2. Medical history
     a. Steroid or alcohol abuse
     b. Frequency of infections
     c. Easy bruising
- Assess for
  1. Fatigue
  2. Muscle weakness
  3. Bone pain and history of fractures
  4. Characteristic physical changes
     a. Buffalo hump
     b. Centripetal obesity
     c. Supraclavicular fat pads
     d. Round or moon face
     e. Large trunk
     f. Thin arms and legs
     g. Generalized muscle wasting and weakness
  5. Characteristic skin changes
     a. Bruises
     b. Thin, translucent skin
     c. Wounds that have not healed properly
     d. Reddish-purple striae on the abdomen and upper thighs
     e. Fine coating of hair over the face and body
     f. Acne
  6. Hypertension
  7. Emotional lability, irritability, confusion, or depression
  8. Increased plasma cortisol level
  9. Increased urinary 17-ketosteroids and 17-hydroxy-corticosteroids

Planning and Implementation

NONSURGICAL MANAGEMENT

- Drug therapy includes
  1. Mitotane (Lysodren) for inoperable adrenal tumors
  2. Aminoglutethimide (Elipten, Cytadren) and metyrapone to decrease cortisol production

- Radiation therapy is not always effective and may destroy normal tissue.

SURGICAL MANAGEMENT

- Transsphenoidal removal of the microadenoma is performed if hyperfunction is caused by increased pituitary secretion of adrenocorticotropic hormone.
- A *hypophysectomy* (surgical removal of the pituitary gland) may be indicated if the microadenoma cannot be located.
- *Adrenalectomy* is indicated if the etiologic agent is an adrenal adenoma or carcinoma.
- Provide preoperative care.
  1. Monitor electrolyte balance; imbalances are corrected before surgery.
  2. Monitor cardiac status for dysrhythmias resulting from potassium imbalance.
  3. Monitor blood glucose levels and report hyperglycemia.
  4. Ensure a high-calorie, high-protein diet.
  5. Administer glucocorticoid preparations as ordered.
- Provide postoperative care.
  1. Provide routine postoperative care according to the critical care unit guidelines, including hemodynamic monitoring per protocol.
  2. Monitor for signs and symptoms of cardiovascular collapse and shock.
  3. Carefully measure intake and output.
  4. Weigh the client daily.
  5. Monitor serum electrolytes daily.
  6. Administer glucocorticoids and mineralocorticoids, if necessary.
  7. Identify the need for and provide pain management.
  8. Prevent complications such as
     a. Skin breakdown
     b. Pathologic fractures
     c. Gastrointestinal bleeding
  9. Observe venipuncture sites for excessive bleeding.
- Teach the client and family
  1. Compliance with medication regimen and its side effects
  2. The importance of wearing a medical alert bracelet
  3. To avoid activities that may lead to skin trauma

4. To use a soft toothbrush and an electric shaver
5. Encourage the client to eliminate or reduce habits that contribute to gastric irritation such as smoking and fasting, and the use of nonsteroidal anti-inflammatory drugs (NSAIDs) or drugs that contain aspirin

- Hypercortisolism results in demineralization of bone and may lead to osteoporosis and fracture.
  1. Consult with a dietitian about diet therapy and ways to increase calcium and vitamin D.
  2. Advise the client to avoid caffeine and alcohol.

Hyperkalemia

OVERVIEW

- Hyperkalemia is a serum potassium level exceeding 5.0 mEq/L (mmol/L).
- The consequences of hyperkalemia can be life threatening, and the imbalance is generally not seen in people with normally functioning kidneys.
- Causes include
  1. Excessive potassium intake from
     a. Potassium-containing foods or medications
     b. Salt substitutes
     c. Potassium chloride (KCl) administration
     d. Rapid infusion of potassium-containing intravenous (IV) solution
  2. Decreased potassium excretion, which may be seen in Addison's disease and renal failure
  3. Movement of potassium from intracellular fluid to extracellular fluid, resulting in
     a. Tissue damage
     b. Acidosis
     c. Hyperuricemia
     d. Hypercatabolism
     e. Uncontrolled diabetes mellitus

COLLABORATIVE MANAGEMENT

- Record client information.
  1. Age (decreased renal function occurs in older persons)
  2. Medical and surgical history
  3. Medication use, particularly diuretics containing potassium
  4. Urinary output and frequency
  5. Diet history, including the use of salt substitutes and methods of preparing food
- Assess for
  1. Cardiovascular manifestations (the most common cause of death)
     a. Irregular heart rate, usually slow and weak
     b. Decreased blood pressure
     c. Electrocardiogram (ECG) abnormalities
        (1) Tall T waves
        (2) Widened QRS complexes
        (3) Prolonged PR intervals
        (4) Flat P waves
     d. Ectopic beats
     e. Late changes
        (1) Dysrhythmias
        (2) Ventricular fibrillation
        (3) Cardiac arrest
  2. Neuromuscular manifestations
     a. Early phase or mild hyperkalemia
        (1) Muscle twitches, cramps
        (2) Paresthesia
     b. Late phase or severe hyperkalemia
        (1) Profound weakness
        (2) Ascending flaccid paralysis in distal to proximal direction involving legs or arms
  3. Gastrointestinal manifestations
     a. Increased motility
     b. Hyperactive bowel sounds
     c. Diarrhea
  4. Respiratory manifestations (profound weakness of skeletal muscles causes respiratory failure in late stage of hyperkalemia)

- Treatment may include all of the following.
  1. Immediately stopping infusions of IV lines containing potassium; leaving the IV line open
  2. Administering
     a. Medications to shift potassium from the extracellular fluid to the intracellular (e.g., dextrose and insulin, calcium chloride, and calcium gluconate)
        (1) Administer these agents through a central line or in a vein with high blood flow to avoid local vein inflammation.
     b. Electrolyte-binding and excreting resins (e.g., oral or rectal sodium polystyrene sulfonate [Kayexalate])
     c. Sodium bicarbonate if hyperkalemia is accompanied by or caused by metabolic acidosis
     d. Potassium-excreting diuretics as ordered, such as furosemide (Lasix, Furoside ♣)
  3. Maintaining potassium restrictions by withholding oral potassium supplements and providing a potassium-restricted diet
  4. Monitoring the client closely for hypokalemia or hypoglycemia
  5. Maintaining strict intake and output
  6. Continuous cardiac monitoring for manifestations of hyperkalemia (e.g., decreased cardiac output, heart block, peaked T waves, fibrillation, systole)
- Dialysis may be necessary when potassium levels reach lethal levels.
- As needed, review diet therapy with the client and family, including
  1. Foods to avoid, including salt substitute
  2. Permissible foods
  3. How to examine medication and food package labels to determine potassium content
- Instruct the client and family to report signs and symptoms of hyperkalemia.

Hypermagnesemia

- Hypermagnesemia is a serum magnesium level exceeding 2.1 mEq/L.
- Common causes of hypermagnesemia include
  1. Increased ingestion of antacids with a high concentration of magnesium
  2. Renal insufficiency
- Assessment findings include
  1. Bradycardia (can lead to cardiac arrest)
  2. Peripheral vasodilation
  3. Hypotension
  4. Electrocardiogram changes
     a. Prolonged PR interval
     b. Widened QRS complex
  5. Drowsiness and lethargy, progressing to coma
  6. Diminished or absent deep tendon reflexes
  7. Respiratory insufficiency can lead to respiratory failure and death
- Interventions for hypermagnesemia include
  1. Discontinuing oral and parenteral magnesium
  2. Administering intravenous fluids (without magnesium)
  3. Administering loop diuretics, such as furosemide (Lasix, Furoside ✦)
  4. Administering calcium for severe cardiac manifestations
  5. Teaching dietary restrictions of meat, nuts, legumes, fish, vegetables, and whole-grain cereal products
  6. Teaching the client to avoid drugs that increase magnesium such as magnesium-containing antacids, laxatives, or commercial enemas

Hypernatremia

H

OVERVIEW

- Hypernatremia is a serum sodium level above 145 mEq/L. Common causes include
  1. Decreased sodium excretion
     a. Hyperaldosteronism
     b. Renal failure
     c. Corticosteroids
     d. Cushing's syndrome
  2. Increased sodium intake
     a. Excessive oral sodium ingestion
     b. Excessive administration of sodium-containing intravenous (IV) fluids
  3. Decreased water intake; nothing by mouth (NPO)
  4. Increased water loss
     a. Increased rate of metabolism
     b. Fever
     c. Hyperventilation
     d. Infection
     e. Excessive diaphoresis
     f. Watery diarrhea
     g. Dehydration

COLLABORATIVE MANAGEMENT

Assessment

- Assess for
  1. Cardiovascular manifestations
     a. Decreased myocardial contractility
     b. Diminished cardiac output
     c. Heart rate and blood pressure responsive to vascular volume
  2. Respiratory manifestations or problems associated with pulmonary edema when hypernatremia is accompanied by hypervolemia
  3. Central nervous system manifestations
     a. Hypernatremia with normovolemia or hypovolemia (agitation, short attention span, confusion, seizures)

    b. Hypernatremia with hypervolemia (lethargy, stupor, coma)

    c. Mild or early manifestations

        (1) Spontaneous muscle twitches

        (2) Irregular contractions

4. Neuromuscular manifestations

    a. Skeletal muscle weakness

    b. Deep tendon reflexes diminished or absent

5. Renal manifestations

    a. Decreased urinary output

    b. Increased specific gravity

6. Integumentary manifestations

    a. Dry, flaky skin

    b. Presence or absence of edema related to accompanying fluid volume changes

7. Psychosocial manifestations (agitation or manic behavior)

Interventions

- Restore fluid balance with IV infusion of isotonic sodium chloride solutions if hypernatremia is caused by fluid and sodium loss.
- Administer diuretics, generally loop diuretics such as furosemide (Lasix, Furoside ✤) or Bumetanide (Bumex) and ethacrynic (Edecrin) if the condition is caused by inadequate renal excretion of sodium.
- Assess the client frequently for symptoms that indicate excessive loss of fluids, dehydration.
- Dietary restriction of sodium is prescribed.
- Fluid restriction may be needed.
- Other nursing interventions include
  1. Checking vital signs
  2. Monitoring for indications of dehydration
  3. Weighing the client daily and monitoring trends
  4. Providing comfort measures to decrease thirst
  5. Recording intake and output
  6. Providing frequent oral hygiene
- Teach the client how to determine sodium content of food, beverages, and medications, including over-the-counter drugs.

Hyperparathyroidism

OVERVIEW

- Hyperparathyroidism results in increased levels of parathyroid hormone (PTH), which acts directly on the kidneys. The result is increased tubular resorption of calcium and phosphate excretion, contributing to hypercalcemia and hypophosphatemia.
- Primary hyperparathyroidism results when one or more parathyroid glands does not respond to the normal feedback of serum calcium, usually caused by a benign, autonomous adenoma in *one* parathyroid gland.
- Secondary hyperparathyroidism is a response to the hypocalcemia in chronic renal disease and in vitamin D deficiency, which results in hyperplasia of the glands.

COLLABORATIVE MANAGEMENT

Assessment

- Ask the client about the following symptoms.
  1. Bone fractures
  2. Recent weight loss
  3. Arthritis
  4. Psychologic distress
  5. History of radiation treatment to the head or neck
- Assess for
  1. Gastrointestinal disturbances such as anorexia, nausea, vomiting, and constipation
  2. Renal calculi and nephrocalcinosis (deposits of calcium in the soft tissue of the kidney)
  3. Hypergastrinemia (elevated serum gastrin levels); hypercalcemia
  4. Fatigue and lethargy
  5. Results of radiographic tests that indicate bone demineralization, bone lesions such as cysts, or fractures
  6. Results of serum parathyroid hormone (PTH), calcium, and phosphate levels and urine cyclic adenosine monophosphate (cAMP)

Interventions

NONSURGICAL MANAGEMENT

- Hydration (usually with intravenous normal saline) and the administration of furosemide (Lasix, Uritol, Furoside) are used to reduce serum calcium levels.
  1. Record strict intake and output measurements.
  2. Observe for changes in blood pressure, rate, or rhythm of pulses and increasing confusion, lethargy, or irritation.
  3. Assess the need for cardiac monitoring.
  4. Monitor for congestive heart failure secondary to fluid overload.
  5. Monitor serum calcium levels frequently.
  6. Instruct the client to report any nausea, vomiting, palpitations, tingling sensations, or numbness.
  7. Administer drug therapy as ordered, including
     a. Phosphates to inhibit bone resorption and interfere with calcium absorption (used only when calcium levels must be lowered rapidly)
     b. Calcitonin to decrease skeletal calcium release and increase the renal clearance of calcium (must be given in conjunction with glucocorticoids)
     c. Mithramycin, a cytotoxic antibiotic, the most effective agent to lower calcium levels (monitor closely for thrombocytopenia and renal and hepatic toxicity)

SURGICAL MANAGEMENT

- The surgery of choice is the removal of the parathyroid glands *(parathyroidectomy)*.
- Partial or total parathyroidectomy may be performed, depending on the cause of the hyperparathyroidism.
- Provide preoperative care.
  1. Provide routine preoperative care.
  2. Stabilize calcium levels per the physician's order.
  3. Monitor bleeding times and coagulation studies.
  4. Monitor complete blood count (CBC).
  5. Explain postoperative care, including pain control, deep breathing and coughing, and neck support technique to elevate the head.
- Provide postoperative care.
  1. Monitor serum calcium levels every 4 hours.

2. Monitor vital signs frequently per protocol.
3. Check neck dressing for abnormal amounts of drainage or bleeding.
4. Observe for respiratory distress caused by hemorrhage or tissue swelling.
5. Have emergency equipment such as a tracheostomy tray, oxygen, and suction at the bedside.
6. Monitor for signs of hypocalcemia, such as tingling and twitching of the extremities and face.
7. Check for Trousseau's and Chvostek's signs.
8. Administer calcium and vitamin D, if needed.

H

Hyperphosphatemia

- Hyperphosphatemia is a serum phosphate level greater than 4.5 mg/dL.
- Elevations of phosphate are well tolerated.
- Problems are associated with hypocalcemia induced as a result of the increase in serum phosphorus levels.
- Common causes include
  1. Renal insufficiency
  2. Aggressive treatment of cancer (tumor lysis syndrome)
  3. Increased intake of phosphorus
  4. Hypoparathyroidism
- Interventions for hyperphosphatemia include management of the underlying hypocalcemia.

Hyperpituitarism

OVERVIEW

- Hyperpituitarism is a condition of hormone oversecretion that occurs when a client has pituitary tumors or hyperplasia.
- Common secretory tumors include the prolactinoma (lactotrophic [PRL]-secreting tumor), causing decreased reproductive functioning, and the somatotrophic-producing

adenoma (growth hormone [GH]), causing gigantism or acromegaly.

1. *Gigantism* occurs before puberty and is characterized by rapid proportional growth in the length of all bones.
2. *Acromegaly* occurs after puberty and is characterized by increased skeletal thickness, hypertrophy of the skin, and enlargement of visceral organs.

- Hypersecretion of adrenocorticotropic hormone results in overstimulation of the adrenal cortex and may lead to the development of Cushing's disease.

COLLABORATIVE MANAGEMENT

Assessment

- Record client information.
  1. Age, sex, and family history
  2. Complaints of change in hat, glove, ring, or shoe size
  3. Complaints of backache and arthralgias (joint pain)
  4. Visual difficulties or headache
  5. Sexual history and functioning
     a. Female clients
        (1) Amenorrhea
        (2) Irregular menses
        (3) Difficulty becoming pregnant
        (4) Decreased libido
        (5) Painful intercourse
     b. Male clients
        (1) Decreased libido
        (2) Impotence
- Assess for
  1. Changes in facial features
     a. Increase in lip and nose size
     b. Prominent supraorbital ridge
  2. Enlarging head, hand, and foot size
  3. Prominent jaw
  4. Dysphagia, difficulty chewing, or dentures that do not fit
  5. Arthritic changes causing pain and decreased mobility
  6. Arrowhead or tufted characteristics on x-ray and a thickened appearance of the distal phalanges
  7. Increased perspiration and oil secretion on the client's skin

8. Increased metabolism and strength (initially with acromegaly and gigantism)
   9. Lethargy and weakness (in later stages of acromegaly and gigantism)
  10. Visual changes
  11. Organomegaly (cardiac or hepatic)
  12. Hypertension
  13. Deepening of the voice because of hypertrophy of the larynx
  14. Hyperprolactinemia (observed with hypogonadism and galactorrhea)
  15. Changes in body image
  16. Depression and emotional distress
  17. Increased adrenocorticotropic hormone (ACTH) or GH

Planning and Implementation

◆**NDx:** Disturbed Body Image

NONSURGICAL MANAGEMENT

- Encourage the client to verbalize concerns and fears related to his or her altered physical appearance.
- Help the client identify his or her strengths and positive characteristics.
- Drug therapy includes
   1. Dopamine agonists stimulate dopamine receptors in the brain and inhibit the release of many pituitary hormones, most specifically GH and PRL. In clients with acromegaly bromocriptine reduces GH levels and decreases tumor size.
   2. Somatostatin analogues inhibit GH release through negative feedback.
- Proton beam or alpha particle radiation therapy is usually effective but slow. Side effects include hypopituitarism, optic nerve damage, oculomotor dysfunction, and visual field defects.

SURGICAL MANAGEMENT

- Surgical removal of the tumor or pituitary gland *(hypophysectomy)* is performed, usually via the transsphenoidal approach.
   1. The client is placed in a semi-sitting position, and an initial incision is made at the inner aspect of the upper lip

2. The sella turcica is entered through the sphenoid sinus, and the gland or tumor is removed.
3. A muscle graft is taken, often from the anterior thigh, to pack the dura and prevent leakage of cerebrospinal fluid (CSF).
4. Nasal packing is inserted, and a dressing is applied under the nose to prevent the packing from dislodging ("moustache" dressing or "drip" pad).

- Preoperative care includes
  1. Explaining to the client that nasal packing will remain in place for 2 to 3 days, which necessitates mouth breathing
  2. Explaining that toothbrushing, coughing, sneezing, nose blowing, and bending must be avoided postoperatively
- Postoperative care includes
  1. Monitoring for changes in neurologic status
  2. Carefully measuring intake and output; weighing the client each day
  3. Observing and reporting signs of diabetes insipidus, such as low urine specific gravity and excessive urinary output
  4. Instructing the client to report postnasal drip
  5. Recording the amount and color of nasal drainage (clear drainage is tested for glucose, whose presence indicates that the fluid is CSF)
  6. Elevating the head of the bed at all times
  7. Reporting a severe persistent headache to the physician immediately (may indicate that CSF has leaked into the sinus area)
  8. Observing the client for indications of meningitis, such as headache, fever, and nuchal rigidity
  9. Instructing client *not* to cough because it increases pressure in the incision area and may lead to a CSF leak
  10. Performing frequent mouth and lip care because the client has to breathe through his or her mouth
  11. Administering glucocorticoid and thyroid hormones if the entire pituitary gland is removed
- A transfrontal craniotomy is performed if the tumor is inaccessible through the transsphenoidal route.

- Identify specific problems and encourage the client to discuss any effect that sexual dysfunction has had on the relationship with his or her sexual partner.
- Drug therapy with bromocriptine may be helpful.
- Inform the client that sexual dysfunction may occur after a hypophysectomy.

Community-Based Care

- Assess the degree of mobility impairment and identify the need for adaptive equipment in the home.
- Teach the client to
  1. Avoid bending over to pick up things or tie shoes.
  2. Avoid straining during a bowel movement; stool softener may be needed.
  3. Rinse the mouth and use dental floss until brushing of teeth can be resumed after the incision has healed.
  4. Expect a decreased sense of smell for 3 to 4 months.
  5. Take hormones, as prescribed, such as vasopressin to maintain fluid balance.

Hypertension

OVERVIEW

- *Hypertension* is defined as systolic blood pressure (SBP) greater than or equal to 140 mm Hg, diastolic blood pressure (DBP) greater than or equal to 90 mm Hg, or both, occurring in a client on at least two separate occasions.
- *Prehypertension* is defined as an SBP of 120 to 139 mm Hg or a DBP of 80 to 89 mm Hg; lifestyle changes are needed to prevent cardiovascular complication.
- Hypertension is the major risk factor for coronary, cerebral, renal, and peripheral vascular disease.
- Four control systems play a major role in maintaining blood pressure.
  1. Arterial baroreceptors
  2. Regulation of body fluid volume

3. Renin-angiotensin system
4. Vascular autoregulation
- There are two major classifications of hypertension.
    1. *Essential,* or primary, with no known cause and associated with risk factors such as a family history of hypertension, older than 60 years of age, hyperlipidemia, stress, and smoking
    2. *Secondary,* from known specific *disease* such as renal vascular and renal parenchymal disease, primary aldosteronism, Cushing's disease, coarctation of the aorta, brain tumors and encephalitis, psychiatric disorders, and some *medications* such as estrogen-containing oral contraceptives, glucocorticoids, mineralocorticoids, cyclosporine, and erythropoietin
- Sustained blood pressure elevation in clients with essential hypertension results in damage to blood vessels in vital organs, causing myocardial infarctions, strokes, peripheral vascular disease, or renal failure.
- *Malignant* hypertension is a severe type of hypertension that progresses rapidly and leads to renal failure, left ventricular failure, and stroke unless intervention occurs promptly.
- *Pulmonary* hypertension involves vasoconstriction and increasing vascular resistance of pulmonary blood vessels. Pulmonary blood pressure rises, leading to poor perfusion, hypoxemia, and right-sided heart failure. Treatment is directed toward improving function and reducing symptoms and includes warfarin therapy, oxygen, and digoxin. Surgical management involves whole lung transplantation.

COLLABORATIVE MANAGEMENT

Assessment

- Record client information.
    1. Age
    2. Race or ethnic origin
    3. Family history of hypertension
    4. Average daily intake of calories, sodium and potassium containing foods
    4. Alcohol intake
    5. Smoking history
    6. Exercise habits

7. Past and present history of renal or cardiovascular disease
8. Medication use (prescribed and over the counter)

■ Assess for
   1. Symptoms of hypertension (although most clients have no obvious symptoms)
      a. Headache, dizziness, or fainting
      b. Edema
      c. Nocturia
      d. Lethargy
      e. Nosebleeds
      f. Vision changes
   2. Blood pressure readings in both arms
   3. Blood pressure readings in supine and erect positions
   4. Peripheral pulse rate, rhythm, and force
   5. Bruits over the carotid and abdominal arteries
   6. Psychosocial stressors
   7. Retinal changes on funduscopic examination
   8. Physical findings related to *secondary* hypertension
      a. Abdominal bruits
      b. Tachycardia, sweating, and pallor
      c. Decreased or absent femoral pulses

H

Planning and Implementation

◈NDx: Deficient Knowledge

■ Interventions include
   1. In collaboration with the dietitian,
      a. Advising the client to decrease sodium intake by not adding table salt to food, not cooking with salt, and not adding seasonings that contain sodium and to limit eating canned, frozen, and other processed foods
      b. Suggesting that the client use spices, herbs, fruits, and other non–salt-containing substances such as powdered garlic and onion or salt substitute to enhance the flavor of food
      c. Advising the client to lose weight
      d. Developing a plan to reduce saturated fat and cholesterol in the diet
   2. Advising the client to restrict alcohol intake and smoking
   3. Collaborating with the physical therapist to assist the client in developing a regular exercise program

4. Teaching or referring the client to stress management programs including yoga, massage, biofeedback, and hypnosis programs
5. Knowing that a stepped-care approach to treat hypertension involves a variety of drug options and protocols used by health care providers
6. Providing drug therapy as prescribed
   a. *Diuretics* are particularly effective for black individuals and for clients with asthma, chronic airway limitation, chronic renal disease, and selected clients with congestive heart failure.
      (1) *Thiazide* diuretics prevent sodium and water reabsorption in the distal tubules of the kidneys while promoting potassium excretion.
      (2) *Loop* diuretics depress sodium reabsorption in the ascending loop of Henle and promote potassium excretion.
      (3) *Potassium-sparing* diuretics act on the distal tubules of the kidneys to inhibit reabsorption of sodium in exchange for potassium ions, thus retaining potassium.
   b. *Calcium channel blockers* lower blood pressure by interfering with transmembrane influx of calcium ions, resulting in vasoconstriction.
   c. *Angiotensin-converting enzyme* (ACE) *inhibitors* convert angiotensin I to angiotensin II. These drugs are most effective in young white adults and are not as effective in black clients.
   d. *Angiotensin II receptor antagonists,* which selectively block the binding of angiotensin II in the vascular and adrenal tissue, are options for clients who complain of cough associated with ACE inhibitors and for those with hyperkalemia.
   e. *Aldosterone receptor antagonists* block the hypertensive effect of the mineralocorticoid hormone aldosterone.
   f. *Cardioselective beta-adrenergic blockers* lower blood pressure by blocking beta receptors in the heart and peripheral vessels, reducing cardiac rate and output.
   g. *Central alpha agonists* act on the central nervous system, preventing reuptake of norepinephrine,

resulting in lower peripheral vascular resistance and blood pressure.

Community-Based Care

- Provide educational information for hypertension control.
    1. Salt restriction
    2. Weight maintenance or reduction
    3. Stress reduction
    4. Alcohol restriction
    5. Exercise program
- Give oral and written information on medication therapy.
    1. Indications
    2. Dosage
    3. Times of administration
    4. Side effects
    5. Drug interactions
    6. The importance of renewing prescriptions
    7. Reporting side effects to the health care provider
    8. The importance of taking the medications even when there are no symptoms
- Instruct the client and family members in the technique of blood pressure monitoring at home.
- Teach the client or family member to record blood pressure readings in a log book or diary.
- Refer the client to home care agency if necessary.
- Refer the client to the American Heart Association for information and support.

Hyperthyroidism

OVERVIEW

- Hyperthyroidism occurs as a result of excessive thyroid hormone secretion.
- The most common cause is Graves' disease (toxic diffuse goiter), which causes the client to have goiter, exophthalmus, and pretibial myxedema (dry, waxy swelling of the front surfaces of the lower legs).

- *Thyrotoxicosis* refers to the signs and symptoms that appear when body tissues are stimulated by increased thyroid hormones.
- Hyperthyroidism produces a state of hypermetabolism with increased sympathetic nervous system activity; it may be transient or permanent.
- *Thyroid storm* or thyroid crisis is a life-threatening event.
    1. Assess for signs and symptoms triggered by a major stressor such as trauma or infection.
        a. Fever
        b. Tachycardia or systolic hypertension
        c. Gastrointestinal symptoms: nausea, vomiting, and diarrhea
        d. Agitation, tremors, and anxiety
        e. Restlessness, confusion, or psychosis
        f. Seizures
    2. Interventions include
        a. Maintaining a patent airway and adequate ventilation
        b. Monitoring continually for cardiac dysrhythmias
        c. Monitoring vital signs every 30 minutes
        d. Reducing fever
        e. Stabilizing hemodynamic status
        f. Correcting dehydration
    3. Medications that may be given include
        a. Antithyroid drugs, such as propyl-thiouracil (PTU) and methimazole (Tapazole), as ordered
        b. Sodium iodide solution
        c. Propranolol (Inderal, Apo-Propranolol) if life-threatening dysrhythmias are present
        d. Glucocorticoids to prevent release of thyroid hormone
        e. Nonsalicylate antipyretics to reduce fever

COLLABORATIVE MANAGEMENT

Assessment

- Record client information.
    1. Age and sex
    2. Weight loss and increased appetite
    3. Heat intolerance or diaphoresis
    4. Palpitations or chest pain

5. Changes in breathing pattern (dyspnea with or without exertion may occur)
6. Changes in vision: blurring, double vision, or eyes tiring easily
7. Changes in ability to perform activities of daily living (ADLs): fatigue, weakness, insomnia
8. Changes in menses (amenorrhea, decreased menstrual flow)
9. Increased libido
10. Medical history
    a. Thyroid surgery
    b. Radiation therapy to the neck (some clients may be resistant to radiation therapy)
    c. Past or current medications, noting the use of thyroid hormones or antithyroid drugs

- Assess for
    1. Two types of ophthalmopathy
        a. Eyelid retraction and eyelid lag
        b. Globe lag
    2. Exophthalmos (seen in Graves' disease)
        a. Impaired vision
        b. Problems with focusing
        c. Possible corneal ulcerations and infections
        d. Excessive tearing
        e. Photophobia
    3. Mass or general enlargement of the thyroid gland
    4. Fine, soft, silky hair and smooth, moist skin
    5. Proximal muscle weakness
    6. Hyperactive deep tendon reflexes or tremors
    7. Restlessness and irritability
    8. Fatigue
    9. Increased serum triiodothyronine (T_3) and serum thyronine (T_4)
    10. Increased radioactive iodine (RAI) uptake on thyroid scan
    11. Electrocardiogram (ECG) changes: tachycardia, atrial fibrillation, and alterations in P and T waveforms

Planning and Implementation

NONSURGICAL MANAGEMENT

- Monitor the effects of the disease on cardiac function.
  1. Monitor vital signs at least every 4 hours.
  2. Instruct the client to report palpitations, dyspnea, vertigo, and/or chest pain immediately.
  3. Provide a quiet, restful environment.
- Drug therapy may include
  1. Antithyroid drugs, such as thioamides, which block thyroid hormone production
  2. Iodide preparations to decrease blood flow through the thyroid gland
  3. Beta-adrenergic blocking agents to relieve diaphoresis, anxiety, and tachycardia
- Teach the client about RAI therapy.
  1. RAI ^{131} I is taken orally (one dose usually on an outpatient basis).
  2. Radiation precautions are generally not required.
  3. Relief of symptoms usually does not occur for 6 to 8 weeks.
  4. Hypothyroidism may occur as a complication.

SURGICAL MANAGEMENT

- All or part of the thyroid gland may be removed (total or subtotal thyroidectomy).
- Preoperative care includes
  1. Providing routine preoperative care
  2. Administering antithyroid drugs and iodine preparations as ordered to place the client in an euthyroid state and to decrease the size and vascularity of the gland
  3. Monitoring cardiac status
  4. Monitoring nutritional status
  5. Teaching the client how to support the neck when coughing or moving
- Postoperative care includes
  1. Providing routine postoperative care
  2. Placing sandbags or pillows to support the client's head and neck
  3. Maintaining the client in a semi-Fowler's position
  4. Administering pain medication as needed

5. Providing humidification
6. Encouraging the client to turn, cough, and deep breathe every 1 to 2 hours
7. Inspecting the neck dressing for drainage (a moderate amount of drainage is expected if a drain is left in place)
8. Keeping equipment for a tracheostomy at the bedside
9. Keeping calcium gluconate or calcium chloride at the bedside for emergency use
10. Administering fluids, as ordered
11. Applying an ice bag to the neck to reduce swelling
12. Observing for complications
    a. Hemorrhage
    b. Respiratory distress
    c. Hypocalcemia and tetany, caused by parathyroid gland injury
       (1) Tingling around the mouth or of the toes and fingers
       (2) Muscular twitching
       (3) Positive Chvostek's and Trousseau's signs
    d. Damage to laryngeal nerves (hoarseness and a weak voice)
- The infiltrative ophthalmopathy of Graves' disease is not influenced by medical therapy.
- Treatment for mild symptoms includes
  1. Elevating the head of the bed at night
  2. Applying eye lubricant or artificial tears
- For severe symptoms
  1. Tape the eyes closed.
  2. Administer short-term steroids, as ordered.
  3. Administer diuretics, as ordered.
- In extreme cases, surgical intervention (orbital decompression) may be necessary.

Community-Based Care

- Teach the client
  1. Pertinent drug information, including side effects
  2. The necessity to report any temperature elevation, sore throat, or symptoms of infection
  3. The signs and symptoms of hyperthyroidism or hypothyroidism

4. Inspection of the incision for redness, tenderness, drainage, and swelling
5. The importance of follow-up visits with physicians
- Home health services may be necessary for the client who has difficulty with ADLs.

Hypocalcemia

OVERVIEW

- Hypocalcemia is a serum calcium level below 9.0 mg/dL or 2.25 mmol/L.
- Small changes in serum calcium levels have major effects on body function.
- Hypocalcemia is usually not a primary disease or condition but a result of other diseases or conditions.
- Common causes of hypocalcemia include
    1. Inhibition of calcium absorption from the gastrointestinal (GI) tract
        a. Inadequate oral intake of calcium
        b. Lactose intolerance
        c. Malabsorption syndromes
            (1) Celiac sprue
            (2) Crohn's disease
        d. Inadequate intake of vitamin D
    2. Increased calcium excretion
        a. Renal failure (polyuric phase)
        b. Diarrhea
        c. Steatorrhea
        d. Wound drainage (especially GI)
    3. Conditions that decrease the ionized fraction of calcium
        a. Alkalosis
        b. Calcium chelators or binders
            (1) Citrate
            (2) Mithramycin (Mithracin)
            (3) Penicillamine
        c. Acute pancreatitis
        d. Hyperphosphatemia
        e. Immobility

4. Endocrine disturbances
    a. Removal or destruction of the parathyroid glands
        (1) Thyroidectomy
        (2) Irradiation of the thyroid
5. Strangulation
6. Neck injuries

||| Cultural Considerations

* Black people with lactose intolerance may have difficulty obtaining enough calcium and vitamin D from other sources to maintain normal calcium levels in the blood and bones.

🔅 Women's Health Considerations

* Postmenopausal women are susceptible to hypocalcemia, which may be related to reduced weight-bearing activities and a decrease in estrogen levels.

🌙 Considerations for Older Adults

* The older adult is more likely than younger persons to be taking medications that affect fluid and electrolyte balance.
* Some older adults may have dietary calcium or vitamin D deficits because of reduced income or problems with obtaining, preparing, or eating food.

COLLABORATIVE MANAGEMENT

Assessment

■ Assess for
    1. Neuromuscular manifestations (the most common manifestations)
        a. Anxiety, irritability, psychosis
        b. Paresthesia followed by numbness
        c. Irritable skeletal muscles: twitches, cramps, tetany, seizures
        d. Hyperactive deep tendon reflexes
        e. Positive Trousseau's sign
            (1) Testing is accomplished by placing a blood pressure cuff around the upper arm, inflating the cuff to greater than systolic pressure, and keeping it there for 1 to 4 minutes

      (2) The hand and fingers spasm in palmar flexion

      (3) Spasms continue for 20 to 30 seconds after the cuff has been released

  f. Positive Chvostek's sign (tapping on the face just below and anterior to the ear—over the facial nerve—triggers facial twitching that includes one side of the mouth, nose, and cheek)

2. Cardiovascular manifestations

  a. Decreased heart rate

  b. Decreased myocardial contractility

  c. Diminished peripheral pulses

  d. Hypotension

  e. Electrocardiogram abnormalities

      (1) Prolonged ST interval

      (2) Prolonged QT interval

3. GI manifestations

  a. Increased gastric motility

  b. Hyperactive bowel sounds

  c. Abdominal cramping

  d. Diarrhea

Interventions

- Drug therapy may be ordered as follows.

  1. Oral supplements of calcium carbonate, calcium citrate, calcium gluconate, or calcium lactate used for mild hypocalcemia

    a. Use with thiazide diuretics can increase risk for hypercalcemia.

    b. Do not give phenytoin within 3 hours of calcium administration.

  2. Parenteral calcium for severe hypocalcemia of calcium acetate, calcium chloride, or calcium gluconate

    a. Give slowly, not to exceed 27 g/min; warm before administration.

    b. Monitor cardiovascular status; the client should be on a cardiac monitor.

    c. There is risk for hypercalcemia and hypomagnesemia.

    d. Assess the infusion site for infiltration.

  3. Agents that increase calcium absorption, including vitamin D, aluminum hydroxide, magnesium chloride, and magnesium sulfate

4. Agents that reduce nerve and skeletal muscle excitability such as magnesium sulfate, methocarbamol, and diazepam
5. Agents that inhibit bone resorption of calcium, including alendronate or estrogen
- Provide a high-calcium diet for mild cases and those with chronic pathologic conditions that put them at risk for hypocalcemia. Foods high in calcium are
  1. Low-fat yogurt
  2. Skim and whole milk
  3. Raw collard greens
  4. Rhubarb
  5. Cheddar and American cheese
  6. Tofu
  7. Broccoli
- Additional interventions include
  1. Minimizing environmental stimuli
  2. Keeping emergency equipment readily available in anticipation of complications
  3. Placing the client on seizure precautions
  4. Using a lift sheet to move the client rather than pulling or grasping the client directly
  5. Observing the client for unusual surface projections or depressions over bony areas, as well as for normal joint motion

Hypofunction, Adrenal

OVERVIEW

- A decreased production of adrenocortical steroids (adrenal hypofunction) may occur secondary to inadequate secretion of adrenocorticotropic hormone (ACTH), dysfunction of the hypothalamic-pituitary control mechanism, or complete or partial destruction of the adrenal glands.
- *Primary* hypofunction, also referred to as *Addison's disease*, occurs when a client's physiologic requirements for glucocorticoid and mineralocorticoid hormones exceed available supply because of autoimmune factors, tuberculosis,

carcinoma, acquired immunodeficiency syndrome (AIDS), hemorrhage, sepsis, radiation, or adrenalectomy.

- The most common cause of *secondary* adrenal hypofunction is the sudden cessation of long-term, high-dose glucocorticoid therapy.
- *Acute* adrenocortical insufficiency (adrenal crisis), is a life-threatening event in which the need for cortisol and aldosterone is greater than available supply. Manifestations may appear suddenly, without warning. Most cases occur in response to a stressful event (surgery, trauma, or severe infection), especially when the adrenal hormone output is already reduced.

COLLABORATIVE MANAGEMENT

Assessment

- Record client information.
  1. Description of symptoms
  2. Activity level
  3. Salt intake (salt craving)
  4. Medical history
     a. Radiation to the head or abdomen
     b. Tuberculosis
     c. Intracranial surgery
     d. Medications such as steroids, anticoagulants, or cytotoxic drugs
- Assess for
  1. Gastrointestinal problems
     a. Anorexia
     b. Nausea, vomiting, diarrhea
     c. Abdominal pain
     d. Weight loss
  2. Increased or decreased skin pigmentation
  3. Hyperpigmentation of the mucous membranes, surgical scars, areolae, skin folds, and area over knuckles on the hand (not seen in secondary disease)
  4. Decreased body hair
  5. Hypoglycemia (cortisol hypersecretion)
     a. Sweating
     b. Headache

    c. Tachycardia

    d. Tremors

6. Volume depletion (cortisol and aldosterone deficiencies)

    a. Postural hypotension

    b. Dehydration

7. Emotional lability, forgetfulness, psychosis

8. Low serum cortisol, decreased fasting blood sugar, low sodium, elevated potassium, and increased blood urea nitrogen (BUN) levels; eosinophil count and ACTH level are elevated in primary disease

Planning and Implementation

- Interventions include
  1. Monitor intake and output.
  2. Weigh the client every day.
  3. Take vital signs to detect postural hypotension and dysrhythmias.
  4. Administer cortisone and hydrocortisone to correct glucocorticoid deficiency.
  5. Administer supplemental mineralocorticoids, such as fludrocortisone (Florinef), as prescribed, to maintain electrolyte balance.
  6. Monitor laboratory values to identify hemoconcentration.
- Teach the client the following.
  1. Medications should be taken with meals or snacks.
  2. Client should consult his or her health care provider regarding increasing dosage during increased stress.
  3. A medical alert bracelet or necklace should be worn at all times.

Hypokalemia

OVERVIEW

- Hypokalemia is defined as a serum potassium ion (K^+) level below 3.5 mEq/L (mmol/L).
- Hypokalemia can be life threatening because every body system can be affected.

- Common causes include
  1. Inappropriate or excessive use of diuretics, digitalis, or corticosteroids
  2. Increased secretion of aldosterone
  3. Diarrhea, vomiting
  4. Wound drainage, excessive drainage from ostomies
  5. Prolonged nasogastric suction
  6. Heat-induced excessive diaphoresis
  7. Inadequate potassium intake, which can occur when the client has nothing by mouth for several days
  8. Cushing's syndrome
  9. Alkalosis
  10. The presence of excess amounts of insulin in the blood, such as during hyperalimentation infusions or during treatment of uncontrolled diabetes
  11. Renal disease impairing resorption of potassium
  12. Dilution of serum potassium that may occur secondary to water intoxication or intravenous (IV) therapy with potassium-poor solutions

COLLABORATIVE MANAGEMENT

Assessment

- Record client information.
  1. Age
  2. Medication use, especially diuretics, corticosteroids, and potassium supplements
  3. Dietary history
  4. Recent illness and medical surgical interventions
- Assess for
  1. Cardiovascular manifestations
     a. Variable pulse rate (more often rapid)
     b. Pulse thready and weak
     c. Peripheral pulses difficult to palpate
     d. Orthostatic hypotension
     e. Electrocardiogram (ECG) abnormalities
     f. ST depression
     g. Inverted T wave
     h. Prominent U wave
     i. Heart block

2. Respiratory manifestations
    a. Shallow, ineffective respirations
    b. Diminished breath sounds and respiratory effort
3. Neurologic changes
    a. Anxiety, lethargy, confusion, coma
    b. Loss of tactile discrimination
4. Musculoskeletal manifestations
    a. General skeletal muscle weakness
    b. Deep tendon hyporeflexia
    c. Eventual flaccid paralysis
5. Gastrointestinal changes
    a. Decreased motility or peristalsis
    b. Hypoactive to absent bowel sounds
    c. Nausea, vomiting
    d. Abdominal distention
    e. Paralytic ileus
    f. Constipation
6. Renal manifestations
    a. Decreased ability to concentrate urine
    b. Polyuria
    c. Decreased specific gravity
7. Psychosocial
    a. Behavioral changes
    b. Lethargy
    c. Inability to perform simple problem-solving tasks

Planning and Implementation

NDx: Risk for Falls

- Provide drug therapy as ordered.
    1. Potassium is a severe tissue irritant and is never administered intramuscularly or subcutaneously.
    2. IV potassium may irritate the veins, causing a chemical phlebitis. It must be diluted well and administered slowly; the maximum infusion rate is 5 to 10 mEq/hr and should never exceed 20 mEq/hr under any circumstances.
        a. Assess the IV site every 2 hours for infiltration; stop the IV solution immediately.
        b. Ask the client about burning or pain at the IV site.
    3. Rapid increases of serum potassium may cause cardiac arrest.

4. Oral potassium has a strong, unpleasant taste; it must not be given on an empty stomach because it may cause nausea and vomiting.
5. Potassium-sparing diuretics that may be appropriate for clients needing diuretic therapy include spironolactone (Aldactone), triamterene (Dyrenium), and amiloride (Midamor).
- Provide diet therapy.
  1. Provide foods high in potassium, including avocados, bananas, cantaloupe, raisins, and whole-wheat bread.
  2. Instruct the client to avoid boiling, poaching, or frying vegetables and fruits in water.
- Safety measures include
  1. Providing frequent rest periods for the client susceptible to skeletal muscle weakness
  2. Maintaining a hazard-free environment
  3. Assisting the client with ambulation

NDx: Constipation

- Treatment includes
  1. Administering laxatives that add bulk or fiber to stimulate peristalsis
  2. Administering drugs such as metoclopramide (Reglan, Maxeran ✦) to enhance gastric emptying and stimulate gastrointestinal motility
  3. Providing a high-fiber diet and encouraging fluids
  4. Encouraging physical activity and exercise to promote gastric motility

NDx: Potential for Respiratory Insufficiency

- Monitor and record
  1. Rate and depth of respiration once each hour
  2. Ability to cough deeply
  3. Indications of cyanosis of the oral mucosa and nail beds

Discharge Planning

- Health teaching includes
  1. Providing drug information, as needed
  2. Teaching early recognition of the signs and symptoms of hypokalemia

3. Providing information on foods rich in potassium and how potassium is lost from the body
4. Teaching the client to measure the rate, rhythm, and quality of his or her peripheral pulses once each day
5. Reinforcing how often serum potassium levels should be checked
6. Referring the client to home health care services as needed
- Focused assessment for home care of the client includes routine system assessment and asking about
  1. 24-hour fluid intake and output
  2. 24-hour diet recall
  3. What over-the-counter medication and prescribed medication has been taken
  4. Any dizziness or light-headedness experienced
  5. Any headaches experienced (including what time of day and what activities are associated)
  6. Presence of muscle twitches, cramps, pain, or spasms

Hypomagnesemia

- Hypomagnesemia is a serum magnesium ion level below 1.2 mg/dL.
- Common causes include
  1. Malnutrition or starvation
  2. Diarrhea or steatorrhea
  3. Celiac disease, Crohn's disease
  4. Certain drugs
     a. Diuretics
     b. Aminoglycoside antibiotics
     c. Cisplatin (Platinol)
     d. Amphotericin B
     e. Citrate (blood products)
     f. Ethanol ingestion
  5. Hyperglycemia
  6. Insulin administration
  7. Sepsis
  8. Alkalosis

- Clinical manifestations include
  1. Cardiac manifestations
     a. Dysrhythmias
     b. Ectopic beats
     c. Ventricular tachycardia
     d. Ventricular fibrillation
  2. Electrocardiogram changes
     a. Tall T waves
     b. Depressed ST segments
  3. Neuromuscular manifestation
     a. Painful paresthesia
     b. Tetanic muscle contractions
     c. Positive Chvostek's and Trousseau's signs
     d. Tetany and seizures
     e. Depression or irritability
     f. Frank psychosis
     g. Confusion
  4. Shallow respirations
  5. Decreased gastric motility with anorexia, nausea, and abdominal distention
- Management of hypomagnesemia includes
  1. Stopping drugs that contribute to the development of hypomagnesemia (loop diuretics, aminoglycosides)
  2. Intravenous infusion of magnesium sulfate
  3. Increasing the client's intake of foods high in magnesium such as meats, nuts, legumes, fish, and vegetables

Hyponatremia

OVERVIEW

- Hyponatremia is a serum sodium level below 136 mEq/L (mmol/L).
- Hyponatremia is usually associated with fluid volume imbalances.
- Common causes include
  1. Increased sodium excretion
     a. Excessive diaphoresis
     b. Diuretics

    c. Wound drainage (especially gastrointestinal)
    d. Decreased secretion of aldosterone
    e. Hyperlipidemia
    f. Renal disease
2. Inadequate sodium intake
    a. Nothing by mouth (NPO)
    b. Low-salt diet
3. Dilution of serum sodium
    a. Excessive ingestion of hypotonic fluids
    b. Psychogenic polydipsia
    c. Freshwater drowning
    d. Renal failure (nephrotic syndrome)
    e. Irrigation with hypotonic fluids
    f. Syndrome of inappropriate antidiuretic hormone (SIADH)
    g. Hyperglycemia
    h. Heart failure

COLLABORATIVE MANAGEMENT

■ Assess for
1. Cardiovascular manifestations
    a. Normovolemic
      (1) Rapid pulse rate
      (2) Normal blood pressure
    b. Hypovolemic
      (1) Rapid pulse rate
      (2) Pulse thready and weak
      (3) Hypotension
      (4) Central venous pressure normal or low
      (5) Flat neck veins
    c. Hypervolemic
      (1) Rapid bounding pulse
      (2) Central venous pressure normal or elevated
      (3) Blood pressure normal or elevated
2. Respiratory changes (secondary to the influence of low serum sodium on cerebral function and circulatory status); late manifestations related to
    a. Skeletal muscle weakness
    b. Shallow, ineffective respiratory movements
    c. Hypervolemia

        d. Pulmonary edema
            (1) Rapid, shallow respirations
            (2) Moist crackles
    3. Neuromuscular manifestations
        a. Generalized muscle weakness
        b. Diminished deep tendon reflexes
        c. Personality changes
        d. Headache
        e. Seizures
    4. Gastrointestinal manifestations
        a. Increased motility; abdominal cramping
        b. Nausea
        c. Hyperactive bowel sounds
        d. Diarrhea
    5. Renal manifestations
        a. Increased urinary output
        b. Decreased specific gravity of urine
- Drug therapy is as follows.
    1. Hyponatremia with a fluid volume deficient (hypovolemia): Intravenous (IV) saline infusions are prescribed to restore both sodium and fluid volume.
    2. Hyponatremia with a fluid excess: Osmotic diuretics that promote excretion of water rather than sodium are given.
    3. Hyponatremia as a result of SIADH may be treated with agents that antagonize such as demeclocycline (Declomycin) or lithium.
    4. Collaborate with the dietitian to provide diet therapy.
        a. Increase oral sodium and restrict oral intake of fluids to some extent.
        b. Common food sources of sodium are table salt, soy sauce, cured pork, cottage cheese, and American cheese.
        c. Accurately measure intake and output.
        d. Reinforce the rationale for fluid restriction.
    5. Weigh the client daily and monitor trends.
- Additional interventions
    1. Monitor for electrolyte imbalances associated with hyponatremia such as hypokalemia, hypoglycemia, and metabolic acidosis.
    2. Monitor for fluid volume overload and retention.
    3. Monitor vital signs and observe for hypovolemic or hypervolemic shock.

Hypoparathyroidism

- Hypoparathyroidism is directly related to the lack of parathyroid hormone (PTH) or decreased effectiveness of PTH on target tissue.
- Hypoparathyroidism always results in hypocalcemia.
- The two forms are
    1. *Iatrogenic,* inadvertently caused by the removal of all viable parathyroid tissue during total thyroidectomy or by surgical removal of hyperplastic parathyroid glands
    2. *Idiopathic,* a rare condition that can occur spontaneously; an autoimmune basis is suspected

COLLABORATIVE MANAGEMENT

- Question the client regarding
    1. Neck surgery or radiation therapy to the head or neck area
    2. Signs and symptoms
        a. Paresthesia
        b. Tetany
        c. Periorbital tingling
        d. Numbness and tingling sensation in the hands and feet
- Assess for
    1. Muscle cramping
    2. Carpopedal spasms
    3. Seizures
    4. Mental changes
    5. Chvostek's or Trousseau's sign
- Management includes
    1. Correcting hypocalcemia, vitamin D deficiency, and hypomagnesemia
    2. Teaching the client the importance of compliance with medication regimen to correct hypocalcemia, vitamin D deficiency, and hypomagnesemia
    3. Encouraging the client to eat food high in calcium and low in phosphorus
    4. Stressing that therapy for hypocalcemia is lifelong
    5. Advising the client to wear a medical alert emblem and to carry a wallet card

Hypophosphatemia

- Hypophosphatemia is a serum phosphate level below 2.7 mg/dL.
- Body functions are not significantly impaired as a result of rapid, wide fluctuations in serum levels.
- Alterations in function are more obvious when hypophosphatemia is chronic.
- Common causes include
  1. Insufficient phosphorus intake
     a. Malnutrition or starvation
     b. Use of aluminum hydroxide–based antacids (ALternaGEL, Amphojel)
     c. Magnesium (BiSoDol, Milk of Magnesia)
  2. Increased phosphorus excretion
     a. Hyperparathyroidism
     b. Hypocalcemia
     c. Renal failure
     d. Malignancy
  3. Intracellular shift
     a. Hyperglycemia
     b. Hyperalimentation
     c. Respiratory alkalosis
     d. Uncontrolled diabetes mellitus
     e. Alcohol abuse
- Clinical manifestations, which do not appear until the decrease in serum phosphate levels is severe or prolonged, include
  1. Decreased stroke volume
  2. Decreased cardiac output
  3. Peripheral pulses slow, difficult to find, and easy to block
  4. Weak, ineffective myocardial contractions
  5. Generalized skeletal muscle weakness; may cause rhabdomyolysis
  6. Ineffective respiratory movements, possibly leading to respiratory failure if skeletal muscle weakness is present
  7. Immunosuppression

8. Prolonged bleeding time in response to relatively slight trauma or tissue injury
9. Decreased platelet aggregation
10. Increased irritability
11. Seizure activity
12. Coma
13. Decreased bone density, alterations in bone shape, fractures

- Treatment of hypophosphatemia includes
  1. Stopping all drugs, such as antacids, osmotic diuretics, and calcium supplements
  2. Administering oral supplements of phosphates and vitamin D
  3. Administering parenteral phosphate only when the serum phosphate level is less than 1 mg/dL and the client is experiencing serious clinical manifestations
  4. Encouraging the client to eat foods high in phosphorus, such as beef, pork, fish, chicken, whole-grain breads, beans, and other legumes and discouraging calcium-rich foods

Hypopituitarism

OVERVIEW

- Hypopituitarism is a deficiency of one or more of the anterior pituitary hormones.
- The clinical features and symptoms vary, depending on the severity of the disease and the number of deficient hormones.
- Growth retardation (in children), metabolic abnormalities, and sexual dysfunction may occur.
- Deficiencies of adrenocorticotropic hormone (ACTH) and thyroid-stimulating hormone (TSH) are life threatening.

COLLABORATIVE MANAGEMENT

Assessment

- Record client information.
    1. Loss of secondary sex characteristics
        a. Adult males may report
            (1) Loss of facial and body hair
            (2) Episodes of impotence
            (3) Decreased libido
        b. Adult females may report
            (1) Amenorrhea
            (2) Difficulty becoming pregnant
            (3) Painful intercourse
            (4) Decreased libido
- Assess for
    1. Neurologic manifestations
        a. Changes in visual acuity and peripheral vision
        b. Bilateral temporal headaches
        c. Diplopia and ocular muscle paralysis secondary to dysfunction of cranial nerves III, IV, and VI
    2. Decrease or loss of facial or body hair
    3. Decrease in muscle mass and tone
    4. Testicular atrophy in males
    5. Loss of or decreased axillary and pubic hair and atrophy of the breasts in females
    6. Changes in body image and self-esteem
    7. Anxiety and ineffective coping skills
    8. Levels of triiodothyronine (T_3), thyroxine (T_4), testosterone, estradiol, and ACTH that are low or in low-normal ranges
    9. Abnormal results of stimulation tests
    10. Changes in the sella turcica
- Management of hypopituitarism focuses on replacement of deficient hormones.
    1. Instruct the client about hormone replacement therapy.
    2. Administer androgens (testosterone) intramuscularly for males.
        a. Instruct the client in self-administration.
        b. Dosage begins at 50 mg, which is gradually increased to 200 mg, based on age.

   c. Teach the client that injections are usually required every 4 to 6 weeks depending on clinical evaluation and recurrence of symptoms.

   d. Teach the side effects of testosterone, which include gynecomastia, baldness, and prostatic hypertrophy.

   e. Alert the client that the maximal effects of treatment include

     (1) Increase in penis size, libido, and muscle mass

     (2) Increased growth of facial, pubic, and axillary hair

     (3) Deepened voice

     (4) Increased bone size and strength

     (5) Increased self-esteem and improved body image

3. Give human chorionic gonadotropin (hCG) therapy for achieving fertility in women.

4. Provide hormone replacement with a combination of estrogen and progesterone administered in a cyclic manner to females, and teach the client about adverse effects of drug therapy, such as hypertension and thrombophlebitis.

Hypothyroidism

OVERVIEW

- Hypothyroidism results from low levels of thyroid hormones.
- *Primary* hypothyroidism is a result of decreased thyroid tissue or decreased synthesis of thyroid hormone.
- *Secondary* hypothyroidism may result from inadequate production of thyroid-stimulating hormone.
- *Goiter* is an enlargement of the thyroid gland resulting from inadequate production of thyroid hormone.
- *Myxedema coma* is a rare but serious presentation of hypothyroidism, manifested by coma, hypotension, hyponatremia, respiratory failure, hypothermia, and hypoglycemia. Emergency care of the client includes

1. Maintaining a patent airway

2. Replacing fluids as needed

3. Administering medications, including levothyroxine sodium, corticosteroids, intravenous glucose

4. Checking the client's temperature frequently

5. Monitoring blood pressure
6. Covering the client with warm blankets
7. Monitoring for changes in mental status

- Hypothyroidism occurs more often in women than in men.
- Endemic goiter occurs in areas where the soil and water are deficient in iodine.

COLLABORATIVE MANAGEMENT

Assessment

- Record client information.
    1. Change in sleep habits (usually significantly increased)
    2. Generalized weakness, anorexia, muscle aches, paresthesia, and cold intolerance
    3. Change in bowel pattern (usually constipation)
    4. Medical history, with special attention to use of drugs such as lithium, aminoglutethimide, sodium or potassium perchlorate, thiocyanates, or cobalt
- Assess for
    1. Integumentary manifestations
        a. Cool, pale, or yellowish dry, coarse, scaly skin
        b. Thick, brittle nails
        c. Decreased hair growth, loss of eyebrow hair
    2. Pulmonary manifestations
        a. Hypoventilation
        b. Pleural effusion
        c. Dyspnea
    3. Cardiovascular manifestations
        a. Bradycardia
        b. Other dysrhythmias
        c. Enlarged heart
        d. Decreased exercise or activity tolerance
        e. Hypotension
    4. Gastrointestinal manifestations
        a. Anorexia
        b. Constipation
        c. Abdominal distention
        d. Weight gain
    5. Musculoskeletal manifestations
        a. Muscle aches and pains
        b. Delayed contraction and relaxation of muscles

6. Neurologic manifestations
   a. Slowing of intellectual functions
   b. Slowness or slurring of speech
   c. Impaired memory
   d. Inattentiveness
   e. Lethargy
   f. Confusion
   g. Paresthesia
   h. Decreased deep tendon reflexes
7. Physiologic and emotional manifestations
   a. Apathy
   b. Agitation
   c. Depression
   d. Paranoia
8. Metabolic manifestations
   a. Decreased basal metabolic rate
   b. Decreased body temperature
   c. Cold intolerance
9. Reproductive manifestations
   a. Females: changes in menses, infertility, decreased libido
   b. Males: decreased libido, impotence
10. Other manifestations
   a. Periorbital edema
   b. Facial puffiness
   c. Nonpitting edema of the hands and feet
   d. Goiter
   e. Anemia
   f. Easy bruising
   g. Decreased serum T_3 and T_4 levels

Planning and Implementation

◄**NDx:** Decreased Cardiac Output

■ Clients with chronic hypothyroidism may have cardiovascular disease.
   1. Monitor blood pressure, heart rate, and rhythm
   2. Observe closely for signs of shock
      a. Hypotension
      b. Decreasing urinary output
      c. Mental status changes

- Teach the client about lifelong replacement of thyroid hormone.
  1. Administer synthetic hormone preparations: levothyroxine sodium (Synthroid, Eltroxin).
  2. Observe closely for chest pain and dyspnea when initiating therapy.
  3. Monitor for signs and symptoms of hyperthyroidism that can occur during replacement therapy.

◆**NDx:** Ineffective Breathing Pattern

- Monitor the client for respiratory difficulty.
  1. Observe and record the rate and depth of respirations.
  2. Auscultate lungs and note abnormalities such as decreased breath sounds.
  3. Recognize that severe respiratory distress may be associated with myxedema coma.
  4. Avoid sedating the client because it may contribute to respiratory distress; if sedation must be used, the usual dosage is decreased because hypothyroidism increases sensitivity to these drugs.

◆**NDx:** Disturbed Thought Processes

- Nursing interventions include
  1. Noting the presence and severity of symptoms such as lethargy, memory deficit, inattentiveness, and difficulty communicating
  2. Orienting the client; explaining procedures slowly and carefully
  3. Encouraging the family to accept the client's mood changes and mental slowness, which should improve with therapy

Community-Based Care

- Client teaching includes
  1. Teaching about the possible need for extra heat or clothing because of cold intolerance if the symptoms have not cleared before discharge
  2. Providing drug information
     a. Emphasizing the need for lifelong administration of medication

    b. Reviewing the signs and symptoms of hyperthyroidism and hypothyroidism

    c. Teaching about the contraindications of over-the-counter medications that may interact with the thyroid medication

    d. Stressing the importance of wearing a medical alert bracelet or necklace because many thyroid medications potentiate and interact with other drugs.

3. Providing the elderly client with additional information about the effects of aging on the thyroid gland

4. Providing diet information to prevent constipation

5. Stressing the importance of adequate rest periods before the client assumes a full schedule

Immunodeficiencies

- An immunodeficiency is a deficient response of the immune system that is due to a missing or damaged immune component.

- The immunodeficient client is susceptible to infections, malignancies, and other diseases.

- Primary or congenital immunodeficiency is present from birth.

- Secondary or acquired immunodeficiency occurs in a person who had a normally functioning immune system at birth but later became immunodeficient as a consequence of disease, injury, exposure to toxins, medical therapy, or unknown causes.

- Types of antibody-mediated immunodeficiency include

    1. Bruton's, or X-linked, agammaglobulinemia

      a. Congenital antibody-mediated immunodeficiency manifested by recurrent otitis, sinusitis, pneumonia, furunculosis, meningitis, and septicemia

      b. Overall good prognosis if antibody replacement begins early in life, except in clients who have poliomyelitis, chronic echovirus infection, or a lymphoreticular malignancy

    c. Treated with intravenous (IV) or intramuscular (IM) immune serum globulin

    d. Antibiotics used for specific infections

2. Common variable immunodeficiency, or acquired hypogammaglobulinemia

    a. Appears in adolescents or young adults

    b. Is characterized by recurrent bacterial infections

    c. Complications of giardiasis, bronchiectasis, gastric carcinoma, lymphoreticular malignancy, and cholelithiasis

    d. Treated by the regular administration of IV or IM immune serum globulin and the use of antibiotics intermittently or long term

3. Immunoglobulin A (IgA) deficiency

    a. May be asymptomatic or have chronic recurrent respiratory tract infections, atopic diseases, or collagen vascular diseases; may have malabsorption syndrome

    b. Treatment limited to appropriate and vigorous treatment of infection

- *Iatrogenic* immunodeficiency is an immunodeficiency or immunosuppressive state induced in the client by medical therapies or procedures.

  1. May be drug induced by

    a. Cytotoxic drugs

    b. Corticosteroids

    c. Cyclosporine

  2. May be radiation induced

  3. Treatment goals: to improve immune function and to protect the client from infections

- Follow and teach the client good handwashing.

Incontinence, Urinary

OVERVIEW

- Urinary incontinence (UI) is the involuntary loss of urine that is severe enough to cause social or hygienic problems. It may be transient or permanent and is *not* a normal change associated with aging.

- Common forms of urinary incontinence include
  1. *Stress* incontinence is characterized by the loss of small amounts of urine during coughing, sneezing, jogging or lifting. Clients are unable to tighten the urethra sufficiently to overcome the increased detrusor pressure, and leakage of urine results.
  2. *Urge* urinary incontinence is the involuntary loss of urine associated with a sudden, strong desire to urinate. Clients are unable to suppress the signal from the bladder muscle to the brain that it is time to urinate.
  3. *Mixed* incontinence is a combination of stress and urge incontinence.
  4. *Overflow* incontinence occurs when the bladder has reached its absolute maximum capacity and some urine must leak out to prevent bladder rupture. The detrusor muscle is underactive and does not send signals to the brain that the bladder is full.
  5. *Functional* incontinence is leakage of urine caused by factors other than pathology of the lower urinary tract.
- In adult clients younger than 65 years of age, incontinence occurs twice as often in women than in men.

COLLABORATIVE MANAGEMENT
Assessment
- Record client information.
  1. History of incontinence
     a. Onset: recent or in the past
     b. Intermittent or continuous
     c. Time of occurrence (day or night)
     d. Contributing factors (e.g., sneezing, coughing)
     e. Circumstances surrounding the problem
     f. Voiding patterns and changes
     g. Perception of bladder fullness
     h. Presence of warning signals
  2. Presence of risk factors for urinary incontinence
     a. Age
     b. Menopausal status
     c. Neurologic disease
        (1) Parkinson disease
        (2) Dementia

　　　　(3) Multiple sclerosis
　　　　(4) Stroke
　　d. Diabetes mellitus
　　e. Childbirth
　　f. Urologic procedures
　　g. Spinal cord injuries
　　h. Medications
　　i. Bowel pattern
　　j. Stress/anxiety level
　3. Mobility
　4. Self-care ability
　5. Cognitive ability
　6. Communication pattern
　7. Barriers to toileting
　　a. Privacy
　　b. Restrictive clothing
　　c. Access to toilet
- Assess as follows:
　1. Palpate the abdominal area for evidence of urinary distention or discomfort.
　2. Percuss the abdomen and listen for the dull sound of a distended bladder.
　3. Observe for urine leakage while the client strains by coughing or bearing down in the standing position.
　4. If ordered, catheterize the client after the client voids to determine the amount of residual urine.
　5. Inspect the external genitalia of female clients to determine whether there is apparent urethral or uterine prolapse or cystocele.
　6. Describe the color, consistency, and odor of any secretions from the genitourinary orifices.
　7. Inspect the urinary meatus of male clients for the presence of discharge or other characteristics.
　8. Query the client regarding the effects of incontinence on socialization, family relationships, and emotional status.
　9. Monitor the urine for the presence of red or white blood cells.
　10. Review the results of the voiding cystourethrogram, which detects the anatomic structure and function of the bladder, as well as the postvoiding residual.

Planning and Implementation

◆NDx: Stress Urinary Incontinence

NONSURGICAL MANAGEMENT

- Provide drug therapy.
  1. Phenylpropanolamine, an alpha-adrenergic agonist
  2. Tricyclic antidepressants: imipramine (Tofranil, Novo-Pramine)
  3. Estrogen for postmenopausal women
  4. Tolterodine
- Collaborate with the dietitian to develop a dietary plan to assist the obese client to lose weight and to encourage the client to avoid alcohol and caffeine (bladder stimulants).
- Provide exercise therapy.
  1. Teach female clients how to do Kegel exercises to strengthen the muscles of the pelvic floor; biofeedback devices may be used to help the client detect the effectiveness of the exercises.
  2. Instruct the client in the correct use of vaginal cones.
     a. The lightest cone is inserted into the vagina with the string to the outside for a 1-minute test period.
     b. If the client is able to hold the first cone in place without its slipping out while she walks around, she proceeds to the second cone and repeats the procedure.
     c. Treatment is begun with the heaviest cone that the client can hold in her vagina for the 1-minute test period.
     d. The treatment is for 15 minutes twice a day; when the client can hold the cone comfortably in her vagina for 15 minutes, proceed to the next heaviest weight.
- Other treatments include behavior modification, psychotherapy, and electrical devices for the inhibition of bladder contraction.
- The Reliance insert is a tampon-like device inserted into the urethra. The client inflates the attached balloon, which prevents urine flow.

SURGICAL MANAGEMENT

- Provide preoperative care.
  1. Provide instruction and clarify events surrounding the surgery.
  2. Prepare the client for any diagnostic testing.

- Operative procedures for women are used to elevate the bladder and urethra into a normal intra-abdominal position, increase the length of the urethra, and decrease hypermobility of the bladder neck. Procedures are as follows:
  1. *Anterior vaginal repair* (colporrhaphy) to elevate the urethral position and repair any cystocele
  2. *Retropubic suspension* to elevate the urethral position and provide longer-lasting results
  3. *Needle bladder neck suspension* (Pereyra or Stamey procedure) to elevate the urethra and provide a longer-lasting result without a long operative time
  4. *Pubovaginal sling procedure* in which a sling made of synthetic material is placed under the urethrovesical junction to elevate the bladder neck
  5. An *artificial sphincter,* a mechanical device that opens and closes the urethra, placed around the anatomic urethra; the procedure is used for men more often than for women
- Provide postoperative care.
  1. Assess and intervene to detect and prevent complications.
  2. Secure the urethral catheter to prevent unnecessary movement or traction on the bladder neck.
  3. Monitor the suprapubic catheter, if present, for leakage of urine and serosanguineous drainage.

◆**NDx:** Urge Urinary Incontinence

- Interventions for urge urinary incontinence include medication and behavioral interventions; surgery is not recommended.
- Drug therapy includes
  1. Anticholinergic agents and anticholinergics with smooth muscle relaxant properties
  2. Tricyclic antidepressants
- Diet therapy includes
  1. Instructing the client to avoid foods that have a bladder-stimulating effect, such as caffeine and alcohol
  2. Instructing the client to space fluids throughout the day and to limit fluids after dinner
- Bladder training is an educational program to help clients gain control of their bladder.

1. Regular schedule of voiding is established.
2. The client is instructed to void during the established time frame and to ignore any urge to urinate that occurs between the mandated interval.
3. Once the client is comfortable with the initial interval, the interval time is increased by 15 to 30 minutes.

- Habit training is a variation of bladder training that is useful for cognitively impaired clients. The caregiver assists the client to void every 2 hours.
- Exercise therapies such as Kegel exercises and vaginal cone therapy are also useful.
- Electrical stimulation with a variety of intravaginal and intrarectal devices has been used to treat both stress and urge urinary incontinence.

COLLABORATIVE PROBLEM:
Reflex (Overflow) Incontinence

- Surgery, which includes removal of the prostate and repair of genital prolapse, may be needed to relieve the obstruction of the bladder outlet.
- Treatment includes
  1. Bethanechol chloride for the short-term management of urinary retention
  2. The Credé maneuver, Valsalva maneuver, or double-voiding technique to assist in promoting bladder contraction
  3. Teaching intermittent self-catheterization to clients with long-term problems of incomplete bladder emptying

NDx: Functional Urinary Incontinence

- The primary focus of the intervention is to treat reversible causes of incontinence. When that is not possible, the goal is to contain the urine and protect the client's skin.
- Interventions include
  1. Teaching the client how to use applied devices such as the intravaginal pessaries for women and urethral clamps for men
  2. Using absorbent pads and briefs to collect urine and keep the client's skin and clothing dry
  3. Inserting a Foley catheter or beginning an intermittent catheterization program as indicated

- Discharge planning includes
  1. Assessing the home environment for barriers that impede access to the toileting facilities
  2. Considering the personal, physical, emotional, and social resources of the client
  3. Considering who the primary caretaker will be and what circumstances or factors exist in the environment that will influence the effectiveness of the plan
  4. Assisting the client to control or manage fears and anxieties related to incontinence while in public
  5. Refering the client to home care agencies
- Teach the client about
  1. The causes of incontinence and treatment options available
  2. Prescribed medications (purpose, dosage, method, route of administration, and expected and potential side effects)
  3. The importance of weight reduction and dietary modification
  4. Options available for external devices or incontinence pads, considering the client's lifestyle and resources
  5. The technique of self-catheterization; ensure that a return demonstration is correct

Infection

OVERVIEW

- The infectious process requires a pathogen (causative agent), portal of exit for the agent, means of transmission, portal of entry to the host (infection recipient), and a susceptible host.
- Reservoirs are sources of infectious agents that includes people, animals, insects, environmental sources such as soil, water.
- Infectious diseases include those that are thought to be communicable (transmitted from person to person) and those that are not communicable (e.g., pancreatitis).
- A *pathogen* is any microorganism that is capable of producing disease.

- *Pathogenicity* is the ability to cause disease.
- *Virulence* refers to the frequency with which a pathogen causes disease (degree of communicability) and its ability to invade and damage a host; it also refers to the severity of the disease.
- *Invasiveness* is the ability of pathogens to spread and grow in tissues of a host after entrance.
- In *colonization* the microorganisms are present in the tissues of the host yet do not cause symptomatic disease.
- Microorganisms that behave as parasites live at the expense of their human host.
- Prevention of the spread of infection is dependent on breaking the chain of infection at any point.
- Host factors that increase the risk of infection include
  1. Congenital or acquired immunodeficiencies (e.g., acquired immunodeficiency syndrome [AIDS])
  2. Alteration of normal flora by antibiotic therapy
  3. Age (especially infants and older adults)
  4. Pregnancy, diabetes, corticosteroid therapy, and adrenal insufficiency
  5. Defective phagocytic function, circulatory disturbances, and neutropenia
  6. Break in skin or mucous membrane integrity
  7. Interference with the flow of urine, tears, or saliva
  8. Impaired cough reflex or ciliary action
  9. Malnutrition and dehydration
  10. Smoking, alcohol consumption, and inhalation of toxic chemicals
  11. Invasive therapy, chemotherapy, radiation therapy, steroid therapy, and surgery
- Common modes of transmission of infection are
  1. Direct contact: source and host have physical contact
  2. Indirect contact: transfer of micro-organisms from a source to a host by passive transfer from an inanimate object such as contaminated equipment or water, or oral-fecal route
  3. Droplet: infection acquired by contact with droplets deposited on the nasal, oral, or conjunctival membrane (e.g., influenza)
  4. Airborne: pathogens suspended in the air for a prolonged time; most often propelled from the respiratory tract by coughing or sneezing (e.g., tuberculosis [TB])

5. Vectors: insects and animals that act as intermediaries between two or more hosts (e.g., ticks, mosquitoes)
- The portal of exit is usually through the portal of entry.
- Human defenses against infection include
   1. Intact skin
   2. Mucous membranes
   3. Respiratory tract
   4. Gastrointestinal (GI) tract
   5. Genitourinary tract
   6. Phagocytosis
   7. Inflammation
   8. Antibody-mediated and cell-mediated immune system
- A nosocomial infection or health care–associated infection is an infection acquired while the client is in an inpatient setting. It occurs while the client is receiving health care.
- Infection or the spread of infection can be controlled by
   1. Hand hygiene
      a. Handwashing
      b. Institutional policy regarding artificial fingernails and extenders and length of fingernails
   2. Barriers including gloves, gowns, and masks
   3. Disinfection/sterilization
- Certain diseases must be reported to the Centers for Disease Control and Prevention (CDC).
- Isolation guidelines from the CDC include Standard, Airborne, Droplet, and Contact Precautions.
   1. *Standard precautions* should be used in the care of *all* clients. These precautions combine body substance and universal precautions and acknowledge that all body secretions, excretions, and moist membranes and tissues (excluding perspiration) are potentially infectious.
   2. *Airborne precautions* are used for clients known to have or suspected of having infections transmitted by small droplet nuclei that are expelled during coughing or sneezing. Tuberculosis (TB), measles (rubeola), and chickenpox (varicella) are examples of airborne diseases. Health care workers must wear HEPA or N-95 respirators to filter inspired air when in the room of a client with known or suspected TB.
   3. *Droplet precautions* are used for clients with known or suspected serious infections transmitted by the droplet

route. Examples include influenza, mumps, meningitis, and pertussis.

4. *Contact precautions* are used to prevent the transmission of organisms that are spread primarily by direct contact or contact with items in the environment. Clients with methicillin-resistant *Staphylococcus aureus* (MRSA) or vancomycin-resistant *Enterococcus* (VRE) are placed on contact isolation.

- Typical complications of infection are relapse, cellulitis, pneumonia, abscess formation, systemic complications, and septic shock.

 Considerations for Older Adults

- Special attention should be given to older adults with an infection.
- Assess for atypical manifestations of infection such as confusion and unusual behavior; fever and pain may not be present.
- Monitor for renal function when the client receives antibiotic therapy.
- Observe for and report adverse side effects of antibiotic therapy because the older client is at risk for these complications.
- Monitor for diarrhea and obtain a specimen for culture, as ordered.
- Keep the client well hydrated unless contraindicated.

COLLABORATIVE MANAGEMENT

Assessment

- Record client information.
  1. Exposure to a person with similar clinical symptoms or to contaminated food or water and date of exposure
  2. Contact with pets and other animals
  3. Travel history
  4. Sexual history
  5. Intravenous (IV) drug use
  6. Transfusion history
  7. Order of onset of symptoms
- Common clinical manifestations are associated with specific sites of infection.

1. Skin manifestations
   a. Redness
   b. Warmth
   c. Swelling
   d. Drainage and pus
   e. Pain
2. Generalized infection manifestations
   a. Fever (temperature above 101° F [38° C] or 99° F [37° C] in the older adult)
   b. Malaise
   c. Fatigue
   d. Muscle aches
   e. Joint pain
   f. Lymphadenopathy
   g. Photophobia
3. GI tract manifestations
   a. Nausea and vomiting
   b. Diarrhea
   c. Pharyngitis
4. Genitourinary tract manifestations
   a. Dysuria
   b. Frequency
   c. Urgency
   d. Hematuria
   e. Fever
   f. Purulent discharge
   g. Pelvic or flank pain
5. Respiratory tract manifestations
   a. Cough
   b. Congestion
   c. Rhinitis
   d. Sore throat
   e. Fever
   f. Chest pain
6. Psychosocial dysfunction
   a. Anxiety and frustration
   b. Social isolation
7. Abnormal laboratory results
   a. Positive culture findings
   b. Serologic testing

    c. White blood cell count
    d. Erythrocyte sedimentation rate
  8. Abnormal radiographic results
    a. Chest x-ray, sinus, or joint films; GI studies
    b. CT or MRI
    c. Ultrasonography
    d. Biopsy

Planning and Implementation

◆NDx: Hyperthermia

- Interventions to reduce fever include
  1. Antimicrobials
  2. Antipyretics
  3. External cooling
  4. Fluid administration
- Effective antibiotic therapy requires
  1. Appropriate antibiotic
  2. Sufficient dosage
  3. Proper rate of administration
  4. Sufficient duration
- Nursing interventions include
  1. Obtaining an allergy history before giving antibiotics
  2. Monitoring the client for side effects of antibiotics, including nausea, vomiting, and rash
  3. Applying a hypothermia blanket and monitoring for shivering
  4. Sponging the client with tepid water
  5. Monitoring for signs of dehydration such as increased thirst, decreased skin turgor, and dry mucous membranes
  6. Encouraging fluid intake
  7. Recording intake and output
  8. Monitoring the client's vital signs and pulse oximetry closely
  9. Monitoring skin color and temperature
  10. Monitoring for decreasing level of consciousness and seizure activity
  11. Monitoring laboratory values
  12. Providing or encouraging oral hygiene

- Aspirin and acetaminophen are generally not given unless the client is extremely uncomfortable or if fever presents a significant risk (e.g., if the client has a history of heart failure, febrile seizures, or head injury).

◆NDx: Social Isolation

- Education is the major intervention to minimize or prevent social isolation.
    1. Educate the client and family about the mode of transmission of the infection and mechanisms that prevent the spread of organisms from the client to others.
    2. Encourage family and friends to visit the client; provide information and instructions on isolation techniques and other precautions needed to prevent transmission of the disease.
    3. Ensure that the client has access to a telephone and radio.
    4. Visit with the client frequently to say "hello" and check if the client needs anything.

Community-Based Care

- Health teaching includes
    1. Encouraging the client to keep immunizations up-to-date
    2. Emphasizing the importance of a clean home environment
    3. Ensuring that the client has proper storage facilities at home for medications and knows how to recognize signs of improper storage
    4. Explaining the importance of handwashing facilities in the home and providing supplies and instruction as needed
    5. Instructing the client about the disease, method of transmission, and how to prevent its transmission
    6. Explaining how to dispose of needles, how to wash clothing soiled with blood or body fluids, and how to clean equipment
    7. Explaining the importance of compliance regarding taking medications at home
        a. Timing of doses
        b. Completion of planned number of days of therapy
        c. Side effects of medications
        d. Allergic manifestations

     e. Importance of notifying the physician if an adverse or allergic reaction occurs
  8. Teaching the client with infusion devices for administration of medications
     a. Care of the device
     b. Indications of device malfunction
     c. Indications of infection of the device or the site of insertion
  9. Refer to home health care agencies as needed

Infections, Chlamydial

OVERVIEW

- *Chlamydia trachomatis* is the most commonly transmitted bacteria in the United States.
- *C. trachomatis* invades columnar epithelial tissues in the reproductive tract and causes clinical manifestations similar to those of gonorrhea.
- The incubation period ranges from 1 to 3 weeks, although the pathogen may be present in the genital tract for months or years without producing symptoms.

COLLABORATIVE MANAGEMENT

Assessment

- Assess for
  1. Men: urethritis, dysuria, frequency of urination, mucoid discharge that is more watery and less copious than gonorrheal discharge
  2. Women (note: 75% are asymptomatic): mucopurulent cervicitis, change in vaginal discharge, dysuria, urinary frequency, soreness in the affected area
- Also assesses for
  1. Sexual history
     a. History of sexually transmitted diseases (STDs)
     b. Sexual partner with history of STDs
     c. Sexual partner with suspicious symptoms

2. Risk factors associated with *C. trachomatis*
   a. Pregnancy
   b. Sexual activity during adolescence
   c. Use of nonbarrier method of birth control
   d. History of multiple sexual partners
3. Exclusion of gonorrhea on Gram stain and culture
4. Diagnostic tests such as enzyme-linked immunoassay and a direct fluorescent antibody test
- Complications include
  1. Men: epididymitis, prostatitis, infertility, and Reiter's syndrome
  2. Women: salpingitis, pelvic inflammatory disease, ectopic pregnancy, and infertility

Interventions

- The treatment of choice is azithromycin (Zithromax) or doxycycline (Monodox, Doxycin ♣).
- Client education includes
  1. Transmission
  2. Signs and symptoms
  3. Medical treatment
  4. Complications of untreated chlamydial infections
  5. Instructing client to avoid sexual activity for 7 days from the start of treatment
  6. Partner treatment
  7. Use of condoms

Infections, Skin

OVERVIEW

- The majority of *cutaneous bacterial* infections are caused by *Staphylococcus* or *Streptococcus.*
- *Folliculitis* is a superficial staphylococcal infection involving the upper portion of the hair follicle and is associated with mild discomfort.
- *Furuncles* (boils) are caused by *Staphylococcus,* but the infection occurs deeper in the hair follicle.

- *Cellulitis* is a generalized nonfollicular infection with either **Staphylococcus** or **Streptococcus**, involving deeper connective tissue.
- *Viral* skin infections include *herpes simplex* virus (HSV) infections (type I virus [classic cold sores] and type II virus [genital herpes]), *herpes zoster* (shingles), and herpetic whitlow.
- Many *fungal* infections may affect the skin.
- Superficial fungal (dermatophyte) infections, or tinea, include
    1. Tinea pedis (athlete's foot)
    2. Tinea manus (hands)
    3. Tinea cruris (groin)
    4. Tinea corporis (ringworm)
    5. Tinea capitis (scalp)
    6. Tinea barbae (beard)
- *Candidiasis* is an opportunistic yeast infection of the skin and mucous membranes.

COLLABORATIVE MANAGEMENT

Assessment

- Record client information.
    1. Recent history of skin trauma
    2. Past or current history of staphylococcal or streptococcal infections
    3. Lesions appearing on the lips, oral cavity, or genitals
    4. Past history of similar lesions
    5. Prodromal symptoms of burning, tingling, or pain
    6. Previous exposure to chickenpox
    7. History of shingles
    8. Anatomic location of dermatophyte infection
    9. Social and environmental factors
    10. History of recent antibiotics or immunosuppressive drugs
    11. Medical history, including diabetes or cancer
    12. Nutritional deficiencies
- Assess for clinical manifestations of common skin infections such as
    1. Redness
    2. Warmth
    3. Edema

4. Tenderness
5. Pain
6. Itching
7. Stinging
8. Localized areas of inflammation
9. Blisters
10. Pustules
11. Papules
12. Vesicles
13. Scaling
14. Single or multiple lesions

Interventions

- Skin care includes
  1. Instructing the client to bathe daily with antibacterial soap for bacterial infection
  2. Applying warm compresses to furuncles or cellulitis
  3. Applying astringent compresses such as Burow's solution to viral lesions
  4. Ensuring that the skin dries between treatments
  5. Positioning the client to promote air circulation
  6. Instructing the client to avoid wearing tight garments
- Isolation precautions include
  1. Using proper handwashing technique to prevent cross-contamination
  2. Maintaining strict isolation for resistant *Staphylococcus*
  3. Teaching the client to avoid sexual contact when recurrent herpes lesions are present
  4. Teaching the client and family to avoid sharing contaminated personal items (e.g., hairbrush, articles of clothing, footwear) of clients with dermatophyte infections
- Drug therapy includes
  1. Antibacterial ointment such as neomycin, gentamicin, chloramphenicol, or povidone-iodine and cream such as silver sulfadiazine
  2. Antifungal ointment and cream, such as imidazole cream for dermatophyte and yeast infections
  3. Antifungal powder such as nystatin or tolnaftate
  4. Antifungal oral preparation such as nystatin or clotrimazole

5. Anti-inflammatory steroid preparations, as ordered, ranging from low to potent fluorinated agents
6. Antiviral ointment such as acyclovir, as ordered, which is the treatment of choice for viral infections
- Incision and drainage of *furuncles* is the primary surgical procedure that is done for skin infections.

Irritable Bowel Syndrome

OVERVIEW

- Irritable bowel syndrome (IBS), is a chronic gastrointestinal (GI) disorder characterized by the presence of chronic or recurrent diarrhea, constipation, or abdominal pain and bloating.
- Factors such as diet, stress, and mental or behavioral illness may precipitate exacerbations.
- Twice as many women as men are affected by IBS.

COLLABORATIVE MANAGEMENT

Assessment

- Assess for symptoms collectively known as the Manning criteria:
  1. Abdominal pain, relieved by defecation or associated with changes in stool frequency or consistency
  2. Abdominal distention
  3. Sensation of incomplete evacuation of stool
  4. Presence of mucus with stool passage
- Other assessment findings include:
  1. Pain in the lower left quadrant of the abdomen that increases after eating and is relieved by a bowel movement
  2. Nausea associated with mealtime and defecation
  3. Diarrhea or constipation
  4. Belching, gas, anorexia, and bloating
  5. Tympanic bowel sounds

Interventions

- Diet therapy includes
  1. Helping the client identify and eliminate offending or upsetting foods
  2. Advising the client to limit caffeine and avoid alcohol and beverages that contain sorbitol or fructose; milk and milk products are avoided if lactose intolerance is suspected
  3. Consulting with the dietitian to teach the client to add 30 to 40 g of fiber to the diet daily
  4. Encouraging the client to eat regular meals and chew food slowly
  5. Teaching the client to drink 8 to 10 cups of liquid per day
- Drug therapy includes
  1. Bulk-forming laxatives for constipation-predominant IBS
  2. Antidiarrheal agents to decrease cramping and frequency of stools
  3. Muscarinic receptor agents to inhibit intestinal motility
  4. Anticholinergic receptor blocking agents or antispasmodics to help relieve abdominal cramping and intestinal spasm
  5. Recently approved 5-HT4 medications for women with constipation-predominant IBS
- Stress management includes
  1. Assisting the client to learn relaxation techniques
  2. Encouraging the client to implement a regular exercise program to promote bowel elimination and reduce stress
  3. Personal counseling
- Complementary and alternative therapies include peppermint and caraway oil combinations, evening primrose oil, chamomile, yoga, hypnosis. and acupuncture.

Kidney Disease, Polycystic

OVERVIEW

- Polycystic kidney disease (PKD) is an inherited kidney disorder of the renal parenchyma that occurs bilaterally.
- The nephron is the primary site of cyst development; cysts develop in the glomeruli and tubules, resulting in less

effective glomerular filtration, tubular reabsorption, and tubular secretion.

- The kidneys become grossly enlarged, cysts become progressively larger, and other abdominal organs may be displaced.

COLLABORATIVE MANAGEMENT

Assessment

- Record client information.
    1. Current health status
    2. Family history of PKD
    3. Age of parents at development of clinical manifestations and related complications
    4. Family history of sudden death from a strokelike phenomenon
    5. History of constipation
    6. Changes in urine or frequency of urination
    7. History of hypertension
    8. History of headaches
- Assess for
    1. Protruding and distended abdomen
    2. Enlarged kidney on palpation
    3. Abdominal pain
    4. Tender tissue and flank pain
    5. Hematuria or cloudy urine
    6. Dysuria
    7. Nocturia
    8. Hypertension
    9. Edema
    10. Uremic symptoms
    11. Anger, resentment
    12. Futility, sadness

Interventions

- Provide drug therapy.
    1. Analgesics for comfort; avoid nonsteroidal anti-inflammatory agents (NSAIDs) and aspirin-containing products
    2. Lipid-soluble antibiotics such as trimethoprim/sulfamethoxazole (Bactrim, Septra, Trimpex) or ciprofloxacin (Cipro) for infectious process

- Provide other interventions.
  1. Apply dry heat to the abdomen or flank.
  2. Teach relaxation techniques.
  3. Teach the client how to prevent constipation.
     a. Nutrition management
     b. Regular exercise
     c. Fluid management
     d. Appropriate use of stool softeners
- Provide hypertension and renal failure management.
  1. Administer antihypertensive agents including angiotensin-converting enzyme (ACE) inhibitors, vasodilators, beta blockers, and calcium channel blockers as ordered.
  2. Administer diuretics, as ordered, for clients with renal insufficiency.
  3. Monitor intake and output.
  4. Record daily weight.
  5. Provide a low-sodium diet initially; diet will change based on the client's condition.
  6. Maintain protein restriction as renal insufficiency progresses.
  7. Provide counseling, support, and teaching about health maintenance.
  8. Discuss coping strategies used successfully in the past.
  9. Encourage the client to verbalize feelings or frustrations.
- Teach the client and family
  1. How to measure and monitor blood pressure and weight
  2. Dietary restrictions, such as a low-sodium or protein-restricted diet
  3. Desired and adverse effects of prescribed medications, including antihypertensive drugs and diuretics
  4. Measures and their rationale for preventing constipation
  5. Resources that are available for research and education, such as the Polycystic Kidney Research Foundation

Labyrinthitis

- Labyrinthitis is an infection of the labyrinth.
- Clinical manifestations include hearing loss, tinnitus, spontaneous nystagmus to the affected side, nausea, vertigo, and vomiting.
- The most common complication is meningitis.
- Treatment includes
  1. Systemic antibiotics
  2. Bedrest in a darkened room
  3. Antiemetics
  4. Antivertiginous medications
  5. Psychological support to cope with hearing loss
  6. Gait training and physical therapy for persistent balance problems

Lacerations, Eye

- The most common areas involved in lacerations of the eye are the eyelids and cornea.
  1. Eye lacerations
     a. Bleed heavily and look more severe than they actually are
     b. Are treated by closing the eye and applying a small ice pack, checking visual acuity, and cleaning and suturing the eyelid
  2. Corneal lacerations
     a. The ocular contents may prolapse through the laceration.
     b. The laceration is manifested by severe eye pain, photophobia, tearing, and decreased visual acuity.
     c. The penetrating object is *never* removed from the eye; it may be holding ocular structures in place.
     d. Treatment includes surgical repair under general anesthesia and antibiotic ointment; an *enucleation*

may be needed if the ocular contents have protruded through the laceration.

e. Complications include scarring, which may alter vision.

Laryngitis

- Laryngitis is an inflammation of mucous membranes lining the larynx with or without edema of the vocal cords.
- Laryngitis is commonly associated with upper respiratory tract infections.
- Clinical manifestations include acute hoarseness, dry cough, and dysphagia; aphonia may occur.
- Management includes
  1. Steam inhalation
  2. Voice rest, which includes whispering
  3. Increased fluid intake
  4. Throat lozenges
  5. Antibiotics
  6. Bronchodilators when sinusitis, bronchitis, or bacterial upper respiratory tract infection is present
- Teach the client to avoid tobacco, alcohol, and pollutants.
- Clients with recurrent bouts of laryngitis require further evaluation for polyps, edema, or tumor.

Leiomyoma, Uterine

OVERVIEW

- Uterine leiomyomas, also called *myomas* and *fibroids* (fibroid tumors), are the most commonly occurring benign pelvic tumors.
- Leiomyomas develop from the uterine myometrium and are attached to it by a pedicle or stalk.
- Leiomyomas are classified according to their position in the layers of the uterus and anatomic position.

- The most common types are
  1. *Intramural,* contained in the uterine wall within the myometrium
  2. *Submucosal,* which protrude into the cavity of the uterus
  3. *Subserosal,* which may grow laterally and extend into the broad ligament

COLLABORATIVE MANAGEMENT

Assessment

- Assessment findings include
  1. Abnormal bleeding
  2. Complaints of a feeling of pelvic pressure
  3. Constipation
  4. Urinary frequency or retention
  5. Increased abdominal size
  6. Dyspareunia (painful intercourse)
  7. Infertility
  8. Abdominal pain occurring with torsion of the fibroid or pedicle
  9. Uterine enlargement on abdominal, vaginal, or rectal examination

Planning and Implementation

COLLABORATIVE PROBLEM: Risk for Hemorrhage

NONSURGICAL MANAGEMENT

- The client who has no symptoms or who desires childbearing is observed and examined for changes in the size of the leiomyoma every 4 to 6 months.
- If the woman is postmenopausal, the fibroids usually shrink.
- Uterine artery embolization, an alternative to surgery, involves the injection of embolic particles into the blood supply of the tumors, thereby occluding the blood supply to the tumors.

SURGICAL MANAGEMENT

- Surgical treatment depends on whether future childbearing is desired, the age of the woman, the size of the fibroid, and associated symptoms.

- A *myomectomy* (removal of the leiomyomas with preservation of the uterus) is done to preserve childbearing capabilities.
- A *transcervical endometrial resection* (TCER), done in cases such as submucosal fibroids and menorrhagia, involves destroying the endometrium with a diathermy resectoscope or with radioablation.
  1. Potential complications include fluid overload (fluid used to distend the abdomen can be absorbed); embolism; hemorrhage; perforation of the uterus, bowel, bladder or ureter injury; persistent increased menstrual bleeding; incomplete suppression of menstruation.
- *Hysterectomy* is the usual surgical management in the older woman who has multiple symptomatic leiomyomas.
- A *total hysterectomy* involves the removal of the uterus by either a vaginal or abdominal approach.
- *Panhysterectomy,* or *total abdominal hysterectomy,* includes the removal of the uterus, ovaries, and fallopian tubes.
- A *radical hysterectomy* involves removal of the uterus, lymph nodes, upper third of the vagina, and the surrounding tissues.
- Preoperative care includes routine measures and a complete psychological evaluation.
  1. Explore the client's feelings about the loss of the uterus, including childbearing, self-image, femininity, and sexual functioning.
  2. Identify the client's support system.
  3. Discuss the client's fear of rejection from her sexual partner.
- Postoperative care for the client undergoing abdominal hysterectomy is similar to that of any other client having abdominal surgery.
  1. Assess for vaginal bleeding (there should be less than one saturated pad in 4 hours).
  2. Assess for bleeding at the incision site.
  3. Assess for intactness of the incision.
  4. Maintain the Foley catheter
- Postoperative care for a client with a vaginal hysterectomy includes
  1. Assessing for vaginal bleeding (there should be less than one saturated pad in 4 hours)

2. Providing perineal care
   a. Sitz baths
   b. Heat lamps
   c. Ice packs
3. Maintaining a Foley catheter
- Complications are as follows:
  1. Abdominal hysterectomy
     a. Intestinal obstruction
     b. Thromboembolism
     c. Atelectasis
     d. Pneumonia
     e. Wound dehiscence
  2. Vaginal hysterectomy
     a. Hemorrhage
     b. Urinary tract problems, especially infection and retention
  3. Both types of hysterectomy
     a. Pulmonary embolism
     b. Depression
     c. Decreased libido

 Considerations for Older Adults

- Older women are more at risk than younger women for all postoperative complications, particularly pulmonary embolism. Obese women are more at risk than others for thromboembolism.

Community-Based Care

- The appropriate health teaching depends on the specific treatment.
- Instruct the client who has had an abdominal or vaginal hysterectomy to
  1. Avoid or limit stair climbing for 1 month.
  2. Avoid tub baths and sitting for long periods.
  3. Avoid strenuous activity or lifting anything weighing more than 5 pounds (2.3 kg).
  4. Expect certain physical changes, including cessation of menses, inability to become pregnant, weakness and fatigue in the convalescence period, and absence of menopausal symptoms unless the ovaries are removed.
  5. Participate in moderate exercise, such as walking.

6. Consume foods that aid in healing, such as foods high in protein, iron, and vitamin C.
7. Avoid sexual intercourse for 3 to 6 weeks.
8. Observe for signs of complications, including infection.
9. Expect emotional reactions and changes.

Leukemia

OVERVIEW

- The leukemias are a group of malignant disorders involving abnormal overproduction of specific cell types, usually at the immature stage, in bone marrow.
- Leukemia may be either acute or chronic.
- The two major types of leukemia are
  1. *Lymphocytic* or *lymphoblastic,* involving abnormal cells coming from the lymphoid pathways (acute and chronic)
  2. *Myelocytic* or *myelogenous,* involving abnormal cells coming from the myeloid maturational pathways (acute and chronic)
- Acute myelogenous leukemia (AML) is the most common type seen in adults.
- Acute promyelocytic leukemia (APL) and chronic myelogenous leukemia (CML) are also seen in adults
- The basic pathologic defect in leukemia is malignant transformation of stem cells or early committed precursor leukocytes, causing an abnormal proliferation of a specific type of leukocyte in the bone marrow that shuts down normal bone marrow production of erythrocytes, platelets, and functionally mature leukocytes.

COLLABORATIVE MANAGEMENT

Assessment

- Record client information.
  1. Age
  2. Environmental exposure

3. Previous illness and exposure to ionizing radiation or medications
4. History of infections, including influenza, cold, pneumonia, bronchitis, and unexplained fever
5. Overt bleeding episodes
6. History of weakness or fatigue
7. Associated symptoms
- Physical assessment may reveal
  1. Integumentary manifestations
     a. Ecchymosis
     b. Petechiae
     c. Pallor of the conjunctiva, nail beds, and palmar creases around the mouth
  2. Gastrointestinal manifestations
     a. Bleeding gums
     b. Anorexia
     c. Weight loss
     d. Enlarged liver and spleen
     e. Rectal bleeding
  3. Renal manifestations: hematuria
  4. Cardiovascular manifestations
     a. Tachycardia at basal activity levels
     b. Orthostatic hypotension
     c. Palpitations
     d. Increased capillary filling times
  5. Respiratory manifestations
     a. Abnormal breath sounds
     b. Dyspnea on exertion
  6. Neurologic manifestations
     a. Fatigue
     b. Headache
     c. Papilledema
  7. Hematologic manifestations
     a. Decreased hemoglobin, hematocrit, and platelet count
     b. Altered (usually elevated) white blood cell (WBC) count
     c. Abnormal coagulation studies
     d. Abnormal bone marrow findings
  8. Musculoskeletal manifestations
     a. Bone pain
     b. Joint swelling and pain

L

9. Laboratory findings
   a. Decreased hemoglobin, hematocrit, and platelet count
   b. Altered WBC count
   c. Bone marrow changes

Planning and Implementation

◄**NDx:** Risk for Infection

- Take infection control measures.
  1. Wash hands often and thoroughly between client contacts.
  2. If you have an upper respiratory infection, wear a mask when entering the client's room.
  3. Place the client in a private room if possible.
  4. Use aseptic technique for dressing changes.
  5. Monitor for signs of infection.
  6. Provide meticulous skin care to maintain skin integrity.
  7. Provide pulmonary toilet to prevent respiratory infections.
  8. Take environmental precautions such as not allowing a standing collection of water in vases, denture cups, or humidifiers in the client's room.
- Chemotherapeutic drugs are ordered to interrupt or halt infectious processes and to control infection.
  1. Induction chemotherapy is intensive and consists of combination chemotherapy started at the time of diagnosis.
  2. Consolidation therapy consists of another course of the same drugs or a different combination of chemotherapeutic agents.
  3. Maintenance may be prescribed for months to years after successful induction and consolidation therapies.
  4. Clinical trials are exploring the use of targeted therapies such as radioimmunotherapy and tumor vaccines.
- Other medications used to treat or prevent infection include
  1. Antibacterial agents (antibiotics including aminoglycosides, a penicillin, or a third-generation cephalosporin), as ordered
  2. Antifungal agents when fungal infections are present (amphotericin B and ketoconazole), as ordered
  3. Antiviral agents used prophylactically (e.g., acyclovir), as ordered

- A bone marrow transplant is the treatment of choice for clients with closely matched donors and who are experiencing temporary remission. A suitable donor is identified after human leukocyte antigen (HLA) typing. The marrow is harvested from the donor and administered by intravenous infusion through a central catheter to the client.
- The client must undergo a conditioning regimen before transplantation that may include intensive chemotherapy and sometimes radiotherapy, usually total body irradiation.
- Complications of bone marrow transplantation include
  1. Infection due to loss of natural immunity
  2. Severe thrombocytopenia
  3. Failure to engraft
  4. Graft-versus-host disease (GVHD)
  5. Veno-occlusive disease
- The immunosuppressive agents required to prevent GVHD increase the client's susceptibility to infection.
- Isolation procedures are required for bone marrow recipients.

NDx: Risk for Injury

- Nursing interventions include
  1. Protecting the client from situations that could lead to bleeding
  2. Assessing for bleeding at least twice per shift for evidence of bleeding such as oozing, enlarging bruises, petechiae, or purpura
  3. Examining stool, urine, nasogastric drainage, and vomiting for blood loss
  4. Measuring any blood loss as accurately as possible
  5. Measuring the client's abdominal girth each shift
  6. Monitoring laboratory values daily

NDx: Fatigue

- Nursing interventions include
  1. Increasing dietary intake with small, frequent meals high in protein and carbohydrates
  2. Administering blood transfusions, if ordered, to increase the oxygen-carrying capacity of the blood
  3. Administering epoetin alpha (Epogen, Procrit), if ordered, and monitoring for side effects

4. Conserving the client's energy by providing rest periods and eliminating or postponing activities

Community-Based Care

- Teach the client and family
  1. Measures to protect the client from infection
  2. The importance of meticulous mouth care
  3. The need to report signs of infection or bleeding immediately to the physician
  4. The necessity of maintaining a healthy diet
  5. The importance of maintaining medical follow-up despite unpleasant side effects
  6. Resources for psychosocial and financial support, and for role and self-esteem adjustment
  7. Safety and bleeding precautions
  8. Care of the central catheter if still in place at discharge
- Assess the need for a home care nurse, aide, or equipment.

Liver, Fatty

- Fatty liver is caused by the accumulation of triglycerides and other fats in the hepatic cells.
- The most common cause is chronic alcoholism.
- Other causes include malnutrition, diabetes mellitus, obesity, pregnancy, prolonged parenteral nutrition, and exposure to toxic drugs.
- The client usually has no symptoms; the typical finding is hepatomegaly (an enlarged liver).
- Assess for
  1. Right upper abdominal pain
  2. Ascites
  3. Edema
  4. Jaundice
  5. Fever
  6. Signs of cirrhosis (see Cirrhosis)
- Liver biopsy confirms the diagnosis.
- Interventions are aimed at removing the underlying cause of the infiltration and dietary restrictions.

Lupus Erythematosus

OVERVIEW

- *Systemic lupus erythematosus* (SLE) is a chronic progressive, inflammatory connective disorder that can cause major body organs and systems to fail; it is characterized by spontaneous remissions and exacerbations.
- *Discoid lupus erythematosus* (DLE) affects only the skin; it is uncommon.
- Lupus typically affects women between 15 and 40 years of age.
- A genetic predisposition is likely.

COLLABORATIVE MANAGEMENT

Assessment

- Extreme variability of symptoms
- Assess the client for
  1. Dry, scaly, raised rash on the face (butterfly rash) or upper body. Individual round discoid lesions are the scaring lesions of discoid lupus.
  2. Articular involvement: *Initial* joint changes are similar to those of rheumatoid arthritis, but severe deformities are not common.
  3. Osteonecrosis
  4. Muscle atrophy
  5. Myalgia
  6. Fever
  7. Various degrees of weakness, fatigue, anorexia, and weight loss
  8. Renal involvement, such as changes in urinary output, proteinuria, hematuria, and fluid retention
  9. Pulmonary effusions or pneumonia
  10. Pericarditis
  11. Neurologic changes, such as psychoses, seizures, paresis, migraine headaches, and cranial nerve palsies
  12. Raynaud's phenomenon
  13. Abdominal pain
  14. Liver enlargement

15. Body image changes
16. Social isolation
17. Fear, anxiety
- Diagnostic tests include
  1. Skin biopsy
  2. Rheumatoid factor
  3. Antinuclear antibody
  4. Erythrocyte sedimentation rate
  5. Serum protein electrophoresis
  6. Anti-Ro (SSA); anti-La (SSB)
  7. Complete blood count, electrolytes
  8. Renal function, cardiac and liver enzymes

Interventions

- Provide drug therapy, including
  1. Topical steroid preparations
  2. Hydroxychloroquine (Plaquenil) to decrease the inflammatory response
  3. Chronic steroid therapy to treat the systemic disease process
  4. Immunosuppressive agents for renal or central nervous system lupus
  5. Antineoplastic agents, including cyclophosphamide (Cytoxan, Procytox ♣) and azathioprine (Imuran)
- Teach measures for skin protection, including
  1. Avoid prolonged exposure to sunlight and other forms of ultraviolet light.
     a. Wear long sleeves and wide-brimmed hats.
     b. Use sun-blocking agents with a sun protection factor (SPF) of 30 or higher.
  2. Clean skin with a mild soap and avoid harsh, perfumed substances.
  3. Use cosmetics with moisturizers and sun protectors.
  4. Use a mild protein shampoo and avoid hair permanents and frosting.
- Reinforce measures for joint protection and energy conservation (see Arthritis, Rheumatoid).
- Help the client identify coping strategies and support systems that can help them deal with the unpredictability of exacerbations.

- Provide health teaching, including
    1. Protection of the skin
    2. The importance of monitoring for fever (the first sign of an exacerbation)
    3. The importance of joint protection and energy conservation
    4. Sexual counseling regarding contraception options and risks of pregnancy
    5. Use of the Lupus Foundation and Arthritis Foundation as resources
    6. Drug information, as needed

Lyme Disease

- Lyme disease is transmitted by infected deer ticks.
- The disease can be prevented by avoiding heavily wooded areas or areas with thick underbrush and by wearing long-sleeved tops and long pants and using an insect repellent on skin and clothes when in an area where infected ticks are likely to be found.
- Stage 1 symptoms begin within 3 to 32 days after the tick bite and include flu-like symptoms, spreading circular rash, malaise, fever, chills, swollen glands, headache, and muscle or joint aches.
    1. Drug therapy includes doxycycline, amoxicillin, or cefuroxime
- Stage 2 symptoms occur 2 to 12 weeks after the tick bite and include cardiac symptoms such as dysrhythmias, dyspnea, dizziness, or palpitations and neurologic manifestations including meningitis, cranial neuropathy, and peripheral neuritis.
    1. Drug therapy includes ceftriaxone and cefotaxime.
- Stage 3, chronic persistent Lyme disease, which occurs weeks to years after the tick bite, may lead to chronic complication such as arthralgias, fatigue and memory or thinking problems, and enlarged lymph nodes. Lyme disease is treated with oral antibiotics such as tetracycline (Achromycin). Severe disease

is treated with intravenous antibiotics such as ceftriaxone or cefotaxime, which may alleviate arthritic, cardiac, and neurologic manifestations.

- Testing for Lyme disease should not be done until 4 to 6 weeks after the tick bite because earlier testing is not reliable.
- Lyme disease vaccination is available for clients over 15 years of age and should be encouraged for those who live in a high-risk area.

Malabsorption Syndrome

- Malabsorption syndrome is associated with a variety of disorders and intestinal surgical procedures and interferes with the ability to absorb nutrients as a result of a generalized flattening of the mucosa of the small intestine.
- Physiologic mechanisms limit absorption because of one or more abnormalities.
  1. Bile salt deficiencies
  2. Enzyme deficiencies
  3. Presence of bacteria
  4. Disruption of the mucosal lining of the small intestine
  5. Alteration in lymphatic or vascular circulation
  6. Decreased gastric or intestinal surface area
- Clinical manifestations of malabsorption include diarrhea, steatorrhea, weight loss, fatigue, bloating and flatus, decreased libido, easy bruising, anemia, bone pain, and edema.
- Interventions focus on avoiding dietary substances that aggravate malabsorption and supplementing nutrients and surgical or nonsurgical management of the primary causative disease.

Malnutrition

- Malnutrition is also known as undernutrition, results from inadequate nutrient intake, increased nutrient loss, and increased nutrient requirements.
- Protein-calorie malnutrition (PCM) affects all aspects of immune function; it causes reduced energy and protein synthesis and an increased risk for infection. The three forms of PCM are
  1. Marasmus, a calorie malnutrition in which body fat and protein are wasted. Serum proteins are often preserved.
  2. Kwashiorkor, a lack of protein quantity and quality in the presence of adequate calories. Body weight is normal and serum proteins are low.
  3. Marasmic-kwashiorkor is a combined protein and energy malnutrition.
- Unrecognized dysphagia is a common problem in nursing homes and can cause malnutrition.
- Anorexia nervosa (self-induced starvation) and bulimia nervosa (binge eating followed by some type of purging behavior such as self-induced vomiting) also lead to malnutrition.
- Clinical manifestations include
  1. Leanness and cachexia
  2. Decreased effort tolerance and lethargy
  3. Intolerance to cold
  4. Ankle edema
  5. Dry, flaking skin and various types of dermatitis
  6. Poor wound healing
  7. A higher than usual incidence of postoperative infection

COLLABORATIVE MANAGEMENT

- Treatment includes
  1. Identify and treat the precipitating cause and supply protein and calories.
  2. Provide high-calorie, high-protein diet.
  3. Offer six small meals. Determine whether the client needs a pureed or dental soft diet.

4. Monitor the client's ability to eat the ordered diet and the amount eaten.
5. Obtain dietary consult. Evaluate whether nutrients consumed are sufficient to meet basal and stress-related energy needs.
6. Provide an environment conducive to eating.
7. Medications such as megestrol acetate (Megace) may be given to stimulate appetite.
8. Provide nutritional supplements or partial enteral nutrition; total parenteral nutrition or peripheral parenteral nutrition.
9. Maintain a daily calorie count and weigh the client daily.
10. Record intake and output.
11. Treat infections and correct fluid and electrolyte imbalance.
12. Measure the client's height and weight.
13. Assess and monitor laboratory values for serum albumin, prealbumin, and leukocyte count.

- Monitor for complications associated with tube feedings.
    1. Development of a clogged tube
    2. Dislodgment of the tube
    3. Fluid excess or dehydration
    4. Increased osmolarity
    5. Electrolyte imbalances
    6. Aspiration

Mastoiditis

- Mastoiditis is a infection of the mastoid air cells caused by an untreated or inadequately treated chronic or acute otitis media.
- Clinical manifestations include swelling behind the ear and pain with minimal movement of the tragus, pinna, or head. Cellulitis develops on the skin or external scalp over the mastoid process.
- Otoscopic examination reveals a reddened, dull, thick, immobile tympanic membrane with or without perforation.

- Other symptoms include low-grade fever; malaise; and anorexia.
- Treatment includes antibiotics or surgical removal of the infected tissue, such as a *tympanoplasty,* or a simple or modified radical *mastoidectomy.*
- Complications of surgery include damage to the abducens and facial nerves (cranial nerves VI and VII, respectively), vertigo, meningitis, brain abscess, chronic purulent otitis media, and wound infection.

Melanoma, Ocular

- Melanoma of the eye is the most common intraocular malignant tumor in adults. Because of its rich blood supply, an ocular melanoma can spread easily.
- Symptoms are not readily obvious, and the lesion may be found during a routine eye examination.
- The melanoma manifests as blurred vision, changes in visual acuity, increased intraocular pressure, change in color of the iris, and sudden change in peripheral vision.
- Treatment includes
  1. *Enucleation* (removal of the entire eyeball) and insertion of a ball implant to maintain conformity of the eye socket until a prosthesis is fitted (approximately 1 month).
  2. Radiation therapy
     a. Complications include vascular changes, retinopathy, glaucoma, necrosis of the sclera, and cataract formation.
     b. Cycloplegic eyedrops and an antibiotic-steroid combination are administered.

Ménière's Disease

- Ménière's disease refers to overproduction or decreased resorption of endolymphatic fluid, causing a distortion of the entire inner-canal system.

- Assess for
  1. Duration, intensity, and time between episodes of the classic triad of symptoms
     a. *Tinnitus*, a continuous, low-pitched roar or a humming sound, is present much of the time but worsens just before and during a severe attack.
     b. *Hearing loss*, initially for low-frequency tones, worsens to include all levels after repeated episodes. Permanent hearing loss develops as the number of attacks increases.
     c. *Vertigo*, described as periods of whirling that might cause the client to fall to the ground, may be so intense that even while lying down, the client holds the bed or ground in an attempt to prevent the whirling. The severe vertigo usually lasts only 3 to 4 hours and is followed by a sense of dizziness.
  2. The presence of a feeling of fullness in the ear before an attack.
  3. Nausea and vomiting
  4. Nystagmus (rapid eye movements)
  5. Severe headache
- Interventions include
  1. Instructing the client to make slow head movements
  2. Teaching dietary changes, such as salt and fluid restriction
  3. Teaching the importance of smoking cessation
- Drug therapy includes
  1. Administering nicotinic acid for its vasodilator effect
  2. Giving antihistamines to reduce the severity of or stop an acute attack
  3. Giving antiemetics to control nausea and vomiting
  4. Giving diazepam (Valium, Apo-Diazepam ✲) to calm the anxious client and help control vertigo, nausea, and vomiting
- Surgical treatment is a last resort because the hearing in the affected ear is sacrificed.
- *Labyrinthectomy* involves the resection of the vestibular nerve or total removal of the labyrinth.
- An endolymphatic drainage and shunt may be performed early in the course of the disease to relieve vertigo.

Meningitis

- Meningitis is an inflammation of the arachnoid and pia mater of the brain, spinal cord, and cerebrospinal fluid.
- *Bacterial meningitis* is a medical emergency; *viral meningitis* is usually self-limiting; *cryptococcal meningitis* is the most common fungal meningitis.

Assessment

- Record client information.
  1. Medical history, including information about viral or respiratory diseases; head trauma; ear, nose, or sinus infection; heart disease; diabetes mellitus; cancer; immunosuppressive therapy; and neurologic surgery or procedures
  2. Exposure to communicable disease
- Assess for
  1. Headache, nausea, vomiting,
  2. Fever and chills
  3. Generalized aches and pains
  4. Nuchal rigidity
  5. Change in level of consciousness
  6. Signs of increased intracranial pressure; change in pupil size and reaction to light, nystagmus, and abnormal eye movement
  7. Dysfunction of cranial nerves III, IV, VI, VII, and VIII
  8. Seizure activity
  9. Presence of all peripheral pulses
  10. Presence of a red macular rash (meningococcal meningitis)
  11. Changes in color and temperature of extremities
  12. Any indicators of abnormal bleeding
  13. Syndrome of inappropriate antidiuretic hormone (SIADH)
  14. Fluid and electrolyte imbalance, particularly hyponatremia
  15. Results of cerebrospinal fluid (CSF) analysis and other diagnostic tests

M

- Interventions include
  1. Assessing and recording the client's vital signs and neurologic checks at least every 4 hours
  2. Performing a vascular assessment every 4 hours
  3. Administering medications such as antibiotics and analgesics, as ordered
  4. Maintaining isolation precautions per hospital policy
  5. Implementing routine seizure precautions
  6. Monitoring for complications such as vascular compromise from septic emboli, shock, coagulation disorders, prolonged fever, and septic complications

Myasthenia Gravis

- Myasthenia gravis (MG) is a chronic neuromuscular autoimmune disease that involves a decrease in the number and effectiveness of acetylcholine (ACh) receptors at the neuromuscular junction.
- In Eaton-Lambert syndrome, a special form of MG often observed in combination with small cell carcinoma of the lung, the muscles of the trunk and the pelvic and shoulder girdles are most commonly affected.

COLLABORATIVE MANAGEMENT
Assessment
- Record client information.
  1. Rapid onset of fatigue
  2. Muscular weakness that increases on exertion or as the day wears on and improves with rest (with a temporary increase in weakness sometimes noted after vaccination, menstruation, and exposure to extremes in environmental temperature)
  3. Inability to perform activities of daily living (ADLs)
  4. Ptosis, diplopia
  5. Respiratory distress
  6. Choking, dysphagia
  7. Weakness of voice

8. Difficulty holding up head, brushing teeth, combing hair, or shaving
9. Paresthesia or aching in weakened muscles
- Assess for
  1. Progressive paresis of affected muscle groups that is resolved by rest, at least in part
  2. Symptoms related to involvement of the levator palpebrae or extraocular muscles
     a. Ocular palsies
     b. Ptosis
     c. Diplopia
     d. Weak or incomplete eye closure
  3. Involvement of muscles for facial expression, chewing, and speech
     a. The client's smile may turn into a snarl.
     b. The jaw hangs.
     c. Difficulty chewing and swallowing may lead to severe nutritional deficits.
  4. Proximal limb weakness; the client has difficulty climbing stairs, lifting heavy objects, or raising arms overhead
  5. Mild or severe neck weakness
  6. Difficulty sustaining a sitting or walking posture
  7. Respiratory distress
  8. Bowel and bladder incontinence
  9. Weakness of the pelvic and shoulder girdles (seen in Eaton-Lambert syndrome, a special form of MG often observed in combination with small cell carcinoma of the lung)
  10. Disturbed body image
  11. Feelings of loss, fear, helplessness, and grief
  12. Usual coping methods
  13. Positive ACh receptor antibodies
  14. Significant improvement after Tensilon testing

Interventions

NONSURGICAL MANAGEMENT

- Interventions include
  1. Assessing motor strength before and after periods of activity

2. Providing assistance with mobilization as necessary
3. Teaching the client to plan activities early in the day or during the energy peaks that follow the administration of medications
4. Planning rest periods for the client to avoid excessive fatigue
5. Performing active and passive range-of-motion (ROM) exercises
6. Using heel and elbow protectors as needed
7. Assessing the need for an egg crate or alternating pressure mattress

- Medications for MG must be given on time and include
  1. Cholinesterase inhibitor drugs, also referred to as anti-cholinesterase drugs such as pyridostigmine (Mestinon, Regonol) to increase the response of muscles to nerve impulses, thus improving strength
     a. The drug is given with a small amount of food to minimize gastrointestinal (GI) side effects; meals are provided 45 minutes to 1 hour after taking medication.
     b. Drugs containing magnesium, morphine or its derivatives, curare, quinine, quinidine, procainamide, hypnotics, or sedatives *are avoided* because they may increase weakness.
     c. Antibiotics such as neomycin, kanamycin, strepto-mycin, polymyxin B, and certain tetracyclines have been shown to *increase myasthenic symptoms.*
  2. Immunosuppression may be accomplished with the use of corticosteroids or with chemotherapeutic agents.

- Observe for *myasthenic crisis*, an exacerbation of the myasthenic symptoms caused by *under*medication with anticholinergic drugs or infection.
  1. Maintain adequate respiratory functioning (ABCs of emergency care); intubation and mechanical ventilation may be needed.
  2. Cholinesterase-inhibiting drugs are withheld because they increase respiratory secretion and are usually ineffective for the first few days after the crisis begins.
  3. Medications are restarted gradually at lower doses.

- Observe for *cholinergic crisis*, an acute exacerbation of muscle weakness caused by *over*medication with cholinergic (anticholinesterase) drugs.
    1. Cholinesterase-inhibiting drugs are withheld while the client is maintained on a ventilator.
    2. Atropine may be given and repeated as necessary, which may thicken secretions, causing more difficulty with airway clearance and possible development of mucous plugs.
- Administration of Tensilon produces a temporary improvement in myasthenic crisis but no improvement or a worsening of symptoms in cholinergic crisis.
- Plasmapheresis is a method by which autoantibodies are removed from the plasma.
- Immunosuppressive drugs are administered concurrently to decrease the formation of additional antibodies. Nursing management includes maintaining the intravenous line or shunt, monitoring vital signs, and assessing neurologic signs.
- Respiratory support includes
    1. Performing a respiratory assessment at least every 8 hours
    2. Monitoring for respiratory distress: dyspnea, shortness of breath, air hunger, and confusion
    3. Encouraging the client to turn, cough, and deep breathe every 2 hours
    4. Performing chest physiotherapy, including postural drainage, percussion, and vibration
    5. Keeping an Ambubag, equipment for oxygen administration, and endotracheal intubation equipment at the bedside in case of respiratory distress
    6. Monitoring the client's response to medications
- Self-care interventions include
    1. Assessing the client's ability to perform ADLs to establish his or her abilities and limitations
    2. Encouraging the client to perform activities as independently as possible; providing assistance as needed
    3. Planning activities to follow the administration of medication to maximize independence and successful attempts at self-care

M

4. Documenting and monitoring the client's response to or tolerance of activity
5. Collaborating with physical and occupational therapists to identify the need for assistive devices
- Collaborate with the speech language pathologist to develop communication strategies as needed.
  1. Instruct the client to speak slowly.
  2. Repeat information to verify that it is correct.
  3. Develop alternative communication systems such as eye blinking or flash cards.
- Ensure adequate nutritional support through small frequent meals and high-calorie snacks. Record calorie counts. Measure intake and output, serum albumin levels, and daily weight.
  1. Assess the client's gag reflex and ability to chew and swallow without undue fatigue or aspiration.
  2. Provide frequent oral hygiene.
  3. Obtain a dietary consultation to identify food preferences and dislikes.
  4. Observe the client for choking, nasal regurgitation, and aspiration.
  5. Give tube feedings if necessary.
- Provide eye protection.
  1. Artificial tears are applied to keep corneas moist and free from abrasion.
  2. A lubricant gel and eye shield may be applied to the eye at bedtime.
  3. To help relieve diplopia, the eye is alternately covered with a patch for 2 to 3 hours at a time.

SURGICAL MANAGEMENT

- Thymectomy is an alternative method of treatment.
- Preoperative care includes
  1. Providing routine preoperative care
  2. Administering pyridostigmine (Mestinon), as ordered, to keep the client stable throughout surgery
  3. If steroids have been used, administering before surgery but tapering postoperatively
  4. Giving antibiotics given before and after surgery
- Postoperative care includes
  1. Providing pulmonary hygiene and suction as necessary

2. Observing for signs of pneumothorax or hemothorax such as chest pain, sudden shortness of breath, diminished or absent breath sounds, and restlessness or a change in vital signs
3. Observing for signs and symptoms of wound infection
4. Providing chest tube care if indicated

Community-Based Care

- Emphasize specific points concerning the disease process.
  1. Episodic nature
  2. Factors that predispose the client to exacerbation, such as infection, stress, surgery, and hard physical exercise
  3. Symptoms of myasthenic crisis and cholinergic crisis
  4. Lifestyle adaptations that may be indicated, such as avoiding heat (sauna, sunbathing), crowds, overeating, and erratic changes in sleep habits
- Provide information concerning the medication regimen and include the name, purpose, dosage, time of administration, administration route, side effects, and the importance of taking medications on time and not missing doses.
- Encourage the client's family to become certified in cardiopulmonary resuscitation (CPR).
- Refer client to home health and other community agencies and support groups such as the Myasthenia Gravis Foundation.

Nephrosclerosis

- Nephrosclerosis is a problem of thickening in the nephron blood vessel, resulting in narrowing of the lumen, decreased renal blood flow, and chronically hypoxic kidney tissue.
- Ischemia and fibrosis develop over time.
- Nephrosclerosis is associated with hypertension, atherosclerosis, and diabetes mellitus.
- Treatment is directed toward control of blood pressure and preservation of renal function.

Nephrotic Syndrome

- Nephrotic syndrome is a condition of increased glomerular permeability that allows larger molecules to pass through the membrane into the urine and be removed from the blood.
- Nephrotic syndrome is commonly caused by changes in an immune or inflammatory process.
- The main features are severe proteinuria, hypoalbuminemia, hyperlipidemia, lipiduria, edema, and hypertension.
- Treatment varies depending on what is causing the disorder (identified by renal biopsy) and may include
  1. Angiotensin-converting enzyme inhibitors
  2. Cholesterol-lowering drugs
  3. Immunosuppressive agents, steroids
  4. Heparin
  5. Mild diuretics
  6. Diet changes; sodium restriction
- Assess the client's hydration status and monitor for dehydration. If plasma volume is depleted, renal problems worsen.

Neuroma, Acoustic

- An acoustic neuroma is a benign tumor of the cranial nerve VII. Damage to hearing, facial movements, and sensation may result.
- Clinical manifestations begin with tinnitus and progress to gradual sensorineural hearing loss; constant mild vertigo occurs later.
- Diagnosis is made by computed tomography (CT) scanning, audiograms, and cerebrospinal fluid analysis (which shows increased pressure and protein).
- Surgical removal of the neuroma by means of a craniotomy is necessary, and hearing may be permanently affected. Extreme care to preserve the function of the facial nerve (cranial nerve VII) is taken. (See Surgical Management under Tumors, Brain for care of the client having a craniotomy.)

Obesity

OVERVIEW

OVERVIEW

- Obesity refers to an excess amount of body fat.
- An obese person weighs at least 20% above the upper limit of the normal range for ideal body weight and has a body mass index (BMI) of 30 or more.
- Morbid obesity refers to weight that has a severely negative effect on health—usually more than 100% above ideal body weight or a body mass index greater than 40.
- Obesity involves complex interrelationships of major factors, including genetic, environmental, psychological, social, cultural, pathologic, and physiologic.
- Causes of obesity include high-fat and high-cholesterol diets, physical inactivity, drug treatment (corticosteroids, NSAIDs), and familial and genetic factors.
- Complications include diabetes mellitus, hypertension, hyperlipidemia, cardiac disease, sleep apnea, cholelithiasis, chronic back pain, early degenerative arthritis, susceptibility to infections, and certain cancers.

COLLABORATIVE MANAGEMENT

- Record client information.
    1. Economic status
    2. Usual food intake
    3. Eating behaviors
    4. Cultural background
    5. Attitude toward food and current weight
    6. Appetite
    7. Medications
    8. Physical activity
    9. Height and weight
    10. Chronic diseases
    11. Family history of obesity
- Management includes
    1. Dietary management developed through close interaction between the client, dietitian, and health care provider

2. Drug therapy
   a. Anorectic drugs suppress appetite, which reduces food intake and over time may result in weight loss.
   b. Orlistat (Xenical) inhibits lipase and leads to partial hydrolysis of triglycerides. Because fats are only partially digested and absorbed, calorie intake is decreased.
   c. Other drugs, which are in the final stage of testing, are directed toward reducing cravings for food and smoking.
3. Exercise program
4. Behavioral treatment including reinforcement techniques and cognitive restructuring

- Surgery is indicated for the client who repeatedly fails at dietary management or is morbidly obese.
  1. Panniculectomy is removal of the panniculus, most often the abdominal apron.
  2. Bariatric surgery is surgical reduction of gastric capacity.
     a. Gastric restrictive surgery: vertical banded gastroplasty or circumgastric banding
     b. Gastric restriction with malabsorption surgery: gastric bypass or Roux-en-Y gastric

- Postoperative care after gastroplasty or intestinal bypass includes
  1. Providing routine postoperative care
  2. Monitoring the patency of the nasogastric (NG) tube and recording the amount of drainage
  3. Applying an abdominal binder to prevent wound dehiscence
  4. Placing the client in semi-Fowler's position or using continuous positive airway pressure (CPAP) ventilation at night to improve ventilation and decrease risk for sleep apnea
  5. Observing skin areas and folds for redness, excoriation, or breakdown and treating these problems early
  6. Using absorbent padding between skin folds to prevent pressure ulcers, particularly from tubes and catheters
  7. Removing the NG tube on the third postoperative day if bowel sounds are present and the client is passing flatus; then beginning clear fluids

8. Giving 1 oz of water in a 1-oz cup and instructing the client to slowly sip the water over a 1-hr period; additional liquids, pureed foods, juice, and soups thinned with broth, water, or milk are added to the diet 24 to 48 hours after clear liquids are tolerated

9. Observing for dumping syndrome

Community-Based Care

- Give the client a list of community resources, such as Weight Watchers, Overeaters Anonymous, and Take Off Pounds Sensibly (TOPS).
- In collaboration with the dietitian, provide health teaching regarding the diet and the importance of maintaining a healthy eating pattern.
- Encourage the client to increase physical activity, decrease fat intake and reliance on medication use, establish a normal eating pattern in response to physiologic hunger, and address medical and psychological problems.

Obstruction, Intestinal

- Intestinal obstruction is partial or complete obstruction of the small or large bowel that impedes the natural progression of digestive processing. It can be either mechanical or nonmechanical (paralytic).
- *Mechanical obstruction* occurs when the bowel is physically obstructed by disorders outside the intestine (adhesions or hernias) or blockages in the lumen of the intestines (tumors, fecal impactions, strictures).
- *Nonmechanical obstruction* (paralytic or adynamic ileus) occurs when peristalsis is decreased or absent, resulting in a slowing of the movement or a backup of intestinal content caused by physiologic, neurogenic, or chemical imbalances.
- Paralytic ileus is associated with trauma, abdominal surgery, hypokalemia, myocardial infarction, or vascular insufficiency.
- Distention results from the inability of the intestine to absorb and mobilize intestinal contents. Increased peristalsis

occurs, leading to additional distention, edema of the bowel, and increased capillary permeability. Absorption of fluid and electrolytes into the vascular space is decreased, and reduced circulatory blood volume and electrolyte imbalances occur. Hypovolemia ranges from mild to extreme.

- *Strangulated obstruction* results when there is obstruction with compromised blood flow.

COLLABORATIVE MANAGEMENT

Assessment

- Record client information.
    1. Medical history, including abdominal surgical procedures; radiation therapy; or bowel diseases such as Crohn's disease, ulcerative colitis, diverticular disease, gallstones, hernias, trauma, and peritonitis
    2. Diet history
    3. Bowel elimination patterns, including the presence of blood in the stool
    4. Familial history of colorectal cancer
- Assess for mechanical intestinal obstruction.
    1. Intermittent abdominal cramping
    2. Peristaltic waves
    3. High-pitched bowel sounds (borborygmi) in *early* obstructive process
    4. Absent bowel sounds in *later* stages
    5. Abdominal distention (hallmark sign)
    6. Nausea and vomiting
        a. Obstruction above the ileum causes early and profuse vomiting of partially digested food and chyme, changing to watery contents containing bile and mucus.
        b. Obstruction in the large intestine produces vomitus with an orange-brown color and a foul odor caused by bacterial overgrowth, which may be fecal contamination.
    7. Obstipation (characteristic of total small and large mechanical obstruction)
- Indications of nonmechanical intestinal obstruction include
    1. Constant, diffuse abdominal discomfort; severe pain in intestinal vascular insufficiency or infarction
    2. Decreased bowel sounds in *early* obstruction

3. Absent bowel sounds in *later* obstruction
4. Vomiting of gastric contents and bile
5. Singultus (hiccups, which are common with all types of intestinal obstruction)

Interventions

- Interventions are aimed at uncovering the cause and relieving the obstruction
- Nasogastric tube management includes
  1. Maintaining the client on nothing by mouth (NPO) status
  2. Monitoring drainage from the nasogastric tube
     a. The Salem sump or Anderson suction tube sits distally in the stomach and is connected to low continuous suction.
     b. Levine tubes are connected to low intermittent suction.
  3. Monitoring for proper placement, patency, and output every 4 hours
  4. Assessing the nasal skin for integrity
  5. Questioning the client regarding the passage of flatus
  6. Recording the passage, amount, and character of bowel movements
  7. Measuring the client's abdominal girth daily
- Nasointestinal tube management includes
  1. Assisting with nasointestinal tube progression by helping the client change position every 2 hours and by advancing the tube 3 to 4 inches at specified times, as ordered (NOTE: Do not tape the intestinal tube to the nose until the desired position is reached in the intestine.)
  2. Monitoring intestinal tube drainage, which occurs by gravity, and instilling 10 mL of air, as ordered, if the drainage stops (NOTE: *Do not* irrigate the tube with fluid.)
  3. Maintaining low intermittent or continuous suction, as ordered, when the tube has reached the desired location
- Obstruction caused by fecal impaction resolves after disimpaction and enema.
- Intussusception (telescoping of bowel) may resolve during hydrostatic pressure changes during a barium enema.
- Administer fluid and electrolyte replacement.
  1. Administer intravenous (IV) fluid because of vascular fluid losses from lack of normal reabsorption in the intestine,

increased intestinal secretions, nasogastric suction, and NPO status (normal saline solutions with potassium replacement are used according to electrolyte results).

2. Provide blood products in case of strangulated obstruction because of blood loss into the bowel or peritoneal cavity.
3. Provide ice chips as prescribed.
4. Monitor vital signs and other measures of fluid status (urinary output, skin turgor, and mucous membrane).
5. Measure intake and output.
6. Assess the client for edema.
7. Weigh the client daily.
8. Administer total parenteral nutrition, as ordered.
9. Provide frequent mouth care.

- Provide pain management.
  1. Report changes in pain to the physician, including pain that significantly increases or changes from a colicky, intermittent type to constant discomfort (changes could indicate perforation or peritonitis).
  2. Opioid analgesics usually are not given in the diagnostic period so that clinical manifestations of perforation or peritonitis are not masked.
  3. Provide a position of comfort, including semi-Fowler's, which helps to relieve the pressure of abdominal distention and facilitates thoracic excursion and normal breathing patterns.
- Broad-spectrum antibiotics are given if strangulation is suspected.

SURGICAL MANAGEMENT

- Surgical management is required for complete mechanical obstruction and for many cases of incomplete mechanical obstruction.
- An exploratory laparotomy is performed to locate the obstruction and determine the nature of the problem.
- The specific surgical procedure performed is dependent on the cause and location of the obstruction. Examples of procedures include lysis of adhesions, colon resection with anastomosis for obstruction resulting from tumor or diverticulitis, and embolectomy or thrombectomy for intestinal infarction.

- Nursing care for abdominal surgery is similar to that described under Cancer, Colorectal.

Community-Based Care

- Client and family education depends on the specific cause and treatment of the obstruction.
    1. Report signs that may indicate recurrent obstruction, including abdominal pain or distention, nausea, vomiting, or constipation (for nonmechanical obstruction after surgery or trauma).
    2. Develop a structured bowel regimen, including a high-fiber diet, daily exercise, and psyllium hydrophilic mucilloid (e.g., Metamucil) with copious amounts of water (for prevention of recurrences of fecal impaction).
- Information about incision care (if surgery was performed), drug therapy, and activity restriction is given to the client and family.

Obstruction, Upper Airway

O

- Upper airway obstruction, a life-threatening emergency, is an interruption in airflow through the nose, pharynx, larynx, or mouth into the lungs.
- The obstruction may be caused by laryngeal edema, peritonsillar abscess, laryngeal carcinoma, stroke, thickened secretions, tongue occlusion, smoke inhalation injury, tracheal and laryngeal trauma, foreign body aspiration, and anaphylaxis.
- Partial airway obstruction may have only subtle or general manifestations such as diaphoresis, tachycardia, and elevated blood pressure.
- Additional manifestations may include hypoxia, hypercapnia, restlessness, increasing anxiety, sternal retractions, seesawing chest, abdominal movements, air hunger, change in level of consciousness, and the universal distress sign for airway obstruction (hands to the neck).
- Management depends on the cause, including
    1. Hyperextension of the neck
    2. Suctioning to remove oral secretions

3. Heimlich maneuver for a foreign body
4. Cricothyroidotomy as an emergency procedure
5. Endotracheal intubation
6. Tracheostomy

Osteoarthritis

OVERVIEW

- Osteoarthritis (OA), formerly referred to as degenerative joint disease (DJD), is characterized by the progressive deterioration of and loss of cartilage in the axial joints.
- Weight-bearing joints, the vertebral column, and the hands are the sites primarily affected.

Considerations for Older Adults

- The prevalence of OA increases with age. Almost everyone older than 55 years of age has some degree of symptomatic involvement.

☼ Women's Health Considerations

- Before 50 years of age, more men than women have OA. It is much more common in women after the age of 50, especially in the hands.
- OA is more common in black women.

COLLABORATIVE MANAGEMENT

Assessment

- Ask questions about the course of the disease.
  1. Nature and location of joint pain
  2. Location and duration of joint stiffness
  3. When and where any joint swelling occurred
  4. What relieves the pain or stiffness
  5. Loss of function or difficulty in accomplishing activities of daily living (ADLs)
- Record the client's risk factors.
  1. Occupation and nature of work
  2. History of trauma

3. Weight history; history of obesity
4. Exercise
5. Current or previous involvement in sports
6. Family history
7. Previous medical condition that may cause joint manifestations

- Assess for
  1. Joint pain, which early in the disease process diminishes after rest and intensifies after activity; later, pain occurs with slight motion or even at rest
  2. Crepitus, which is a continuous grating sensation that may be felt or heard as the joint is put through range of motion
  3. Joint enlargement from bony atrophy
  4. Heberden's nodes (at the distal interphalangeal joints) or Bouchard's nodes (at the proximal interphalangeal joints) if the hands are involved; nodes are hard and cause tenderness when palpated
  5. Joint effusions, which are common when the knees are involved
  6. Skeletal muscle atrophy adjacent to the involved area
  7. Compression of the spinal nerve roots manifested by radiating pain, stiffness, and muscle spasms in one or both extremities
  8. Compression of spinal and vertebral arteries
  9. Level of mobility and function
  10. Ability to perform ADLs
  11. Anger, depression, and body image changes

- Diagnostic tests include
  1. Erythrocyte sedimentation rate (ESR)
  2. High-sensitivity C-reactive protein (hsCRP)
  3. Standard x-rays, computed tomography, or magnetic resonance imaging

Planning and Implementation

◆**NDx:** Chronic Pain

- Pain assessment
  1. Determine pain location, characteristics, quality, and severity (obtain pain score).
  2. Document response to pain medication and other comfort measures.

- Drug therapy includes
  1. Acetaminophen (Tylenol, Atasol ✦), primary drug of choice
     a. Client is at risk for liver damage if they take more than 4000 mg/day, have current alcoholism, or have pre-existing liver disease.
  2. Topical salicylates, such as over-the-counter Aspercreme, capsaicin
  3. Nonsteroidal anti-inflammatory drugs (NSAIDs)
  4. Corticosteroid injections into single joints
  5. Local agents such as hyaluronate (Hyalgan and hylan GF 20 [Synvisc]) for OA of the knee
  6. Muscle relaxants for severe muscle spasms
     a. Remind the client not to drive or operate dangerous machinery when taking muscle relaxants.
- Other interventions include
  1. Resting the joint when it is painful but exercising it to maintain mobility and tone
  2. Immobilizing the affected joint with a splint or brace (local rest)
  3. Obtaining 8 to 10 hours of sleep at night and a 1- or 2-hour nap in the afternoon if possible (systemic rest)
  4. Relieving daily stress that can enhance pain (psychological rest)
  5. Placing the affected joints in functional positions
     a. Avoid large pillows under the head or knees.
     b. Apply or teach the importance of a moist heating pad, a hot shower or bath, hot packs or compresses, paraffin dips, diathermy, and ultrasound.
  6. Implementing cold applications for acutely inflamed joints
  7. Encouraging the obese client to reduce weight; refer to dietitian as needed
- Complementary or alternative therapies include
  1. Transcutaneous electrical nerve stimulator (TENS)
  2. Imagery, music therapy, and relaxation techniques to reduce pain
  3. Acupressure, acupuncture, tai chi
  4. Dietary supplements, herbal medicines, or ointments (The client should ask his or her health care provider before using these supplements.)
  5. Therapeutic touch, hypnotherapy

SURGICAL MANAGEMENT

- An *osteotomy* (bone resection) is performed to correct joint deformity.
- A *total joint arthroplasty* (TJA), also called total joint *replacement* (TJR), is the surgical creation of a joint. TJA is used when all other measures of pain relief have failed; hips and knees are most commonly replaced.
- TJA is contraindicated in the presence of infection, advanced osteoporosis, or severe inflammation. However, if the infection or inflammation can be fully treated, TJA may be performed.
- Total hip replacement (THR)
  1. Provide preoperative care, reinforcing the information concerning the surgery. Preoperative care teaching may be done by a team including the nurse, physical therapist, and occupational therapist.
     a. Explain postoperative care such as transfers, precautions, ambulation, and postoperative exercises.
     b. Explain the option for blood transfusion such as an autologous blood transfusion and cell savers.
     c. Epoetin alpha may be given to prevent the need for postoperative blood transfusion.
     d. Determine risk factors for clotting problems such as previous clotting problems, obesity, and advanced age.
  2. Provide routine postoperative care.
  3. Prevent dislocation.
     a. Place the client in a supine position with the head slightly elevated.
     b. Place the affected leg in a neutral rotation. The use of abduction devices depends on facility policy.
     c. Keep the client's heels off the bed to prevent pressure sores.
     d. Follow surgeon preference regarding turning. Generally, the client can be turned to either side as long as the leg remains abducted.
     e. Observe for and report to the surgeon signs of hip dislocation, including hip pain, shortening of the affected leg, and leg rotation.
     f. If dislocation occurs, the surgeon manipulates and relocates the affected hip, after the client receives an analgesic or is anesthetized. The hip is then

immobilized by an abduction splint or other device until healing occurs, usually in about 6 weeks.

4. Monitor the client for venous thromboembolism (VTE), which includes deep vein thrombosis and pulmonary embolism. Institute preventive measures; anticoagulants are prescribed to prevent VTE.

5. Apply thigh-high antiembolism stockings, sequential compression devices, and/or foot sole pumps (A-V Impulse System).

6. Encourage the client to perform the leg exercises taught by the physical therapist.
   a. Plantar flexion and dorsiflexion (heel pumping)
   b. Circumduction (circles) of the feet
   c. Gluteal and quadriceps muscle setting
   d. Straight leg raises

7. Assess for wound infection.
   a. Check vital signs every 4 hours.
   b. Observe for excessive or foul-smelling drainage from the incision; send drainage for culture and sensitivity testing.
   c. Older clients may not have fever with infection but may have altered mental status.

8. Assess for bleeding and manage anemia.
   a. Observe the surgical hip dressing for bleeding and other drainage. Empty and record the amount of drainage in any drainage device every 4 hours. The total amount of drainage is usually less than 50 mL every 8 hours.
   b. Check laboratory values such as hemoglobin and hematocrit.
   c. Blood pressure may be lower than usual because of blood loss during surgery or because cement (which tends to dilate blood vessels) was used during surgery.

9. Perform neurovascular assessments at the same time as vital signs are checked.

10. Provide pain management.
    a. Patient-controlled analgesia, epidural analgesia
    b. Pain Buster, a small pump that continuously infuses a local anesthetic directly into the surgical site
    c. Oral medication

11. Assist the client on his or her first attempt to get out of bed, usually the day after surgery.
    a. Stand on the same side of the bed as the client's affected leg.
    b. Assist the client to a sitting position.
    c. Have the client stand on the unaffected leg and pivot to the chair.
    d. Do not allow the client to flex the hip more than 90 degrees.
    e. To prevent hyperflexion, raised toilet seats, straight-backed chairs, and reclining wheelchairs may be used.
12. Weight bearing on the affected leg depends of the type of prosthesis and the surgical approach.
13. The occupational therapist may recommend assistive-adaptive devices to help with ADLs.
14. Typical length of stay is 3 days. The client may be discharged to a rehabilitation unit, transitional care unit, long-term care unit, or home.

- Total knee arthroplasty (TKA)
  1. Provide preoperative care.
  2. Provide routine postoperative care.
     a. Provide care similar to that for hip replacement although maintaining abduction is not necessary. Maintain the knee in a neutral position.
     b. Apply ice packs or a Hot/Ice Machine to decrease swelling.
     c. Monitor and maintain the continuous passive motion (CPM) machine, which keeps the knee in motion and prevents formation of scar tissue, which could impede mobility of the knee and exacerbate postoperative pain.
        (1) CPM is generally used intermittently for several hours at a time.
        (2) Check the cycle and range-of-motion settings every 8 hours or more.
        (3) Ensure that the joint being moved is correctly positioned on the machine.
        (4) Assess and document the client's response to the machine.
        (5) Turn the machine off while the client is having a meal in bed.

3. Monitor for complications.
   a. VTE
   b. Infection
   c. Bleeding
- Shoulder arthroplasty (TSA). A hemiarthroplasty, typically of the humeral component, may be performed as an alternative to TSA.
   1. The Neer prosthesis is the most commonly used.
   2. Provide postoperative care.
      a. Monitor the CPM machine or perform passive range-of-motion exercises.
      b. Perform frequent neurovascular assessments.
      c. Monitor for subluxation and pulmonary embolism.
- Total elbow arthroplasty (TEA)
   1. Total elbow replacement is successful in increasing range of motion, but infection and loosening may occur because of extensive cutting during surgery.
   2. The CPM device may be used postoperatively or passive exercises are prescribed.
- Finger and wrist replacements
   1. A bulky dressing is used for 2 to 3 days after surgery, followed by a dynamic splint, brace, or cast.
   2. The arm is elevated as much as possible.
   3. A splint or short arm cast may be applied.
- Total ankle arthroplasty (TAA)
   1. When an ankle is replaced, an arthrodesis (bone fusion) is usually performed for added stability.
   2. Monitor for infection, delayed wound healing, nerve injuries, and loosening.

NDx: Impaired Physical Mobility

- Reinforce the techniques and principles of the exercise, ambulation, and ADL program developed by occupational and physical therapists as well as the use of assistive-adaptive devices.
- The ideal time for exercise is immediately after the application of heat.

- Client education includes
  1. Do the exercise specifically prescribed for you.
  2. Do the exercises on good and bad days; consistency is important.
  3. If pain increases with exercise, stop and notify your physician.
  4. Use active rather than active-assist or passive exercises whenever possible.
  5. Do not substitute normal activities or household tasks for the prescribed exercises.
  6. Avoid resistive exercises when your joints are severely inflamed.

Community-Based Care

HOME CARE MANAGEMENT

- Collaborate with discharge planner and physician to determine the best placement for the client at discharge.
- Health teaching
  1. Explain the general rules of joint protection.
     a. Use large joints rather than small ones.
     b. Do not turn a doorknob clockwise; turn it counterclockwise.
     c. Sit in a chair that has a high, straight back.
     d. Use two hands instead of one to hold objects.
     e. When getting into bed, do not push off with your fingers; use the entire palm of your hand.
     f. Do not bend at the waist; bend with the knees while keeping the back straight.
     g. Use long-handled devices.
     h. Use assistive-adaptive devices, such as Velcro closures and built-up utensil handles.
     i. Do not use pillows in bed, except a small one under your head.
     j. Avoid twisting or wringing your hands.
  2. Instruct the client to check with the Arthritis Foundation about new treatments that propose to cure the disease.

Osteomalacia

- Osteomalacia, described as softening of the bone tissue, is characterized by inadequate mineralization of bone as a result of vitamin D deficiency.

COLLABORATIVE MANAGEMENT

Assessment

- Record client information.
  1. Age
  2. Exposure to sunlight
  3. Skin pigmentation (Clients with dark skin are at a greater risk than clients with light skin.)
  4. Dietary habits
  5. Current medical problems and prescribed and over-the-counter medications
  6. History of fractures and when they occurred
- Assess for
  1. Muscle weakness in the lower extremities, which may progress to a waddling and unsteady gait, which contributes to falls
  2. Bone pain and muscle cramps (Pain is aggravated by activity and is worse at night.)
  3. Bone tenderness
  4. Skeletal malalignment, such as long-bone bowing or spinal deformity
  5. Indications of hypocalcemia or hypophosphatemia
  6. Anxiety regarding the suspected diagnosis or the possible occurrence of a fracture or deformity
  7. Changes in x-ray examination findings, such as the presence of radiolucent bands called Looser's lines or transformation zones (pseudofractures)

Interventions

- Encourage increased dietary intake of vitamin D through dietary intake, sun exposure, and drug supplementation.
- Refer to Osteoporosis for additional nursing diagnoses and interventions.

Osteomyelitis

OVERVIEW

- *Osteomyelitis* is the term used to describe any infection of the bone.
- Categories of osteomyelitis include
  1. Exogenous, in which infectious organisms enter from outside the body as in an open fracture
  2. Endogenous (hematogenous osteomyelitis), in which organisms are carried by the bloodstream from other areas of infection in the body
  3. Continuous, in which bone infection results from skin infection of adjacent tissue
- Two major types of osteomyelitis are acute and chronic.
- Common causes of osteomyelitis include penetrating trauma, infection elsewhere in the body, vascular compromise or insufficiency, drug abuse, or long-term catheter use.

 Considerations for Older Adults

- Clients with diabetes mellitus or peripheral vascular disease who have foot ulcers commonly acquire osteomyelitis.
- Multiple organisms are responsible for osteomyelitis in these clients.

COLLABORATIVE MANAGEMENT

Assessment

- Assess for
  1. Bone pain that is described as a constant, localized, pulsating sensation that intensifies with movement
  2. Fever
  3. Swelling, tenderness, and erythema around the site of infection
  4. Draining ulcers on the feet or hands
  5. An elevated white blood cell count and erythrocyte sedimentation rate
  6. A positive result on a blood culture

- Interventions include
  1. Administering intravenous (IV) antibiotics specific for the involved organism for several weeks (may require up to 3 months of oral antibiotics)
  2. Teaching the client and family the importance of strict adherence to the antibiotic regimen and the complications that could occur as a result of inadequate treatment or failure to follow up with health care providers
  3. Irrigating the wound with antibiotic solution
  4. Implementing drainage precautions for all open wounds
  5. Implementing a pain management program
  6. Covering the wound and using strict aseptic technique when changing dressings
     a. Wounds may be managed through the window of a cast, which must remain dry during dressing or irrigation procedures.
  7. Using hyperbaric oxygen therapy to increase tissue perfusion
  8. Performing *sequestrectomy* to debride the infected bone and allow revascularization of tissue
  9. Using *bone grafts* to obliterate bone defects
  10. Using *bone segment transfers,* which consists of reconstruction with microvascular bone transfers, when the infected bone is extensively resected
  11. Using *muscle flaps* to treat relatively small bony defects
  12. *Amputating* the affected limb if the surgical procedure is ineffective or inappropriate

Osteoporosis

OVERVIEW

- Osteoporosis is a metabolic disease in which bone demineralization results in decreased density and subsequent fractures, most commonly in the wrist, hip, and vertebral column.
- Generalized osteoporosis involves many structures in the skeleton and is further divided into

1. *Primary osteoporosis*, which occurs in both genders at any age but most often affects women after menopause and men in their later years.
2. *Secondary osteoporosis*, which results from an associated medical condition such as hyperparathyroidism, long-term use of corticosteroids, or prolonged immobility
- Regional osteoporosis occurs when a limb is immobilized (greater than 8 to 12 weeks) related to a fracture, injury, paralysis, or joint inflammation.
- Vertebral fractures occur in both categories.

COLLABORATIVE MANAGEMENT

Assessment

- Record client information.
  1. Age, sex, race, body build, height, and weight
  2. Usual exposure to sunlight
  3. Cigarette, alcohol, and caffeine use
  4. Daily calcium and vitamin D intake
  5. Usual exercise pattern
  6. Current medical problems and prescribed and over-the-counter medications
  7. History of falls, fractures, and other injuries
  8. Family history of osteoporosis
  9. Daily routine
- Assess for
  1. Classic dowager's hump (kyphosis of the dorsal spine) by inspection and palpation of the vertebral column
  2. Back pain after lifting, bending, or stooping
  3. Back pain that increases with palpation, particularly of the lower thoracic and lumbar vertebrae
  4. Back pain with tenderness and voluntary restriction of spinal movement, which indicates compression fractures, usually of T8 to L3
  5. Fractures in the distal end of the radius or at the upper third of the femur
  6. Constipation, abdominal distention, and respiratory compromise from movement restriction and spinal deformity
  7. Disturbed body image, especially if the client is severely kyphotic

8. The threat of fractures that could occur during activities, creating fear and anxiety and resulting in limitations of social or physical activities

Interventions

- Drug therapy includes hormone replacement, calcium supplements, biphosphonates, selective estrogen receptor modulators, calcitonin, vitamin D, or a combination of several drugs.
- Instruct the client to
  1. Increase his or her dietary intake of calcium and vitamin D.
  2. Avoid alcohol and caffeine.
  3. Increase dietary protein, vitamin C, and iron to promote bone healing in clients with fractures.
  4. Create a hazard-free environment; hip protectors are inexpensive devices that can prevent hip fractures if the client experiences falls.
  5. Exercise to strengthen the abdominal and back muscles to improve posture and provide support for the spine (in collaboration with physical therapy).
  6. Perform abdominal isometrics, deep breathing, and pectoral stretching to increase pulmonary capacity.
  7. Perform extremity exercises.
     a. Isometric
     b. Resistive
     c. Active range of motion (ROM) to improve joint mobility and increase muscle tone
  8. Walk daily, both slow and fast, and bicycle.
  9. Avoid recreational activities that could cause vertebral compression, such as bowling and horseback riding.
- Drug therapy for pain relief includes
  1. Analgesics, opioids, and non-narcotics for the acute phase
  2. Muscle relaxants to ease the discomfort of muscle spasms
  3. Anti-inflammatory agents for pain and spinal nerve root inflammation; monitor the client (particularly the elderly) for problems associated with nonsteroidal anti-inflammatory drugs (NSAIDs), such as gastrointestinal bleeding and heart failure
- Back braces may be used to immobilize the spine during the acute phase and to provide spinal column support. (Because

elderly clients tolerate these devices poorly, carefully ensure proper fit and assess client tolerance.)

Community-Based Care

- Discharge planning includes
  1. Helping the client and family to identify and correct hazards in the home before discharge
  2. Ensuring that the client can correctly use all assistive devices ordered for home use
  3. Teaching measures to prevent falls, such as use of orthotic and ambulatory aids
  4. Reviewing the prescribed exercise regimen
  5. Referring the client to a home health agency and support groups such as the National Osteoporosis Foundation

Otitis Media

OVERVIEW

- Otitis media is an infection in the middle ear that causes an inflammatory process within the mucosa.
- This inflammatory process leads to swelling and irritation of the bones, or ossicles, within the middle ear, resulting in the formation of purulent inflammatory exudate.
- Otitis media may be *acute, chronic,* or *serious.*

COLLABORATIVE MANAGEMENT

- Assess for the symptoms of acute or chronic otitis media.
  1. Ear pain (is relieved if the tympanic membrane ruptures)
  2. Feeling of fullness in the ear
  3. Slightly retracted tympanic membrane initially. (Later, the membrane is red, thickened, and bulging, with a loss of landmarks; exudate may be seen behind the membrane.)
  4. Conductive hearing loss
  5. Headache
  6. Malaise
  7. Fever

8. Nausea and vomiting
9. Slight dizziness or vertigo
- If the disease progresses, the eardrum spontaneously perforates and pus or blood drains from the ear.
- Treatment includes
  1. Bedrest to limit head movement and thus decrease pain
  2. Localized heat and occasional application of cold
  3. Systemic antibiotic therapy
  4. Analgesics such as acetylsalicylic acid (aspirin, Entrophen ♣) or acetaminophen (Tylenol, Abenol ♣), or treat severe pain with opioid
  5. Oral and nasal decongestants
- *Myringotomy* is the surgical procedure performed after initial antibiotic therapy if the tympanic membrane continues to bulge.
- Postoperative care consists of antibiotic eardrops such as neomycin sulfate or bacitracin.
- Care must be taken to keep the external ear and canal free from other substances while the incision is healing; the client should avoid showering and washing his or her hair.

Otosclerosis

- Otosclerosis is a disease of the labyrinthine capsule of the middle ear, resulting in the development of irregular areas of new bone formation.
- It has a familial tendency, and the incidence of disease in women is twice that in men.

COLLABORATIVE MANAGEMENT

- Assess for
  1. Slowly progressive conductive hearing loss
     a. The loss is bilateral, although the progression of the disease is different in each ear, which gives the effect of one "good" ear and one "bad" ear.
     b. Initial hearing loss is of the lower frequencies but progresses to all frequencies.

2. Roaring or ringing type of constant tinnitus
3. Normal tympanic membrane; occasionally, the eardrum has a pinkish discoloration
- Treatment is directed toward improving hearing through amplification with a hearing aid.
- Surgical procedures used to correct hearing loss include a partial or complete *stapedectomy* (removal of stapes) and a prosthesis.

Overhydration

OVERVIEW

- Overhydration, also called fluid overload, is not an actual disease but a sign of a problem in which fluid intake or retention is greater than the body's fluid need.
- The three types of overhydration are
  1. *Isotonic,* or hypervolemia, which occurs as a result of excess fluid in the extracellular fluid (ECF) space; may result in circulatory overload and edema if severe
  2. *Hypotonic* (water intoxication), in which the excess fluid is hypotonic to normal body fluids; electrolyte imbalances may occur
  3. *Hypertonic* overhydration, which is rare and which is caused by excessive sodium intake

COLLABORATIVE MANAGEMENT

Assessment

- Assess for
  1. Cardiovascular changes
     a. Increased pulse rate, bounding pulse
     b. Full peripheral pulses
     c. Elevated blood pressure, decreased pulse pressure
     d. Elevated central venous pressure
     e. Distended neck and hand veins
     f. Engorged venous varicosities
  2. Respiratory changes
     a. Increased respiratory rate with shallow respirations

    b. Dyspnea that increases with exertion or in the supine position

    c. Moist crackles present on auscultation

    d. Integumentary changes

    e. Pitting edema

    f. Skin pale and cool to touch

3. Neuromuscular changes

    a. Altered level of consciousness

    b. Headache

    c. Visual disturbances

    d. Skeletal muscle weakness

    e. Paresthesia

4. Gastrointestinal changes: increased motility

    a. Manifestations of isotonic overhydration

    b. Liver enlargement

    c. Ascites formation

    d. Manifestations of hypotonic overhydration

    e. Polyuria

    f. Diarrhea

    g. Nonpitting edema

    h. Cardiac dysrhythmias associated with electrolyte dilution

    i. Projectile vomiting

Interventions

- Administer diuretics (as long as renal failure is not the cause of the overhydration).
- Osmotic diuretics are used first to prevent severe electrolyte imbalance.
- High-ceiling (loop) diuretics are given if osmotic diuretics are not effective.
- Monitor the client for response to medications, especially weight loss and increased urinary output.
- Observe for signs and symptoms of fluid and electrolyte imbalance and assess laboratory findings.
  1. Use diet therapy to control fluid volume through restrictions of both fluids and sodium.
  2. Measure intake and output.
  3. Weigh the client at the same time and on the same scale each day.
  4. Monitor urine for color, character, and specific gravity.

5. Monitor for increased fluid overload.
   a. Increased pulse quality
   b. Increased neck vein distention
   c. Presence of crackles in lungs
   d. Increased peripheral edema

Paget's Disease

OVERVIEW

- Paget's disease, or osteitis deformans, is a metabolic disorder of bone remodeling, or turnover, in which increased resorption or loss results in bone deposits that are weak, enlarged, and disorganized.
- Three phases of the disease are
  1. *Active*, in which a prolific increase in osteoclasts causes massive bone destruction and deformity
  2. *Mixed*, in which the osteoblasts react in a compensatory manner to form new bone, and bone is disorganized and chaotic in structure
  3. *Inactive*, in which the newly formed bone becomes sclerotic and ivory hard
- Common sites include the vertebrae, femur, skull, sternum, and pelvis.

COLLABORATIVE MANAGEMENT

Assessment

- Assess for
  1. Bone pain, described as deep and aching, and aggravated by weight bearing and pressure; severe bone pain may indicate complications such as osteogenic sarcoma
  2. Back pain and headache
  3. Arthritis at the joints of affected bones
  4. Nerve impingement, particularly in the lumbosacral area of the vertebral column
  5. Posture, stance, and gait to identify gross bony deformities
  6. Flexion contracture of the hips

7. Size and shape of the skull, which is soft, thick, and enlarged
8. Deafness and vertigo
9. Cranial nerve compression
10. Warm and flushed skin
11. Apathy, lethargy, and fatigue
12. Pathologic fractures
13. Hyperparathyroidism and gout
14. Hydrocephalus from bony enlargement of the skull, which blocks the cerebrospinal fluid
15. Increase in serum alkaline phosphatase
16. Ability to cope with pain and the effects of having a chronic disorder
17. Fear associated with the potential development of bone cancer

Interventions

- Drug therapy includes
  1. Nonsteroidal anti-inflammatory drugs (NSAIDs) for pain
  2. Calcitonin, a thyroid hormone, which seems to retard bone resorption and subsequently relieve pain. It may be used in conjunction with etidronate disodium (Didronel) which is prescribed for 6 months on and 6 months off.
  3. Mithramycin (Mithracin), a potent anticarcinogen and antibiotic reserved for clients with marked hypercalcemia or severe disease and neurologic compromise
  4. Alendronate (Fosamax) or tiludronate (Skelid)
- Other pain relief measures include
  1. Applying heat and giving a massage
  2. Collaborating with physical therapy to institute an exercise program
  3. Teaching the client to perform range-of-motion and gentle stretching
  4. Applying and teaching the application of orthotic devices for support and immobilization
  5. Encouraging the client to eat a diet rich in calcium
  6. Providing the client with the address of the Paget's Disease Foundation and the local chapter of the Arthritis Foundation
- A partial or total joint replacement may be needed to treat secondary arthritis and uncontrolled pain.

Pain, Back

OVERVIEW

- The areas of the back most commonly affected by back pain are the cervical and lumbar vertebrae.
- *Acute lumbosacral (low back) pain (LBP)* is typically caused by a muscle strain, spasm, ligament sprain, disc degeneration, or herniated nucleus pulposus (usually between the fourth and fifth lumbar vertebra).
- If back pain continues for 3 months, or if repeated episodes occur, the client has *chronic* back pain.
- Risk factors for *acute* back pain include
  1. Trauma (twisting or hyperflexion during lifting)
  2. Obesity
  3. Congenital spinal problems, such as scoliosis
  4. Smoking (causes premature disk degeneration)
- Risk factors for *chronic* back pain in women include
  1. Poor posture
  2. Wearing high-heeled shoes

Considerations for Older Adults

- In older adult clients, back pain is usually caused by osteoarthritis.
- Cervical pain is also common in clients with advanced rheumatoid arthritis who experience cervical disk subluxation, most often at the C1-2 level (first and second cervical vertebrae).
- Physiologic changes associated with aging, such as spinal stenosis, vertebral malalignment, and vascular changes, also contribute to back pain in the older adult.

COLLABORATIVE MANAGEMENT

Assessment

- Assess for
  1. Pain: location, quality, radiation, severity, treatment
  2. Posture and gait
  3. Vertebral alignment and swelling
  4. Muscle spasm

5. Tenderness of the back and involved extremity
6. Sensory changes: paresthesia, numbness
7. Muscle tone and strength
8. Limitations in movement
9. Reaction to illness
10. Vertebral changes seen on x-ray, computed tomography (CT) scan, or magnetic resonance imaging scan
11. Abnormal electromyography and nerve conduction studies

Interventions

NONSURGICAL MANAGEMENT

- To treat *acute* LBP
  1. Have the client use the Williams position when in bed (semi-Fowler's bed position with the knees flexed). A bed board or firm mattress may be useful for clients with a muscle injury. For clients with a herniated disk, a flat position may aggravate the pain.
  2. Collaborate with the physical therapist to develop an individualized exercise program.
  3. Drug therapy includes muscle relaxants and nonsteroidal anti-inflammatory drugs (NSAIDs).
  4. Epidural or local steroid injection may be helpful in some cases.
  5. Apply ice and heat therapy.
     a. Apply moist heat in the form of heat packs or hot towels for 20 to 30 min four times daily, as well as hot showers or baths, which are beneficial for some clients.
     b. Apply ice therapy using ice packs or ice massage over the affected area for 10 to 15 minutes every 1 to 2 hours.
     c. Some clients prefer alternating ice and heat therapy.
     d. Deep heat therapy such as ultrasound treatments and diathermy may be administered by the physical therapist.
- Approaches for treating *chronic* back pain include
  1. Collaborate with the dietitian to implement a weight loss program if appropriate.

2. Have the client use a custom-fitted lumbosacral brace or corset for LBP.
3. Have the client use ergonomic office furniture.
4. Have the client use shoe inserts or insoles.
5. Have the client use distraction, imagery, and music therapy.

SURGICAL MANAGEMENT

- *Traditional* operative procedures include
  1. *Percutaneous laser disk decompression,* which relieves the pain of a herniated disk by drawing the herniated portion away from the nerve root
  2. *Diskectomy,* in which the spinal nerve is usually lifted to remove the offending portion of the disk
  3. *Laminectomy,* which is the removal of one or more vertebral laminae, plus osteophytes, and the herniated nucleus pulposus through a 3-inch (7.5-cm) incision
  4. *Spinal fusion,* which stabilizes the spine if repeated laminectomies are performed
- *Alternative* operative procedures have varying degrees of popularity. Hospital stays are shorter than with traditional operative procedures, and spinal cord complications are less likely.
  1. Percutaneous lumbar diskectomy
     a. A metal cannula is inserted adjacent to the affected disk under fluoroscopy and a special cutting tool is threaded through the cannula for removal of pieces of the disk that are compressing the nerve root (laser surgery may be used). In-patient hospitalization is not necessary.
     b. Possible complications: infection and nerve root injury
  2. Microdiskectomy
     a. Microscopic surgery is performed through a 1-inch (2.5-cm) incision.
     b. Possible complications: infection, dural tears, and missed disk fragments
  3. Laser-assisted laparoscopic lumbar diskectomy
     a. A laser with modified standard disk instruments is inserted periumbilically through the laparoscope.
     b. Possible complications: infection and nerve root injury

P

  4. *Disk prosthesis* involves placing a hard plastic prosthesis that replaces the client's natural disk and is shaped to allow full spinal movement.
- Preoperative care for back surgery includes
  1. Providing routine preoperative care
  2. Explaining to the client that various sensations may be experienced in the affected leg or both legs (for lumbar surgery) because of manipulation of nerves and muscles during surgery
  3. Teaching the client what to expect postoperatively and how to move in bed
  4. Addressing the need for a postoperative brace and bone grafting if the client is having a spinal fusion
- Postoperative care for back surgery includes
  1. Take vital signs and do neurologic checks every 4 hours during the first 24 hours.
  2. Assess for fever and hypotension.
  3. Check the dressing for any drainage. (Clear drainage may indicate a cerebrospinal fluid leak.)
  4. Check the client's ability to void. An inability to void may indicate damage to sacral spinal nerves. Opioid analgesics have been associated with difficulty voiding.
  5. Manage pain with opioid analgesics or patient-controlled anesthesia, as ordered.
  6. Graduated compression stocking, sequential compression devices (SCDs), or pneumatic compression boots (PCBs) may be used until the client can ambulate independently to prevent deep vein thrombosis and possible pulmonary emboli.
  7. Assist the client to get out of bed, usually the evening of surgery. (NOTE: Bedrest for 24 to 48 hours may be necessary for clients with a spinal fusion.)
  8. Empty any surgical drains that are placed and record the amount of drainage.
  9. Log roll the client every 2 hours.
  10. Encourage the client to deep breathe every 2 hours to prevent atelectasis and pneumonia.
  11. Ensure that a brace or other type of thoracolumbar support is worn when the client is out of bed (for spinal fusion).

Community-Based Care

- Health teaching includes
  1. The prescribed exercise program (Client mastery is ensured by observing correct performance on return demonstration, in collaboration with physical therapy.)
  2. Importance of daily walking
  3. Restrictions on climbing stairs, lifting and bending, and activities such as driving
  4. Principles of body mechanics
  5. The use of a firm mattress or bed board, if appropriate
  6. Drug information
  7. A weight-reduction diet, if needed
  8. The use of moist heat
  9. The importance of stopping smoking
  10. The possibility of recurrence of back pain
  11. For unresolved pain, referral to a pain specialist or clinic

Pain, Cervical Spine

P

- *Cervical back pain* is usually related to a herniation of the nucleus pulposus in an intervertebral disk (ruptured disk) between the fifth and sixth vertebrae or to nerve compression caused by osteophyte formation; it may also occur from muscle strain or ligament sprain.

COLLABORATIVE MANAGEMENT

Assessment

- Assess for
  1. Pain that radiates to the scapula and down the arm when the client moves his or her neck
  2. Sleep disturbances from pain
  3. Headache
  4. Numbness and tingling in the affected arm
  5. Vertebral changes seen on computed tomography or magnetic resonance imaging

Interventions

NONSURGICAL MANAGEMENT

- Nonsurgical management of neck pain is the same as described for back pain except that the exercises focus on the neck and shoulder.
- A soft collar may be prescribed for the client to wear at night; it should not be worn for more than 10 days or it can lead to increased pain and decreased muscle strength and range of motion.

SURGICAL MANAGEMENT

- Depending on the causative factors, either an anterior or posterior approach can be used.
- Postoperatively, the client will wear some type of cervical collar.
- In addition to the postoperative care described under Surgical Management for Back Pain, nursing interventions include
  1. Assessing airway breathing and circulation
  2. Checking for swallowing ability
  3. Assessing the client's ability to void
  4. Monitoring intake and output
  5. Assisting the client with ambulation, usually the evening of surgery unless a multilevel fusion was performed
  6. Monitoring for complications
     a. Hoarseness due to laryngeal injury
     b. Dysphagia
     c. Esophageal, tracheal, or vertebral artery injury
     d. Graft extrusion and screw loosening if a fusion was performed

Pancreatitis, Acute

OVERVIEW

- Acute pancreatitis is a serious and, at times, life-threatening inflammatory process of the pancreas brought on by premature activation of pancreatic enzymes and resulting in autodigestion and fibrosis of the pancreas.

- The extent of the inflammation and tissue destruction ranges from mild involvement, characterized by edema and inflammation, to severe, necrotizing hemorrhagic pancreatitis, characterized by diffusely bleeding pancreatic tissue with fibrosis and tissue death.
- Many factors can cause injury to the pancreas.
  1. Biliary tract disease with gallstones
  2. Excessive alcohol ingestion
  3. Postoperative trauma from surgical manipulation after biliary tract, pancreatic, gastric, and duodenal procedures
  4. External blunt trauma
  5. Metabolic disturbances
  6. Renal failure or renal transplant
  7. Drug toxicities, including opiates, sulfonamides, thiazides, steroids, and oral contraceptives
  8. Other medical diseases
- Complications include transient hyperglycemia, pleural effusions, atelectasis, pneumonia, multisystem organ failure, acute respiratory distress syndrome (ARDS), shock, and coagulation defects.

COLLABORATIVE MANAGEMENT

Assessment

- Record client information.
  1. History of abdominal pain related to alcohol ingestion or high fat intake
  2. Individual and family history of alcoholism, pancreatitis, or biliary tract disease
  3. Previous abdominal surgeries or diagnostic procedures
  4. Medical history, including peptic ulcer disease, renal failure, vascular disorders, hyperparathyroidism, and hyperlipidemia
  5. Recent viral infection
  6. Use of prescription and over-the-counter drugs
- Assess for
  1. Abdominal pain (the most frequent symptom), including a sudden onset, midepigastric, or left upper quadrant location with radiation to the back, aggravated by a fatty meal, ingestion of a large amount of alcohol, or lying in the recumbent position

2. Weight loss, with nausea and vomiting
3. Jaundice
4. Gray-blue discoloration of the abdomen and periumbilical area (Cullen's sign)
5. Gray-blue discoloration of the flanks (Turner's sign)
6. Absent or decreased bowel sounds
7. Abdominal tenderness, rigidity, and guarding
8. Dull sound on abdominal percussion, indicating ascites
9. Elevated temperature with tachycardia and decreased blood pressure
10. Adventitious breath sounds, dyspnea, or orthopnea
11. Elevated serum amylase and lipase levels

Planning and Implementation

◆NDx: Acute Pain

NONSURGICAL MANAGEMENT

- Fasting includes
  1. Withholding food and fluids in the acute period; hydration is maintained with intravenous fluids
  2. Maintaining nasogastric intubation to decrease gastric distention and suppress pancreatic secretion
  3. Assessing frequently for the presence of bowel sounds
- Drug therapy may include
  1. Meperidine hydrochloride (Demerol), the drug of choice for pain because it is less likely than other drugs to cause spasm of the smooth musculature of the pancreatic ducts and the sphincter of Oddi
  2. Histamine receptor–blocking drugs to decrease hydrochloric acid production
  3. Anticholinergics to decrease vagal stimulation and decrease gastrointestinal motility
  4. Antibiotics for clients with acute necrotizing pancreatitis
- Comfort measures include
  1. Helping the client assume a fetal position to decrease abdominal pain
  2. Providing frequent oral hygiene
  3. Encouraging the client to express the emotions and responses he or she is feeling
  4. Providing reassurances and diversional activities

SURGICAL MANAGEMENT

- Surgical management is usually not indicated for acute pancreatitis.
- The client with complications such as pancreatic pseudocyst and abscess may require surgical drainage.
- Postoperative care includes
  1. Monitoring drainage tubes for patency and recording output
  2. Maintaining suction to drainage tubes
  3. Providing meticulous skin care because pancreatic drainage is particularly excoriating to the skin
  4. Collaborating with the enterostomal therapist to promote skin integrity; possibilities include the use of ostomy appliances and the application of topical ointments

◀NDx: Imbalanced Nutrition: Less than Body Requirements

- Interventions include
  1. Withholding food and fluids in the early stages of the disease
  2. Providing total parenteral nutrition (TPN) or total enteral nutrition (TEN) for severe nutritional depletion and for clients who are unable to eat for 7 to 10 days
  3. When food is tolerated, providing small, frequent, high-carbohydrate and high-protein feedings with limited fats
  4. Providing supplemental liquid diet preparations and vitamins and minerals to boost caloric intake, if needed

Community-Based Care

- Client and family health teaching is aimed at preventing future episodes and preventing disease progression to chronic pancreatitis.
  1. Encourage alcohol abstinence to prevent further pain and extension of the inflammation and insufficiency.
  2. Teach the client to notify the physician if he or she is experiencing acute abdominal pain or symptoms of biliary tract disease such as jaundice, clay-colored stools, and dark urine.
  3. Emphasize the importance of follow-up visits with the physicians.

4. Refer the client with an alcohol abuse problem to support groups such as Alcoholics Anonymous.
5. Refer the client to home health nursing as needed.

Pancreatitis, Chronic

OVERVIEW

- Chronic pancreatitis is a progressive, destructive disease of the pancreas characterized by remissions and exacerbations.
- Inflammation and fibrosis of the tissue contribute to pancreatic insufficiency and diminished organ function.
- The disease usually develops after repeated episodes of alcohol-induced acute pancreatitis, also known as *chronic calcifying pancreatitis;* it may also be associated with chronic obstruction of the common bile duct.
- Chronic pancreatitis is characterized by protein precipitates that plug the ducts and lead to ductal obstruction, atrophy, and dilation, causing metaplasia and ulceration, and resulting in fibrosis of the pancreatic tissue.
- The pancreas becomes hard and firm because of cell atrophy and pancreatic insufficiency.
- *Chronic obstructive pancreatitis* develops from inflammation, spasm, and obstruction of the sphincter of Oddi.
- Inflammatory and sclerotic lesions develop in the head of the pancreas and around the ducts, causing an obstruction and backflow of pancreatic secretions and enzymes.
- *Pancreatic insufficiency* is characterized by the loss of exocrine function, which causes a decreased output of enzymes and bicarbonate; loss of endocrine function results in diabetes mellitus.

COLLABORATIVE MANAGEMENT

Assessment

- Record client information.
  1. History of abdominal pain related to alcohol ingestion or high fat intake with specific information about

alcohol intake, including time, amount, and relationship of alcohol to pain development

2. Individual and family history of alcoholism, pancreatitis, or biliary tract disease
3. Previous abdominal surgeries or diagnostic procedures
4. Medical history, including peptic ulcer disease, renal failure, vascular disorders, hyperparathyroidism, and hyperlipidemia
5. Recent viral infections
6. Use of prescription or over-the-counter drugs

- Assess for
    1. Abdominal pain (major clinical manifestation): continuous, burning, or gnawing dullness with intense and relentless exacerbations
    2. Abdominal tenderness
    3. Left upper quadrant mass, indicating a pseudocyst or abscess
    4. Dullness on abdominal percussion, indicating pancreatic ascites
    5. Steatorrhea, foul-smelling stools that may increase in volume as pancreatic insufficiency progresses
    6. Weight loss and muscle wasting
    7. Jaundice and dark urine
    8. Signs and symptoms of diabetes mellitus
    9. Elevated serum alkaline phosphatase and amylase levels
    10. Elevated serum bilirubin and alkaline phosphatase levels if the intrahepatic bile duct is obstructed
    11. Identification of calcification of pancreatic tissue in biopsy specimen

Interventions

NONSURGICAL MANAGEMENT

- Drug therapy includes
    1. Opioid analgesia with meperidine hydrochloride (Demerol, the drug most often used), as ordered (NOTE: The client may become dependent on opioids with long-term use.)
    2. Non-opioid analgesics

3. Pancreatic enzyme replacements given with meals or snacks to aid in digestion and absorption of fat and protein
   a. Record the number and consistency of stools per day to monitor the effectiveness of enzyme therapy.
4. Insulin or oral hypoglycemic agents to control diabetes
5. Histamine receptor antagonists to decrease gastric acid
- Diet therapy includes
  1. Withholding food and fluids to avoid recurrent pain exacerbated by eating
  2. Providing TPN for severe nutritional depletion
  3. Providing small, frequent, high-carbohydrate and high-protein feedings with limited fats, when tolerated

SURGICAL MANAGEMENT

- Surgical management is not the primary intervention for chronic pancreatitis. Surgery may be indicated for intractable pain, incapacitating pain relapses, or complications such as pseudocyst and abscess.
- Surgical procedures include
  1. *Incision* and *drainage* for abscesses or pseudocysts
  2. *Laparoscopic cholecystectomy* or *choledochotomy* for underlying biliary tract disease
  3. *Sphincterotomy* (incision of the sphincter) for fibrosis
  4. *Pancreatojejunostomy* (the pancreatic duct is opened and anastomosed to the jejunum, relieving obstruction) to relieve pain and preserve pancreatic tissue and function
  5. *Partial pancreatectomy,* which may be performed for advanced pancreatitis or disabling pain
  6. *Vagotomy* with gastric antrectomy to alter nerve stimulation and decrease pancreatic secretion
- For preoperative and postoperative care, see Cancer, Pancreatic, for care of the client undergoing a Whipple procedure.

Community-Based Care

- Health teaching is aimed at preventing further exacerbations.
  1. Avoid known precipitating factors, such as alcohol, caffeinated beverages, and irritating foods.
  2. Comply with diet instructions: bland, low-fat, frequent meals with avoidance of rich, fatty foods.

3. Follow written instructions and prescriptions for pancreatic enzyme therapy.
   a. How and when to take enzymes
   b. The importance of maintaining therapy
   c. The importance of notifying the physician of increased steatorrhea, abdominal distention, cramping, and skin breakdown
4. Comply with elevated glucose management, including either oral hypoglycemic drugs or insulin injections and monitoring of blood glucose levels.
5. Keep follow-up visits with the physicians.

■ Refer the client to financial counseling, social services, vocational rehabilitation, home health services, and Alcoholics Anonymous as needed.

Paralysis, Facial

■ Facial paralysis, or *Bell's palsy*, is an acute paralysis of cranial nerve VII, with maximal paralysis reached within 2 to 5 days.
■ Pain behind the face or ear may precede paralysis by a few hours or days.
■ The disorder is characterized by a drawing sensation and an inability to close the eye, wrinkle the forehead, smile, whistle, or grimace; the face appears masklike and sags.

COLLABORATIVE MANAGEMENT

■ Treatment includes
1. Administering prednisone (Deltasone✦, Winpred) to decrease inflammation
2. Administering analgesics for pain
3. Protecting the eye from corneal abrasion or ulceration by patching and administering artificial tears
4. Providing emotional support
5. Providing small, frequent soft meals
6. Teaching the client to use warm, moist heat, massage, and facial exercises such as whistling, grimacing, and blowing air out of the cheeks three or four times a day

Parkinson's Disease

- Parkinson's disease, also referred to as *paralysis agitans*, is a debilitating neurologic disorder involving the basal ganglia and substantia nigra.
- The disease is characterized by muscle rigidity, akinesia (slow movements), postural instability, and tremors.
- The disease involves five stages.
  Stage 1: mild disease with unilateral limb involvement
  Stage 2: bilateral limb involvement
  Stage 3: significant gait disturbances and moderate generalized disability
  Stage 4: severe disability, akinesia, and muscle rigidity
  Stage 5: completely dependent in all aspects of activities of daily living
- The use of ibuprofen and other nonsteroidal anti-inflammatory drugs has been demonstrated to reduce the risk of developing Parkinson's disease if taken years before symptoms develop. However, the long-term use of these agents may result in significant complications and should not be taken unless prescribed by the client's health care provider.

COLLABORATIVE MANAGEMENT

Assessment

- Record client information.
  1. Time and progression of symptoms
  2. Bradykinesia: problems performing two activities at once
  3. History of slight tremor, fatigue, and loss of manual dexterity
  4. Changes in handwriting, which typically becomes small and can be accomplished only slowly
- Assess for
  1. Rigidity, which is present early in the disease process and progresses over time
     a. Cogwheel rigidity, manifested by a rhythmic interruption of the muscles of movement

    b. Plastic rigidity: mildly restrictive movements

    c. Lead-pipe rigidity: total resistance to movement

2. Posture
   a. Stooped posture
   b. Flexed trunk
   c. Fingers adducted and flexed at the metacarpophalangeal joint
   d. Wrists slightly dorsiflexed

3. Gait
   a. Slow and shuffling
   b. Short, hesitant steps
   c. Propulsive gait
   d. Difficulty stopping quickly

4. Speech
   a. Soft, low-pitched voice
   b. Dysarthria
   c. Echolalia: automatic repetition of what another person says
   d. Repetition of sentences
   e. Change in voice volume, phonation, or articulation

5. Motor
   a. Bradykinesia
   b. Akinesia
   c. Tremors
   d. "Pill-rolling" movement
   e. Masklike facies
   f. Difficulty chewing and swallowing
   g. Uncontrolled drooling, especially at night
   h. Difficulty getting into and out of bed
   i. Little arm swinging when walking
   j. Change in handwriting, micrographia

6. Autonomic dysfunction
   a. Orthostatic hypotension
   b. Excessive perspiration and oily skin
   c. Flushing, changes in skin texture
   d. Blepharospasm

7. Psychosocial
   a. Emotional lability
   b. Depression
   c. Paranoia

P

d. Easily upset
e. Rapid mood swings
f. Cognitive impairments
g. Delayed reaction time
h. Sleep disturbances

Interventions

- Provide drug therapy.
    1. Administer drug therapy on time to maintain continuous therapeutic drug levels.
        a. Anticholinergic drugs, if the client's primary symptom is tremor
        b. Dopamine agonists
        c. Levodopa combinations
        d. Monoamine oxidase inhibitors
        e. Catechol O methyltransferase inhibitors
        f. Variety of investigational drugs
    2. Monitor the client for drug toxicity and side effects such as delirium, cognitive impairment, decreased effectiveness of the drug, or hallucination.
    3. Treatment of drug toxicity or tolerance includes
        a. Reduction in medication dosage
        b. Change in medications or in the frequency of administration
        c. Drug holiday (particularly with levodopa therapy)
- Other interventions include
    1. Physical therapy (PT) and occupational therapy (OT) consultations to plan and implement an active and passive range-of-motion mobility program and muscle-stretching program such as traditional exercise programs, yoga, and tai chi; exercises for the muscles of the face and tongue to facilitate swallowing and speech
    2. Participation in activities of daily living (ADLs); PT and OT consultation to provide training in ADLs and the use of adaptive devices
    3. Teaching the client and family to monitor the client's sleeping pattern and to discuss whether or not the client is safe to operate machinery or perform other potentially dangerous tasks
    4. Monitoring the client's ability to eat and swallow; monitoring food and fluid intake; collaborating with the

registered dietitian for caloric calculation and diet planning

5. Assessing the need for a speech-language pathologist consultation for evaluation of swallowing dysfunction and communication problems

6. Teaching the client to speak slowly and clearly; using alternative communication methods such as a communication board

7. Referring the client and family to a social worker to help with financial and health insurance agencies as well as referring the client to state and social agencies and support groups

8. Instructing the client with orthostatic hypotension to wear an elastic stocking and change position slowly, especially when moving from a sitting to a standing position

9. Allowing sufficient time for the client to complete activities; scheduling appointments and activities for late in the morning to prevent rushing the client or scheduling them at the time of the client's optimal level of functioning

10. Implementing interventions to prevent complications of immobility such as constipation, pressure ulcers, contractures, and atelectasis

- *Stereotactic pallidotomy* can be a very effective treatment for Parkinson's disease. Using a probe, the target area in the brain receives a mild electrical stimulation to decrease tremor and rigidity. When the probe is in the ideal location, a temporary lesion is made. If this is successful, a permanent lesion is made.

- *Unilateral thalamotomy* is a treatment of tremor through thermocoagulation of brain cells.

- *Deep brain stimulation* involves placing a thin electrode in the thalamus or subthalamus which is connected to a "pacemaker" that delivers electrical current to interfere with "tremor" cells. The electrodes are connected to an implantable pulse generator that is placed underneath the skin in the client's chest, something like a cardiac pacemaker.

- Experimental surgical treatment includes brain graft surgery, which consists of transplanting small pieces of the client's own adrenal gland into the caudate nucleus of the brain; fetal tissue transplant, and gene therapy, to name a few.

Pediculosis

- Pediculosis is infestation by human lice and includes *pediculosis capitis* (head lice), *pediculosis corporis* (body lice), and *pediculosis pubis* (pubic or crab lice).
- The oval-shaped lice measure approximately 2 to 4 mm in length.
- The female louse lays hundreds of eggs, called *nits*, which are deposited at the base of the hair shaft.
- The most common symptom is pruritus, which may or may not be accompanied by excoriation.
- The treatment is chemical killing with agents such as lindane (Kwell, Hexit ♣) or topical malathion.
- Clothing and bed linens must be thoroughly washed in hot water.

Pelvic Inflammatory Disease

- Pelvic inflammatory disease (PID) is a complex infectious process in which organisms from the lower genital tract migrate from the endocervix upward through the uterine cavity into the fallopian tubes.
- PID is most often caused by sexually transmitted organisms especially *Chlamydia* and *Neisseria gonorrhoeae.*
- The infection may spread to other organs or tissues such as the uterus, fallopian tubes, and pelvic structures.
- Resultant infections include
  1. Endometritis (infection of the endometrial cavity)
  2. Salpingitis (infection of the fallopian tubes)
  3. Oophoritis (infection of the ovary)
  4. Parametritis (infection of the parametrium)
  5. Peritonitis (infection of the peritoneal cavity)
  6. Tubal or tubo-ovarian abscess
- Manifestations include tenderness in the tubes and ovaries and low, dull abdominal pain; some women experience only

mild discomfort or menstrual irregularity; others have no symptoms at all.

- Interventions include
  1. Pain management
  2. Antibiotics
  3. Rest
  4. Instructing the client to refrain from sexual intercourse and to take her temperature twice per day
  5. Providing support to the client who may be anxious and concerned about infertility
  6. Reminding the client of the importance of keeping appointments with her health care provider
  7. Instructing the client on signs of persistent or recurrent infection and education to prevent exposure to and infection with all sexually transmitted diseases
  8. Discussing contraception and the client's need or desire for it
  9. Counseling the client to contact her sexual partners for examination and treatment

Pericarditis

OVERVIEW

- Acute pericarditis is an inflammation or alteration of the pericardium, the membranous sac enclosing the heart.
- The two types of pericarditis are
  1. *Acute pericarditis,* which is most commonly associated with infective organisms (bacteria, viruses, fungi), malignant neoplasms, postmyocardial infarction syndrome, postpericardiotomy syndrome, systemic connective tissue diseases, renal failure, and idiopathic causes
  2. *Chronic constrictive pericarditis,* which is caused by tuberculosis, radiation therapy, trauma, renal failure, and metastatic cancer, with the pericardium becoming rigid, preventing adequate ventricular filling, and resulting in cardiac failure

COLLABORATIVE MANAGEMENT

- Assess for
  1. Substernal precordial pain that can radiate to the left neck, shoulder, and back that is aggravated by breathing, coughing, and swallowing
  2. Pericardial friction rub
  3. Acute pericarditis
     a. Elevated white blood cell count
     b. ST-T wave elevation on electrocardiography (ECG)
     c. Fever (infectious cause)
  4. Chronic constrictive pericarditis
     a. Right-sided heart failure, including dyspnea, exertional fatigue, and orthopnea
     b. Pericardial thickening on echocardiogram and computed tomography (CT) scan
     c. Inverted or flat T waves on ECG
     d. Atrial fibrillation
- Treatment depends on the type of pericarditis.
- Acute pericarditis is treated by
  1. Administering nonsteroidal anti-inflammatory agents
  2. Administering corticosteroid therapy
  3. Administering antibiotics
  4. Encouraging rest
- For chronic constrictive pericarditis, the definitive treatment is surgical excision of the pericardium (pericardiectomy)
- Complications of pericarditis include pericardial effusions and cardiac tamponade, which is manifested by jugular venous distention, paradoxical pulse (systolic blood pressure at least 10 mm Hg higher on expiration than on inspiration), decreased cardiac output, muffled heart sounds, and circulatory collapse.
- Treatment of cardiac tamponade includes pericardiocentesis, in which a needle is inserted into the pericardial space. When the needle is properly positioned, a catheter is inserted and the pericardial fluid is withdrawn. Intravenous fluids are administered to improve cardiac output.
- For recurrent tamponade or effusions or adhesions from chronic pericarditis, a portion or all of the pericardium may be removed to allow adequate ventricular filling and contraction.

- In severe cases, removal of the toughened encasing pericardium (pericardectomy) may be necessary.

Peritonitis

- Peritonitis is an acute inflammation of the visceral or peritoneal peritoneum and endothelial lining of the abdominal cavity or peritoneum.
- *Primary peritonitis* is an acute bacterial infection that develops as a result of contamination of the peritoneum through the vascular system.
- *Secondary peritonitis* is caused by bacterial invasion as a result of an acute abdominal disorder such as gangrenous bowel, perforation of the viscera by blunt or penetrating trauma, or bile leakage.
- Complications of peritonitis include shock, respiratory problems, and paralytic ileus.

COLLABORATIVE MANAGEMENT

Assessment

- Record client information.
  1. History of abdominal pain that is aggravated by coughing or movement of any type and that is relieved by knee flexion
  2. Abdominal distention
  3. Anorexia, nausea, or vomiting
  4. Hiccups
  5. Low-grade fever or recent spikes in temperature
- Assess for
  1. Pain, which may be sharp and localized or poorly localized and referred to either the shoulder or thoracic areas
  2. Abdominal rigidity ("boardlike") or distention with rebound tenderness
  3. Absent bowel sounds
  4. Fever with tachycardia

5. Dehydration as evidenced by dry mucous membranes, poor skin turgor, and decreased urinary output
6. Compromised respiratory status; arterial blood gas results
7. Elevated white blood cell count
8. Dilation, edema, and inflammation of the small and large intestine as seen on abdominal x-ray

Interventions

NONSURGICAL MANAGEMENT

- Administer intravenous (IV) fluids and broad-spectrum antibiotics.
- Monitor daily weight.
- Record intake and output.
- Keep the client on nothing by mouth status.
- Monitor and record drainage from the nasogastric tube used for gastric and intestinal decompression.
- Provide pain management with IV analgesics; administer through patient-controlled analgesia (PCA) pump if available.
- Administer oxygen as prescribed according to the client's respiratory status.

SURGICAL MANAGEMENT

- Surgical management may be necessary to identify and repair the underlying cause of the peritonitis.
- Surgery is focused on controlling the contamination, removing foreign material from the peritoneal cavity, and draining fluid collections.
- During surgery, the peritoneum is irrigated with antibiotic solutions, and drainage catheters are inserted.
- Postoperative care includes
  1. Monitoring the client's
     a. Level of consciousness
     b. Vital signs
     c. Fluid and electrolyte status
     d. Intake and output

    e. Weight

    f. Skin turgor

    g. Edema

2. Maintaining the client in a semi-Fowler's position

3. Providing meticulous wound care; irrigating and packing the wound as prescribed

4. Assisting the client to gradually increase activity level

Considerations for Older Adults

- The only signs and symptoms of dehydration in the older adult may be a change in mental status.
- Assess for skin turgor using the skin over the forehead or sternum.
- Provide frequent mouth care to help maintain moist mucous membranes.

Community-Based Care

- The client may be discharged home or to a transitional care unit to complete antibiotic therapy and recovery.
- If the client is discharged home, collaborate with the case manager to determine the need for home care nursing or a home care aide.
- Provide written and oral postoperative instructions, including

    1. The necessity to report any redness, swelling, tenderness, drainage, or unusual or foul-smelling drainage from the wound

    2. Care of the incision and dressing; ensure that the client has the necessary equipment to perform wound care (dressings, solutions, catheter, tipped syringe); stress the importance of handwashing

    3. The need to report temperature higher than 101° F (38.2° C) or abdominal pain to the physician

    4. Pain medication administration and monitoring

    5. Dietary limitations, if necessary

    6. Activity limitations, including avoidance of heavy lifting until healing has occurred

P

Pharyngitis

- Pharyngitis or "sore throat" is an inflammation of the mucous membranes of the pharynx, usually occurring with acute rhinitis or sinusitis.
- Causes of acute pharyngitis include bacteria, viruses, and physical and chemical influences.
- Pharyngitis is characterized by throat soreness and dryness, throat pain, pain on swallowing, dysphagia, fever, and severe hyperemia (redness).
- Viral sore throats usually have a gradual onset and are accompanied by rhinorrhea, headache, mild hoarseness, and low-grade fever.
- Bacterial infections, such as group A streptococcal, can lead to acute glomerulonephritis and rheumatic fever carditis.
- Viral and bacterial pharyngitis may be associated with mild to severe hyperemia, with or without enlarged tonsils and with or without exudates, and lymph node enlargement in the neck.
- Nasal discharge varies from thin and watery to purulent.
- Management of *viral pharyngitis* includes
  1. Rest
  2. Increased fluid intake
  3. Analgesics for pain
  4. Warm saline throat gargles
  5. Mild antiseptic throat lozenges
- Management of *bacterial pharyngitis* includes antibiotics and supportive care measures.
- Rare complication of pharyngitis is epiglottitis, which may cause a partial or complete airway obstruction.

Pheochromocytoma

OVERVIEW

- A pheochromocytoma is a catecholamine-producing tumor that arises in the chromaffin cells of the adrenal medulla.
- Most of these tumors are benign, but they can occur in a malignant form.

COLLABORATIVE MANAGEMENT

- Assess for
  1. Paroxysmal hypertensive episodes, which vary in length from a few minutes to several hours
  2. Palpitations
  3. Severe headache
  4. Profuse diaphoresis
  5. Flushing
  6. Apprehension or a feeling of impending doom
  7. Pain in the chest or abdomen
  8. Nausea and vomiting
  9. Heat intolerance
  10. Weight loss
  11. Tremors
  12. Elevated vanillylmandelic acid and free catecholamines during a 24-hour urine collection
- Surgery is performed to remove the tumor and the affected adrenal glands.
- Preoperative care includes
  1. Identifying factors that contribute to hypertensive crisis; monitoring blood pressure
  2. Instructing the client not to smoke, drink caffeine-containing beverages, or change position suddenly
  3. Providing a diet rich in calories, vitamins, and minerals
  4. Ensuring adequate hydration
  5. Administering alpha-adrenergic blocking agents, as ordered, to decrease the risk of hypertension during surgery
  6. Providing a calm, restful environment

- Postoperative care includes
    1. Providing the same care as that for an adrenalectomy (see Hyperaldosteronism)
    2. Monitoring for hypotension and hypovolemia
    3. Monitoring for shock and hemorrhage
- If inoperable, the tumor is managed with alpha- and beta-adrenergic blocking agents.
- Clients who are managed medically must be instructed in the correct technique to monitor their own blood pressure.

Phlebitis

- Phlebitis is an inflammation of the superficial veins caused by an irritant, commonly intravenous therapy.
- Phlebitis is manifested as a reddened, warm area radiating up an extremity.
- The client may experience pain, soreness, and swelling of the extremity.
- Treatment involves application of warm, moist soaks, which dilate the vein and promote circulation.

Pneumonia

OVERVIEW

- Pneumonia is an excess of fluid in the lung resulting from an inflammatory process.
- It can be caused by infectious or noninfectious irritating agents such as inhaled fumes or aspirated food or fluids.
- Pneumonia is classified as community acquired or hospital acquired (nosocomial).
- Prevention is aimed at immunizing against the causative agents whenever possible and reducing the risks of exposure.

COLLABORATIVE MANAGEMENT

Assessment

- Record client information.
    1. Age
    2. Living and work or school environment
    3. Diet, exercise, and sleep routines
    4. Tobacco and alcohol use
    5. Medications: prescribed, over-the-counter, drug addiction, or intravenous drug use
    6. Chronic pulmonary illness
    7. Recent medical history (influenza, pneumonia, viral infections)
    8. History of rashes, insect bites, or exposure to animals
    9. Home respiratory equipment use and cleaning regimen
    10. Current symptoms
- Assess for
    1. General appearance
    2. Breathing pattern; use of accessory muscles
    3. Chest or pleuritic pain or discomfort
    4. Dyspnea, cyanosis
    5. Crackles, rhonchi, and wheezes on auscultation
    6. Bronchial breath sounds over areas of density or consolidation
    7. Character of cough
    8. Sputum production, including amount, color, and odor
    9. Fever, chills, headache
    10. Mental status changes (especially in the older adult)
    11. Gastrointestinal symptoms
    12. Fatigue anxiety
    13. Leukocytosis and hypoxia (especially in the older adult)
    14. Positive sputum culture
    15. Positive chest x-ray examination
    16. Hypotension and tachycardia
    17. Changes in arterial blood gases, pulse oximetry

Planning and Implementation

◆**NDx:** Impaired Gas Exchange and Ineffective Airway Clearance

- Monitor rate, rhythm, depth, and effort of respirations.
- Assess client's oxygen status and administer oxygen as indicated.
- Instruct the client on the correct use of incentive spirometry (sustained maximal inspiration) and encourage him or her to perform 5 to 10 breaths per session every hour while awake.
- Assess the client's ability to cough effectively.
- Encourage coughing and deep breathing.
- Monitor intake and output and ensure adequate hydration.
- Encourage the client to ambulate and get out of bed and into a chair, as tolerated.
- Perform nasotracheal suctioning if the client is unable to clear secretions.
- Administer aerosolized bronchodilators, such as beta$_2$ agonists, when bronchospasm is part of the disease process.
- Monitor for complications such as hypoxemia, ventilatory failure, atelectasis, pleural effusion, and pleurisy.

◆**NDx:** Potential for Sepsis

- Administer antibiotic therapy as determined by sputum analysis.
- Use steroids and nonsteroidal anti-inflammatory drugs in conjunction with antibiotics for the client with aspiration pneumonia.
- Septicemia may develop if the invading organism obtains access to the bloodstream.

Community-Based Care

- Provide health teaching.
    1. Stress the importance of avoiding upper respiratory infections by
        a. Avoiding crowds
        b. Avoiding persons who have a cold or influenza
    2. Recommend an annual influenza vaccine and the pneumococcal vaccine once every 5 years unless contraindicated.
    3. Stress the importance of completing medication regimen.
    4. Stress the importance of eating a balanced diet.

5. Instruct the client to notify the physician of chills, fever, dyspnea, hemoptysis, or increasing fatigue if symptoms fail to resolve.
6. Encourage the client to get plenty of rest and to gradually increase level of activity.
7. Encourage the client to quit smoking, as appropriate. Warn the client of the danger of myocardial infarction if smoking is continued while nicotine patches are in place.

Pneumothorax

- Pneumothorax is an accumulation of atmospheric air in the pleural space, resulting in a rise in intrathoracic pressure and reduced vital capacity.
- Assess for
  1. Reduced breath sounds
  2. Hyperresonance on percussion
  3. Prominence of the involved side of the chest, which moves poorly with respiration
  4. Pleuritic chest pain
  5. Tachypnea
  6. Subcutaneous emphysema
  7. Deviation of the trachea away from (closed) or toward (open) the affected side
- Interventions are aimed at rapid removal of trapped atmospheric air, including insertion of a large-bore needle and chest tubes to ensure lung inflation.

Pneumothorax, Tension

- Tension pneumothorax results from an air leak into the lung or chest wall.
- Air forced into the thoracic cavity causes complete collapse of the affected lung.

- Air entering the pleural space during expiration does not exit during inspiration; therefore the air accumulates under pressure, compressing blood vessels and limiting venous return, and decreasing cardiac output.
- Assess for
  1. Tracheal deviation to the unaffected side
  2. Respiratory distress
  3. Unilateral absence of breath sounds
  4. Distended neck veins
  5. Cyanosis
  6. Hypertympanic sound over the affected side
  7. Asymmetry of the thorax
- Initial treatment includes emergency insertion of a large-bore needle into the second intercostal space in the midclavicular line on the affected side to relieve pressure.
- Chest tube placement into the fourth intercostal space of the midaxillary line follows; underwater seal drainage is maintained until the lung is fully expanded.

Poliomyelitis

- Poliomyelitis (polio) is an acute viral disease characterized by destruction of the motor cells of the anterior horn of the spinal cord, the brainstem, and the motor strip of the frontal lobe.
- Polio is transmitted through droplet infection or by the fecal or oral route and the gastrointestinal tract.
- The disease is rare in North America because immunization during childhood is prevalent.
- Polio is characterized by fever, chills, excessive perspiration, severe muscle aches and weakness, increased deep tendon reflexes, abdominal tenderness, dysphagia, and irritability.
- Treatment is symptomatic.
- Analgesics are used to relieve pain, and respiratory status is monitored carefully.

Polyneuritis and Polyneuropathy

OVERVIEW

- Both inflammatory and noninflammatory processes can damage cranial and peripheral nerves.
- The terms *polyneuritis*, *polyneuropathy*, and *peripheral neuropathy* may be used interchangeably.
- The disorder is characterized by muscle weakness with or without atrophy, pain that is described as stabbing, cutting or searing, paresthesia or loss of sensation, impaired reflexes, autonomic manifestations, or a combination of these symptoms.
- The most common type of this disorder is a symmetric polyneuropathy in which the client experiences decreased sensation, along with a feeling that the extremity is asleep. Tingling, burning, tightness, or aching sensations usually start in the feet and progress to the level of the knee before being noted in the hands ("glove and stocking" neuropathy).
- Factors associated with polyneuropathy include diabetes; renal or hepatic failure; alcoholism; vascular disease; vitamin B_1, B_6, and B_{12} deficiency; and exposure to heavy metals or industrial solvents.

P

COLLABORATIVE MANAGEMENT

- Assess for
  1. Light touch sensation and pain in the distal extremities
  2. Position sense and kinesthetic sensation
  3. Sensitivity to vibration by placing a tuning fork on a bony prominence
  4. Any signs of injury
  5. Indications of autonomic dysfunctions, such as orthostatic hypotension, abnormal sweating, and miosis
- Treatment consists of removal or treatment of the underlying cause and symptomatic therapy.
  1. Treat the underlying cause.
  2. Supplement the client's diet with vitamins.
  3. Provide pain management as needed.

4. Provide health teaching, including the importance of foot care and inspecting the extremities for injuries.
5. Stress the importance of wearing shoes at all times and of purchasing well-fitting shoes.
6. Teach the client how to recognize potential hazards, such as exposure to extremes of environmental temperature.
7. Discourage smoking.
8. Establish a trusting nurse-client relationship.

Polyps, Cervical

- Cervical polyps are pedunculated (on stalks) tumors arising from the mucosa and extending to the cervical os.
- The polyps result from a hyperplastic condition of the endocervical epithelium or inflammation and are the most common neoplastic growth of the cervix.
- Clinical findings include
  1. Premenstrual or postmenstrual bleeding
  2. Postcoital bleeding
  3. Small, single, or multiple bright red polyps that are soft with fragile consistency and may bleed when touched
- Polyps are easily removed in the physician's office.
- Immediate postprocedural instructions include avoidance of
  1. Tampons
  2. Douching
  3. Sexual intercourse

Polyps, Gastrointestinal

- Gastrointestinal tract polyps are small growths covered with mucosa and attached to the intestinal surface; most are benign but have the potential to become malignant.
- Adenomas require medical consultation because of their malignant potential.

- Familial adenomatous polyposis (FAP) and hereditary nonpolyposis colorectal cancer (HNPCC) are inherited syndromes characterized by progressive development of colorectal adenomas. Left untreated, colorectal cancer will occur.
- Pedunculated polyps are stalklike, with a thin stem attaching them to the intestinal wall.
- Polyps are usually asymptomatic but can cause rectal bleeding, intestinal obstruction, and intussusception.
- Polyps can usually be removed by *polypectomy* with an electrocautery snare that fits through a colonoscope, eliminating the need for abdominal surgery.
- Postoperatively, monitor for
  1. Abdominal distention and pain
  2. Rectal bleeding
  3. Mucopurulent rectal drainage
  4. Fever
- Teach the client about the nature of the polyp, clinical manifestations to report to the health care provider, and the need for regular, routine monitoring.

Postpolio Syndrome

- Postpolio syndrome is a new onset of weakness, pain, and fatigue in persons who had poliomyelitis 30 or more years previously.
- Physical and emotional stressors are contributing factors.
- Treatment is symptomatic and includes lifestyle modifications to preserve energy and physiologic function.
- Adaptive and orthotic devices may be needed.

Premenstrual Syndrome

- Premenstrual syndrome (PMS) is a collection of symptoms that are cyclic in nature, occurring each month during the luteal phase of the menstrual cycle, followed by relief with menses and a symptom-free phase.
- The cause is not well understood, but many theories have been reported in the literature.
- Three elements are found in defining PMS: symptoms, severity level, and timing.
- Clinical manifestations are highly variable and include
  1. Behavioral manifestations
     a. Lowered work performance
     b. Appetite increase and food cravings
     c. Insomnia
     d. Alcohol and drug overindulgence
     e. Child abuse
     f. Assaultive behavior
  2. Emotional or psychological manifestations
     a. Anxiety
     b. Easily precipitated crying spells
     c. Depression
     d. Panic attacks
     e. Irritability, tension
     f. Change in libido
     g. Mood swings
  3. Dermatologic manifestations
     a. Acne
     b. Urticaria
     c. Herpes
  4. Metabolic manifestations
     a. Breast tenderness
     b. Edema
  5. Neurologic manifestations
     a. Headache, migraine
     b. Syncope, vertigo

    c. Numbness of hands and feet

    d. Short-term memory problems

    e. Difficulty concentrating

    f. Unclear thinking

    g. Epilepsy (if susceptible)

6. Respiratory manifestations

    a. Sinusitis

    b. Asthma

    c. Rhinitis

    d. Colds

7. Urologic manifestations

    a. Oliguria

    b. Cystitis

    c. Enuresis

    d. Urethritis

8. Other manifestations

    a. Allergies

    b. Hypoglycemia

    c. Joint pain

    d. Backache

    e. Palpitations

    f. Water retention

- Management is focused on eliminating uncomfortable symptoms and is highly individualized.

  1. Instruct the client to keep a menstrual chart for three consecutive menstrual cycles, showing the length of the menstrual cycle, duration of bleeding, and occurrence of symptoms

  2. Dietary measures may help, such as limiting sugar, red meat, alcohol, coffee, tea, chocolate, caffeine, and salt. Calcium, magnesium, and vitamins A, B_6, and C are used to relieve symptoms.

  3. Drug therapy, which is controversial, includes diuretics, progesterone therapy, bromocriptine mesylate (Parlodel), birth control pills, antidepressants, and nonsteroidal anti-inflammatory drugs.

  4. Provide education about PMS and its symptoms.

  5. Refer the client to self-help and support groups.

Prolapse, Mitral Valve

- Mitral valve prolapse occurs because the mitral valve leaflets enlarge and prolapse into the left atrium during systole.
- Mitral valve prolapse is usually benign but may progress to pronounced mitral regurgitation.
- Most client's are asymptomatic.
- A familial occurrence is well established; it is associated with Marfan syndrome and other congenital cardiac defects.
- Assess for
  1. Atypical chest pain; sharp pain localized in the left side of the chest
  2. Dizziness and syncope
  3. Palpitations
  4. Midsystolic click or a late systolic murmur that may be audible at the apex
- Valve replacement surgery is indicated only when pronounced mitral regurgitation follows.

Prolapse, Uterine

- Uterine prolapse is caused by congenital defects, persistent high intra-abdominal pressure related to heavy physical labor or exertion, or any cause that weakens pelvic support.
- Three grades are described, according to the degree of descent of the uterus.
  Grade I: The uterus bulges into the vagina, but the cervix does not protrude through the entrance to the vagina.
  Grade II: The uterus bulges further into the vagina, and the cervix protrudes through the entrance to the vagina.
  Grade III: The body of the uterus and cervix protrudes through the vaginal entrance; the vagina is turned inside out.
- Uterine prolapse physical findings include
  1. Client's report of "something in the vagina"
  2. Dyspareunia

3. Backache
4. Feeling of heaviness or pressure in the pelvis
5. Bowel or bladder problems, such as incontinence
6. Protrusion of the cervix during pelvic examination
- Interventions are based on the degree of prolapse.
   1. Insertion of a pessary
   2. Surgical vaginal hysterectomy

Prostatic Hyperplasia, Benign

OVERVIEW

- Glandular units in the prostate undergo tissue hyperplasia, resulting in benign prostatic hypertrophy (BPH).
- The enlarged prostate extends upward into the bladder and inward, narrowing the prostatic urethral channel.
- The prostate obstructs urine flow by encroaching on the bladder opening, resulting in a hyperirritable bladder and producing urgency and frequency, bladder wall hypertrophy, and hydronephrosis and hydroureter.
- Urinary retention or incomplete bladder emptying results in urinary tract infections.

P

 Considerations for Older Adults

- The development of BPH is a nearly universal condition in older men.

COLLABORATIVE MANAGEMENT

Assessment

- Record client information.
   1. Age
   2. Urinary pattern and symptoms (prostatism)
      a. Frequency
      b. Nocturia
      c. Hesitancy
      d. Intermittency
      e. Diminished force and caliber of stream

    f. Sensation of incomplete bladder emptying

    g. Postvoid dribbling (overflow incontinence)

    h. Hematuria

- Assess for
  1. Distended bladder
  2. A uniform, elastic, nontender prostate enlargement (NOTE: Cancer causes the prostate to become stone hard and nodular.)
  3. Laboratory findings, including possible urinary tract infection

Interventions

- Drug therapy includes
  1. Finasteride (Proscar), which may be used to shrink the prostate gland and improve urine flow
     a. Finasteride lowers dihydrotestosterone, a major cause of prostate growth.
     b. The major side effects are impotence and decreased libido, although they are uncommon.
  2. Alpha-blocking agents, such as terazosin (Hytrin), doxazosin (Cardura), and tamsulosin (Flomax)
- Prostatic fluid may be released by prostatic massage, regular intercourse, and masturbation.
- Teach the client to
  1. Avoid drinking large amounts of fluid in a short period
  2. Avoid alcohol and diuretics
  3. Void as soon as the urge is felt
  4. Avoid medications that increase urinary retention, such as anticholinergics, antihistamines, and decongestants

SURGICAL MANAGEMENT

- Surgery is performed for acute urinary retention, chronic urinary tract infections secondary to residual urine in the bladder, hematuria, hydronephrosis, and bladder neck obstruction symptoms such as urinary frequency and nocturia.
- The usual surgical interventions to treat BPH include
  1. *Transurethral resection of the prostate (TURP),* which involves the insertion of a resectoscope though the urethra and resection of the enlarged portion of the prostate. This is the safest procedure.

2. *Suprapubic* (or *transvesical*) *prostatectomy,* which involves a low abdominal incision to expose the bladder. The prostate gland is enucleated through the bladder cavity, and repair to the bladder is done, if required.

3. *Retropubic* (or *extravesical*) *prostatectomy,* which is accomplished by an abdominal incision above the symphysis pubis. A small incision is made into the prostate gland, and the gland is enucleated.

4. *Perineal prostatectomy,* which is used primarily to remove prostate glands filled with calculi, to treat prostatic abscesses, to repair complications, or to treat poor surgical risks. The surgeon makes a U-shaped incision between the ischial tuberosities, the scrotum, and the rectum; the prostatic capsule is opened and enucleated.

- Preoperative care includes
  1. Informing the client to expect an indwelling bladder catheter and possibly continuous bladder irrigation
  2. Informing the client to expect hematuria and blood clots
  3. Providing information about sexual functioning and continence

- Postoperative care includes
  1. Informing the client that he may feel the urge to void because of the large diameter of the three-way Foley catheter and the pressure of the balloon on the internal sphincter
  2. Instructing the client to try not to void around the catheter, which will cause the bladder to spasm
  3. Maintaining continuous bladder irrigation with normal saline solutions, as ordered
  4. Monitoring the color of the output and adjusting the rate of the irrigation accordingly to keep the urine clear
  5. Hand irrigating the catheter, as ordered, to remove obstructive blood clots
  6. Monitoring for frank bleeding, hyponatremia, and anemia
  7. Assessing the suprapubic catheter (in suprapubic prostatectomy), the catheter site, and the drainage system, if necessary
  8. After removal of the catheter, instructing the client to increase fluid intake
  9. Observing voided urine for clots, color, and consistency

10. Administering antispasmodics and analgesics, as ordered
11. Monitoring the dressing and drains (in open surgical procedures)
12. Avoiding rectal procedures (in perineal prostatectomy)

Considerations for Older Adults

- Even if the postoperative client becomes restless and confused, use of restraints should be avoided; familiar personal objects can be given to the client for distraction.
- The older adult who is susceptible to heart failure may not be able to tolerate large amounts of fluid.

Community-Based Care

- Inform the client that temporary loss of control of urination is normal and will improve.
- Provide the following discharge instructions for the client.
    1. Contract and relax the urinary sphincter frequently to re-establish urinary control (Kegel exercises).
    2. Increase water intake to keep urine flowing freely.
    3. Avoid strenuous activities to prevent injury.
    4. Notify the physician of persistent hematuria.
    5. Consume alcohol, soft drinks, and spicy foods in moderation to prevent irritation to remaining prostatic tissue and overstimulation of the bladder.
    6. Keep the area around the suprapubic catheter clean and report decreased drainage or redness at the catheter insertion site (in suprapubic prostatectomy).

Prostatitis

- Prostatitis is an inflammatory condition of the prostate.
- Abacterial prostatitis can occur after a viral illness or may be associated with sexually transmitted diseases.
- Bacterial prostatitis is usually associated with urethritis or an infection of the lower urinary tract.
- Common causative organisms include *Escherichia coli, Enterobacter, Proteus,* and group D streptococci.

- Bacterial prostatitis is manifested by
  1. Fever and chills
  2. Dysuria
  3. Urethral discharge
  4. Boggy, tender prostate
  5. Decreased sexual function
  6. Urinary tract infections
  7. White blood cells in the prostatic secretions
- *Chronic prostatitis* is manifested by
  1. Backache
  2. Perineal pain
  3. Mild dysuria
  4. Urinary frequency
  5. Hematuria (possible)
  6. An irregularly enlarged, firm, and lightly tender prostate
- Complications include epididymitis and cystitis.
- Treatment includes antimicrobials, such as carbenicillin indanyl sodium (Geocillin) or fluoroquinolones (ciprofloxacin), and comfort measures such as sitz baths, stool softeners, and analgesia.
- Health teaching includes measures that will drain the prostate, including intercourse, masturbation, and prostatic massage.
- Teach the client with chronic prostatitis the importance of increasing fluid intake and of long-term antibiotic therapy, such as trimethoprim (Protrin).

Pseudocysts, Pancreatic

- Pancreatic pseudocysts develop as a complication of acute or chronic pancreatitis.
- Of clients with pancreatitis, 10% to 20% experience pseudocysts, with a 10% mortality rate.
- These "false cysts" do not have an epithelial lining and are encapsulated saclike structures that form on or surround the pancreas.
- The pancreatic wall is inflamed, vascular, and fibrotic, containing large amounts of straw-colored or dark brown viscous fluid (enzyme exudate from the pancreas).

- The pseudocyst may be palpated as an epigastric mass in 50% of cases.
- The primary symptoms are epigastric pain radiating to the back, abdominal fullness, nausea, vomiting, and jaundice.
- Complications include hemorrhage; infection; obstruction of the bowel, biliary tract, or splenic vein; abscess or fistula formation; and pancreatic ascites.
- A pseudocyst may spontaneously resolve or may rupture and cause hemorrhage.
- Surgical intervention with internal drainage is accomplished by creating an ostomy between the pseudocyst and the stomach, jejunum, or duodenum; external drainage is provided by insertion of a sump drainage tube to remove pancreatic exudate and secretions.
- Pancreatic fistulas with skin breakdown are a common postoperative complication.

Psoriasis

OVERVIEW

- Psoriasis is a scaling skin disorder with underlying dermal inflammation characterized by exacerbations and remissions.
- Abnormal proliferation of epidermal cells in the outer skin areas results in cell shedding every 4 to 5 days.

COLLABORATIVE MANAGEMENT

Assessment

- Record client information.
  1. Precipitating factors, including skin trauma, upper respiratory tract infections, operation, past and current medications, and stress
  2. Family history of psoriasis
  3. Age at onset
  4. Description of progression and patterns of recurrences
  5. Gradual or sudden onset of episode
  6. Description of lesion location

7. Associated symptoms such as fever and pruritus
8. Previous treatment modalities
- *Psoriasis vulgaris* is the most common type of psoriasis and is characterized by
  1. Thick erythematous papules or plaques surmounted by silvery-white scales
  2. Sharply defined borders between lesions and normal skin distributed symmetrically, with the scalp, elbows, trunk, knees, sacrum, and extensor surfaces of the limbs commonly involved
  3. Associated nail involvement
- *Exfoliative psoriasis* (erythrodermic psoriasis) is characterized by generalized erythema and scaling without obvious lesions.

Interventions

- Topical therapy includes
  1. Topical steroids applied to skin lesions, followed by warm, moist dressings to increase absorption
  2. Tar preparations, which contain crude coal tar and derivations and are available in solution, ointment, lotion, gel, and shampoo
- Ultraviolet light therapy decreases epidermal growth rate.
- Systemic treatment with a cytotoxic agent is given for severe, debilitating psoriasis.
- Some systemic agents that induce immunosuppression are used when lesions do not respond to other therapies.
- The client's self-esteem often suffers because of the presence of skin lesions and the treatment modalities.
  1. Encourage the client to meet and talk with other people with psoriasis.
  2. Use touch to communicate acceptance of the client and the skin problem.
- Additional interventions include
  1. Identifying precipitating factors
  2. Explaining the rationale of the treatment plan and the importance of compliance
  3. Teaching the proper application and side effects of the therapeutic agents
  4. Emphasizing the control of symptoms by identifying precipitators and encouraging compliance with treatment

5. Emphasizing the importance of follow-up visits with the physicians

Ptosis

- Ptosis is the drooping of, or the inability to use, the upper eyelid.
- Causes of ptosis are
  1. Congenital, resulting from muscle dysfunction
  2. Mechanical, caused by abnormal weight of the eyelid from edema
  3. Inflammation, tumors, or injury to the third cranial nerve
- Treatment is palliative; surgery may be indicated if visual acuity or appearance is adversely affected.
- Nursing management after surgery consists of
  1. Assessing the eye for drainage and infection
  2. Applying cool compresses, ophthalmic antibiotic, or an antibiotic-steroid combination ointment
  3. Teaching the client
     a. The procedure to instill the ointment
     b. To keep the eye as clean as possible
     c. To avoid rubbing the eye

Pulmonary Disease, Occupational (OPD)

- OPD results from exposure to occupational or environmental fumes, dust, vapors, gases, bacterial or fungal antigens, and allergens.
- Consider an occupational cause for all clients with new-onset asthma or dyspnea.
- There are several occupational pulmonary diseases.
  1. *Occupational asthma (OA)* is divided into two types.
     a. *Latency (allergic) OA* is characterized by airflow limitation that develops after a period of exposure (a

few weeks to several years) and usually resolves when exposure ceases.

   b. *Irritant-induced OA* usually occurs within 24 hours of exposure to, most commonly, chlorine, ammonia, or phosgene. Exposure to massive concentrations can result in pulmonary edema, acute respiratory distress syndrome, and death. Symptoms include cough, wheeze, and dyspnea.

2. *Pneumoconiosis* refers to chronic respiratory diseases related to the inhalation of dust. Two types are

   a. *Silicosis,* a chronic fibrosing disease of the lungs caused by long-term inhalation of silica dust. Clinical manifestations include dyspnea on exertion, reduced lung volume, fatigue, weight loss; and upper lobe fibrosis.

   b. *Coal miner's pneumoconiosis,* also known as *black lung disease,* which results from deposits of coal dust in the lung. Initial symptoms are similar to bronchitis with eventual development of emphysema.

3. *Diffuse interstitial fibrosis* results in a restrictive problem interfering with alveolar gas exchange. The most common types are

   a. *Asbestosis,* characterized by diffuse pleural thickening and diaphragmatic calcification caused by exposure to asbestos. At risk are asbestos miners, building construction and remodeling workers, and shipyard workers.

   b. *Talcosis,* a fibrosis occurring after years of exposure to high concentrations of talc dust in the production of paints, ceramics, roofing materials, cosmetics, and rubber goods

   c. *Berylliosis,* which is caused by exposure to beryllium during processes in which metals are heated to fumes or machined creating dust

   d. *Extrinsic allergic alveolitis,* which causes a hypersensitivity pneumonitis as an immunologic response to inhaling dust or chemicals that contain bacterial or fungal antigens. It is characterized by the formation of granulomas with central necrosis in the alveoli and surrounding blood vessels.

■ Preventive measures include wearing special respirators and ensuring adequate ventilation.

- Refer to the section on asthma for nursing care of the client with occupational asthma.
- Refer to the section on emphysema for nursing care of the client with restrictive disease.
- Oxygen therapy is indicated for hypoxemic clients.
- Respiratory therapy to promote sputum clearance is essential.

Pyelonephritis

OVERVIEW

- Pyelonephritis is an infection of the renal pelvis and refers to the active presence of microorganisms or the effects remaining from previous infections within the kidney.
- Microorganisms enter the renal pelvis and activate the inflammatory response, which results in mobilization of white blood cells (WBCs) and local edema.
- The infection is generally classified as acute or chronic.
- Complications include renal abscess, perinephric abscess, emphysematous pyelonephritis, and septicemia.
- Pregnancy, diabetes mellitus, and chronic renal calculi increase the risk for pyelonephritis.
- Stones, obstruction, and neurogenic impairment involving the voiding mechanism often lead to chronic pyelonephritis.

COLLABORATIVE MANAGEMENT

Assessment

- Record client information.
  1. History of pyelonephritis
  2. History of urinary tract infections, especially if associated with pregnancy
  3. History of diabetes mellitus, stone disease, or other structural or functional abnormalities of the genitourinary tract
- Assess for
  1. Flank or abdominal discomfort
  2. Hematuria, cloudy urine
  3. General malaise
  4. Chills and fever

5. Asymmetry, edema, or erythema of the costovertebral angle
6. Anxiety, embarrassment, or guilt
7. Presence of WBCs and bacteria in the urine

Planning and Implementation

NDx: Acute Pain

- Drug therapy initially includes broad-spectrum antibiotics. With urine and blood culture sensitivity results, a specific antibiotic may be ordered.
- Encourage the client to eat a balanced diet and to drink 2 to 3 L of fluids per day.
- Surgical procedures include
  1. Pyelolithotomy, removal of a stone from the renal pelvis
  2. Nephrectomy, removal of a kidney
  3. Ureteral diversion or reimplantation of the ureter to restore the bladder drainage mechanism

COLLABORATIVE PROBLEM: Potential for Renal Failure

- Provide antibiotic therapy specifically for the causative organism.
- Control blood pressure to minimize the progression to renal failure.
- Encourage the client to drink at least 2 L of fluid each day unless contraindicated.
- Refer to the dietitian for diet counseling as necessary.
- Assess for signs of impending renal failure, such as decreased urinary output.

Community-Based Care

- Health teaching includes
  1. Medication administration
  2. Nutrition and fluid intake
  3. Balance between rest and activity
  4. Limitations after surgery
  5. Manifestations of disease reoccurrence, such as *functional* incontinence, which is leakage of urine caused by factors other than pathology of the lower urinary tract

Raynaud's Phenomenon and Raynaud's Disease

- Raynaud's phenomenon is caused by vasospasm of the arterioles and arteries of the upper and lower extremities.
- *Raynaud's phenomenon* usually occurs unilaterally in people of either sex who are older than 30 years of age.
- *Raynaud's disease* occurs in both men and women between 17 and 50 years of age, but is more common in females.
- Cutaneous vessels are constricted, causing blanching of the extremities, followed by cyanosis.
- When the vasospasm is relieved, the tissue becomes reddened or hyperemic.
- Assess for
  1. Color changes in the extremity or digits, ranging from blanched to reddened to cyanotic
  2. Numbness of the extremity or digits
  3. Coldness of the extremity or digits
  4. Pain
  5. Swelling
  6. Ulcerations
  7. Aggravation of symptoms by cold or stress
  8. Gangrene of digits in severe cases
- Interventions include
  1. Drug therapy to prevent vasoconstriction
  2. Lumbar sympathectomy to relieve symptoms in the feet
  3. Sympathetic ganglionectomy to relieve symptoms in the upper extremities
- Health teaching emphasizes methods to minimize vasoconstriction.
  1. Decreasing exposure to cold
  2. Decreasing stress
  3. Wearing warm clothes, socks, and gloves
  4. Keeping the home at a comfortable, warm temperature

Rectocele

- A rectocele is a protrusion of the rectum through a weakened vaginal wall.
- A rectocele may develop as a result of the pressure of a baby's head during a difficult delivery, a traumatic forceps delivery, or a congenital defect of the pelvic support tissues.
- Assess for
  1. Constipation
  2. Hemorrhoids
  3. Fecal impaction
  4. Feelings of vaginal or rectal fullness
  5. Bulge of the posterior vaginal wall during pelvic examination
- Management is focused on promoting bowel elimination through the use of
  1. High-fiber diet
  2. Stool softeners
  3. Laxatives
- The surgical intervention is a posterior colporrhaphy or posterior repair.
- Care is similar to that for rectal surgeries.
- If both a cystocele and a rectocele are repaired, the client has an anterior and posterior repair.

R

Refractive Errors

- Refractive errors result from problems in the ability of the eye to focus images on the retina.
- Types of refractive errors include
  1. *Myopia* (nearsightedness), a defect in which distant objects appear blurred
  2. *Hyperopia* (farsightedness), a defect in which close objects appear blurred
  3. *Presbyopia*, the inability of the lens to alter its shape to focus the eye for close work

4. *Astigmatism,* a refractive defect that prevents focusing of sharp, distinct images
- Treatment of refractive errors includes
  1. Eyeglasses
  2. Contact lenses (complications include corneal edema, corneal abrasions, and giant papillary cell conjunctivitis)
  3. Surgery
     a. *Radial keratotomy* treats mild to moderate myopia. Complications include overcorrection or undercorrection of the refractive error, corneal scars, and chronic dry eyes.
     b. *Photorefractive keratectomy* is an alternative for clients with mild to moderate stable myopia and low astigmatism. The eyes are treated one at a time, 3 months apart. Expected postoperative side effects include pain, hazy vision, light sensitivity, tearing, and pupil enlargement. Complications include difficulty with night vision, corneal clouding, undercorrection, farsightedness, increased intraocular pressure, and chronic dry eyes and glare.
     c. *Laser in-situ keratomileusis (LASIK)* corrects nearsightedness, farsightedness, and astigmatism using the excimer laser. Usually both eyes are treated at the same time. Most clients have improved functional vision within an hour of surgery. Compared with other surgical methods, LASIK is associated with less postoperative pain and fewer occurrences of complications (which include corneal clouding and chronic dry eyes).
     d. *Intacs corneal ring placement,* a reversible procedure, is the most recent vision-enhancing procedure for nearsightedness. Healing to best vision is immediate. Overcorrection or undercorrection of refraction is possible, but removal, readjustment, or replacement of the ring can be done.

Regurgitation, Aortic (Insufficiency)

- In *aortic regurgitation* (insufficiency), the aortic valve leaflets do not close properly during diastole, and the annulus may become dilated, loose, or deformed.
- Regurgitation of blood from the aorta into the left ventricle occurs during diastole; the left ventricle dilates to accommodate the greater blood volume and hypertrophies.
- Nonrheumatic causes include infective endocarditis, congenital anatomic aortic valvular abnormalities, hypertension, and Marfan syndrome, a generalized, systemic connective tissue disease.
- Clients with aortic insufficiency remain asymptomatic for many years because of the compensatory mechanisms of the left ventricle.
- Signs and symptoms include
  1. Palpitations (severe disease)
  2. Dyspnea on exertion
  3. Orthopnea
  4. Paroxysmal nocturnal dyspnea
  5. Nocturnal angina with diaphoresis
  6. Bounding arterial pulse
  7. Widened pulse pressure
  8. High-pitched, blowing, decrescendo diastolic murmur
- Nonsurgical therapy focuses on drug therapy and rest.
- Surgical treatment is performed after symptoms of left ventricular failure have developed but before irreversible dysfunction occurs.
- Aortic valve replacement surgery is the treatment of choice; the valve is excised during cardiopulmonary bypass surgery then replaced with a prosthetic (synthetic) or biologic (tissue) valve.
- The postoperative client requires lifetime anticoagulation therapy to prevent thrombus formation on the valve.
- For preoperative and postoperative care, see Surgical Management under Coronary Artery Disease.

R

Regurgitation, Mitral

- *Mitral regurgitation* (insufficiency) results from fibrotic and calcific changes that prevent the mitral valve from closing completely during systole, allowing backflow of blood into the left atrium when the left ventricle contracts.
- During diastole, regurgitant output again flows from the left atrium to the left ventricle along with normal blood flow, increasing the volume of blood to be ejected during the next systole.
- To compensate for the increased volume and pressure, the left atrium and ventricle dilate and hypertrophy.
- Rheumatic heart disease is the predominant factor, usually coexisting with mitral stenosis.
- Signs and symptoms include
  1. Fatigue and weakness
  2. Dyspnea on exertion
  3. Orthopnea
  4. Anxiety
  5. Atypical chest pains and palpitations
  6. Atrial fibrillation
  7. Neck vein distention
  8. Pitting edema
  9. High-pitched, systolic murmur
- Drug therapy is instituted to maintain normal cardiac output.
- The reparative surgical procedure is mitral annuloplasty, which is performed during cardiopulmonary bypass surgery. Mitral valve leaflets and annuli are reconstructed to narrow the valve orifice.
- The postoperative client requires lifetime anticoagulation therapy to prevent thrombus formation on the valve.
- For preoperative and postoperative care, see care of the client undergoing a coronary artery bypass grafting procedure under Coronary Artery Disease.
- Discharge planning includes
  1. Providing health teaching information regarding
     a. Medications
     b. Oral hygiene
     c. Plan of work, activity, and rest to conserve energy

d. The importance of antibiotics before any procedure (e.g., dental work, surgery)

2. Referring the client to community resources such as the American Heart Association

Renal Failure, Acute

- Acute renal failure (ARF) is the rapid decrease in renal function leading to the accumulation of metabolic wastes in the body.
- The three types of ARF are
  1. *Prerenal failure* (prerenal azotemia) from inadequate tissue perfusion
     a. This can be reversed by correcting blood volume, increasing blood pressure, and improving cardiac output.
     b. Prolonged hypoperfusion can lead to tubular necrosis and ARF.
  2. *Intrarenal/intrinsic ARF* from damage to the glomeruli, interstitial tissue, or tubules
     a. Synonyms include acute tubular necrosis (ATN) and lower nephron nephrosis.
     b. Causes include exposure to nephrotoxins, acute glomerulonephritis, vasculitis, and renal artery or vein stenosis.
  3. *Postrenal failure* from obstruction. Failure results from an obstruction of formed urine anywhere in the genitourinary tract.
- The following are the four phases of ARF:
  1. The *onset phase,* which lasts from hours to several days, begins with the precipitating event and continues until oliguria is observed. Clinical manifestations are rising blood urea nitrogen (BUN) and creatinine levels.
  2. During the *oliguric phase,* urine output is 100 to 400 mL/24 hours, usually lasting 8 to 15 days but possibly lasting several weeks, especially in older clients.
  3. The *diuretic phase* begins when the BUN level starts to fall and lasts until a normal level is reached. Normal renal

tubular function is re-established. Diuresis can result in an output of up to 10 L/day.

4. During the recovery/*convalescence phase,* the client returns to normal activities but functions at a lower energy level.

COLLABORATIVE MANAGEMENT

Assessment

- Record client information.
  1. Exposure to nephrotoxins
  2. Recent surgery or trauma
  3. Transfusions
  4. Drug history, especially treatment with antibiotics, angiotensin-converting enzyme inhibitors and nonsteroidal anti-inflammatory drugs
  5. History of contrast dye used with x-ray
  6. History of diabetes mellitus, systemic lupus erythematosus, and chronic malignant hypertension
  7. History of acute illnesses, including influenza, colds, gastroenteritis, and sore throat or pharyngitis
  8. History of intravascular volume depletion
  9. History of urinary obstructive disease
- Assess for prerenal azotemia
  1. Hypotension
  2. Tachycardia
  3. Decreased urine output
  4. Decreased cardiac output
  5. Decreased central venous pressure
  6. Lethargy
- Assess for intrarenal (intrinsic) ARF
  1. Genitourinary manifestations
     a. Decreased urinary output (oliguria)
     b. Absence of urine (anuria)
  2. Cardiovascular manifestations
     a. Tachycardia
     b. Hypertension
     c. Distended neck veins
     d. Elevated central venous pressure
     e. Peripheral edema
     f. Electrocardiogram changes

3. Respiratory manifestations
   a. Shortness of breath
   b. Pulmonary edema
   c. Friction rub
   d. Rales or crackles
4. Neurologic manifestations
   a. Lethargy
   b. Varying levels of consciousness
5. Gastrointestinal manifestations
   a. Nausea and vomiting
   b. Anorexia
   c. Flank pain
6. Other
   a. Electrolyte imbalance; changes in BUN and creatinine
- Assess for postrenal failure
  1. Oliguria
  2. Intermittent anuria
  3. Symptoms of uremia
  4. Lethargy

Interventions

- The client may move from the oliguric phase (fluids and electrolytes are retained) to the diuretic phase in which hypovolemia and electrolyte loss are the main problems.
- The client with ARF receives multiple medications.
  1. As kidney function changes, drug dosages are modified.
  2. Monitor for drug side effects and interactions.
- Fluid challenges and diuretics are commonly used to promote renal perfusion.
  1. Monitor for fluid overload.
- A low-dose dopamine infusion may be used to promote renal perfusion.
- Hypercatabolism results in the breakdown of muscle for protein, which leads to increased azotemia. Clients require increased calories. Total parenteral nutrition with intralipid infusion may be required to reduce catabolism.
- Indications for hemodialysis or peritoneal dialysis in clients with ARF are symptoms of uremia, persistent hyperkalemia, uncompensated metabolic acidosis, excess fluid volume, uremic pericarditis, and uremic encephalopathy. (See Renal Failure, Chronic, for a discussion of dialysis.)

R

ntinuous arteriovenous *hemofiltration* (CAVH), and continuous arteriovenous hemodialysis and filtration (CAVHD), alternatives to dialysis, may be used.

- CAVH is indicated for clients who are fluid volume overloaded, resistant to diuretics, and hemodynamically unstable.
- CAVHD uses a dialysate delivery system to remove nitrogenous or other waste products in clients with limited cardiac output or significant hypotension, or who do not respond to diuretic therapy.

Community-Based Care

- The needs of the client vary depending on the status of the disease on discharge. Refer to Community-Based Care under Renal Failure, Chronic.
- Follow-up care may include medical visits, laboratory tests, consultation with a dietitian, temporary dialysis, home nursing care, and social work assistance.

Renal Failure, Chronic

OVERVIEW

- Chronic renal failure (CRF) is a progressive, irreversible kidney injury; kidney function does not recover.
- The progression toward CRF occurs in three stages.
  Stage I: diminished renal reserve
    a. There is a reduction in renal functioning without accumulation of metabolic wastes.
    b. The unaffected kidney may compensate for the affected kidney.
  Stage II: renal insufficiency
    a. Metabolic wastes begin to accumulate in the blood because the unaffected nephrons no longer compensate.
    b. Levels of blood urea nitrogen (BUN), serum creatinine, uric acid, and phosphorus are elevated in proportion to the amount of nephrons lost.
  3. Stage III: end-stage renal disease (ESRD)
    a. ESRD occurs when excessive amounts of urea and creatinine accumulate in the blood.

    b. The kidneys are unable to maintain homeostasis and require dialysis.

- Pathologic alterations include disruptions in the glomerular filtration rate (GFR), abnormal urine production, poor water excretion, electrolyte imbalance, and metabolic anomalies.
- When less than 20% of nephrons are functional, hyposthenuria (loss of urine concentrating ability) and polyuria occur; left untreated severe dehydration occurs.
- *Urea* is the primary product of protein metabolism and is normally excreted by the kidney; BUN varies with dietary intake of protein.
- *Creatinine* is derived from creatine and phosphocreatine; the normal rate of excretion depends on muscle mass, physical activity, and diet.
- *Azotemia* is the increased accumulation of nitrogenous waste in the blood and is a classic indicator of renal failure.
- Variations in sodium excretion occur, depending on the stage of CRF.
- *Hyponatremia*, or sodium depletion, in early CRF is due to obligatory loss.
- Hyponatremia occurs because the reduced number of functional nephrons are insufficient to reabsorb sodium, thus sodium is lost in the urine.
- *Hyperkalemia* results from an increase in potassium load, including ingestion of potassium in medications, failure to restrict potassium in the diet, blood transfusions, and excess bleeding.
- Other pathologic occurrences include numerous metabolic disturbances such as changes in pH (metabolic acidosis), calcium (hypercalcemia) and phosphorus (hyperphosphatemia) imbalances, and vitamin D insufficiency.
- Renal osteodystrophy caused by hypocalcemia and phosphorus retention results in skeletal demineralization manifested by bone pain, pseudofractures, sclerosis of the spine, skull demineralization, osteomalacia, reabsorption of bone, and loss of tooth lamina.
- Cardiovascular alterations include anemia, hypertension, heart failure, and pericarditis.
- Gastrointestinal (GI) alterations include uremic stomatitis, anorexia, nausea, and vomiting.

COLLABORATIVE MANAGEMENT

Assessment

- Record client information.
  1. Age and gender
  2. Height and weight
  3. Current and past medical conditions
  4. Medications, prescription and nonprescription
  5. Family history of renal disease
  6. Dietary and nutritional habits
  7. Change in food tastes
  8. History of GI problems such as nausea, vomiting, anorexia, diarrhea, or constipation
  9. Current energy level
  10. Recent injuries and abnormal bruising or bleeding
  11. Weakness
  12. Shortness of breath
  13. Detailed urinary elimination history
- Assess for
  1. Cardiovascular abnormalities
     a. Hypertension
     b. Cardiomyopathy
     c. Uremic pericarditis
     d. Peripheral edema
     e. Congestive heart failure
     f. Pericardial friction rub or effusion
  2. Respiratory manifestations
     a. Breath that smells like urine (uremic fetor or halitosis)
     b. Deep sighing or yawning
     c. Tachypnea
     d. Pulmonary edema or pleural effusion
     e. Kussmaul's respiration
     f. Uremic lung or hilar pneumonitis
  3. Neurologic manifestations
     a. Lethargy or daytime drowsiness
     b. Insomnia
     c. Shortened attention span
     d. Paresthesia
     e. Slurred speech
     f. Muscle twitching, tremors, jerky movements

g. Seizures
h. Coma
4. GI disruptions
    a. Anorexia
    b. Nausea
    c. Vomiting
    d. Unpleasant or metallic taste
    e. Constipation
    f. Diarrhea
    g. Uremic gastritis (possible GI bleeding)
5. Genitourinary findings
    a. Change in urinary frequency
    b. Hematuria
    c. Change in urine appearance
    d. Proteinuria
6. Integumentary or dermatologic manifestations
    a. Pale, yellow skin
    b. Uremic frost (urea crystals on the face and eyebrows–rare)
    c. Severe itching (pruritus)
    d. Dry skin
    e. Purpura
    f. Ecchymoses
7. Hematologic findings
    a. Anemia
    b. Abnormal bleeding
8. Immunologic considerations: susceptibility to infections

Planning and Implementation

◆**NDx:** Imbalanced Nutrition: Less than Body Requirements

- Dietary principles are based on the regulation of protein intake; limitation of fluid intake; restriction of potassium, sodium, and phosphorus intake; administration of vitamin and mineral supplements; and providing adequate calories.
- The dietitian provides dietary teaching and planning, and assists the client in adapting the diet to food preferences, ethnic background, and budget.
- Monitor and restrict sodium intake.
- Monitor potassium intake and serum potassium levels.

- Monitor phosphorus levels in clients with renal failure to avoid osteodystrophy.
- Administer vitamin and mineral supplements, as ordered.

NDx: Excess Fluid Volume

- Interventions include
  1. Administering diuretics (diuretics are not given to clients with ESRD)
  2. Weighing the client daily on the same scale and at the same time
  3. Measuring and recording intake and output
  4. Maintaining fluid restriction, as ordered

NDx: Decreased Cardiac Output

- Interventions include
  1. Administering calcium channel blockers, angiotensin-converting enzyme (ACE) inhibitors, alpha- and beta-adrenergic blockers, and vasodilators
  2. Teaching the family to measure the client's blood pressure and weight daily and to bring these records when visiting the physician, nurse, or dietitian
  3. Monitoring the client for decreased cardiac output, heart failure, congestive heart failure, and dysrhythmias

NDx: Risk for Infection

- Interventions include notifying the physician of signs and symptoms of the effects of medications or drug toxicity.

NDx: Risk for Injury

- Interventions include
  1. Monitoring the client closely for drug-related complications
  2. Teaching the client to avoid certain medications that can increase renal damage
  3. Teaching the client to avoid medications that contain magnesium
  4. Administering cardiotonic drugs such as digoxin or digitoxin and monitoring the client for signs of toxicity, including nausea, vomiting, anorexia, visual disturbances, cardiac irregularities, and bradycardia

5. Administering agents to control phosphorus excess, such as calcium acetate, calcium carbonate, and aluminum hydroxide
6. Monitoring the client for hypercalcemia and hypophosphatemia
7. Instructing the client to avoid compounds containing magnesium
8. Administering opioid analgesics cautiously because the effects may last longer and uremic clients are sensitive to the respiratory depressant effects

◆NDx: Fatigue

- Vitamin and mineral supplements are given, and the anemic client receives recombinant erythropoietin.
  1. Monitor for hypertension.
  2. Monitor dietary intake; improved appetite challenges clients in their attempts to maintain protein, potassium, and fluid restriction.

◆NDx: Anxiety

- Interventions include
  1. Observing the client's behavior for signs of anxiety
  2. Evaluating the client's support system
  3. Explaining all procedures, tests, and treatments
  4. Providing instruction on ESRD appropriate to the client's needs and ability to understand
  5. Encouraging the client to discuss current problems, fears, or concerns and to ask questions
  6. Facilitating discussion with family members concerning the client's prognosis and potential impacts on the client's lifestyle

◆COLLABORATIVE PROBLEM:
Potential for Pulmonary Edema

- Assess for early signs of pulmonary edema such as restlessness, dyspnea, and crackles.
  1. Place the client in a high Fowler's position and give oxygen to maximize lung expansion and improve gas exchange.
  2. Insert Foley catheter.
  3. Measure and record intake and output.

4. Assess breath and heart sounds.
5. Monitor serum chemistry results for electrolyte imbalance.
6. Monitor pulse oximetry.
- Provide drug therapy.
  1. Loop diuretics; monitor for ototoxicity
  2. Morphine sulfate to reduce myocardial oxygen demands; monitor for respiratory depression
  3. Vasodilators such as nitroglycerin
- *Renal replacement therapy* is required when the clinical and laboratory manifestations of renal failure present complications that are potentially life-threatening or that pose continuing discomfort to the client.
- *Hemodialysis* removes excess fluid and waste products and restores chemical and electrolyte balance. It is based on the principle of diffusion, in which the client's blood is circulated through a semipermeable membrane that acts as an artificial kidney.
- Dialysis settings include acute care facility, free-standing centers, and the home.
- Total dialysis time is usually 12 hours per week, generally divided into three 4-hour treatments.
- Vascular access route is needed to perform hemodialysis.
- Long-term vascular access for hemodialysis is accomplished by
  1. Arteriovenous (AV) fistula
  2. AV graft
- Complications of vascular access include
  1. Thrombosis or stenosis
  2. Infection
  3. Ischemia
  4. High-output heart failure
  5. Aneurysm formation
- Temporary vascular access for hemodialysis is accomplished by an AV shunt or specially designed catheter inserted into the subclavian, internal jugular, or temporal vein.
- Nurses are specially trained to perform hemodialysis.
- Postdialysis care includes
  1. Closely monitoring for side effects
     a. Hypotension
     b. Headache
     c. Nausea

    d. Malaise

    e. Vomiting

    f. Dizziness

    g. Muscle cramps

  2. Obtaining the client's weight and vital signs

  3. Avoiding invasive procedures for 4 to 6 hours because of heparinization of the dialysate

  4. Monitoring for signs of bleeding

  5. Monitoring laboratory results

■ Complications of hemodialysis include

  1. Dialysis disequilibrium

  2. Infectious disease

  3. Hepatitis infection

  4. Human immunodeficiency virus (HIV) infection

 Considerations for Older Adults

♦ ESRD occurs most often in people 65 to 69 years of age.

♦ Clients older than 65 years of age receiving dialysis are more at risk than younger clients for dialysis-induced hypotension.

■ *Peritoneal dialysis* (PD), an alternative and slower dialysis method, is accomplished by the surgical insertion of a silicone rubber catheter (Tenckhoff catheter) into the abdominal cavity to instill dialysis solution into the abdominal cavity.

■ Candidates for PD include

  1. Clients who are hemodynamically unstable

  2. Clients who are unable to tolerate anticoagulation

  3. Clients who lack vascular access

  4. Pediatric or older adult clients

■ The PD process occurs by means of a transfer of fluid and solutes from the bloodstream through the peritoneum.

■ The types of PD are

  1. Intermittent

  2. Continuous ambulatory (CAPD)

  3. Continuous cycle

  4. Multiple bag-continuous

  5. Automated

■ Complications of PD include

  1. Peritonitis

  2. Pain

  3. Poor dialysate flow

4. Leakage of the dialysate
5. Exit site and tunnel infection
- Nursing interventions include
  1. Implementing and monitoring PD therapy and instilling, dwelling, and draining the solution, as ordered
  2. Maintaining PD flow data and monitoring for negative or positive fluid balances
  3. Obtaining baseline and daily weights
  4. Monitoring laboratory results to measure the effectiveness of the treatment
  5. Maintaining accurate intake and output records
  6. Taking vital signs every 15 to 30 minutes
  7. Performing an ongoing assessment for signs of respiratory distress or pain
- *Renal transplantation* is appropriate for select clients.
- Candidates for a kidney transplant are free from medical problems that could increase risk, such as
  1. Advanced uncorrectable cardiac disease
  2. Active infection
  3. Intravenous drug abuse
  4. Malignancies
  5. Severe obesity
  6. Active vasculitis
  7. Severe psychological problems
  8. Long-standing pulmonary disease
- Treatment of the following diseases must be completed before transplantation occurs.
  1. Gastrointestinal system disorders, peptic ulcer, diverticulitis
  2. Ureteral or bladder abnormalities
  3. Metabolic diseases such as diabetes mellitus, gout, or hyperparathyroidism
- Donor kidneys are obtained from a living related donor or a cadaver.
- After a suitable donor kidney is found, the client undergoes a *nephrectomy,* removal of the diseased kidney, with reimplantation of the donor organ.
- Postoperative care of the renal transplant recipient is similar to that for other abdominal surgeries.
  1. Monitor for the return of renal function by assessing hourly urine output.

2. Examine urine color; it is pink and bloody urine right after surgery and gradually returns to normal over several days to weeks.
3. Obtain daily urinalysis, glucose level, presence of acetone, specific gravity, and culture (if needed).
4. Monitor the client for oliguria.
   a. Administer diuretic and osmotic agents to increase urinary output.
   b. Weigh the client daily.
   c. Observe for fluid overload, which could lead to hypertension, heart failure, and pulmonary edema.
5. Monitor the client for diuresis.
   a. Observe for electrolyte imbalance, such as hypokalemia or hyponatremia.
   b. Hypotension episodes reduces blood flow and oxygen to the kidney.
6. Monitor the client for complications.
   a. Rejection
      (1) Hyperacute rejection occurs immediately after transplantation surgery.
      (2) Acute rejection occurs from 1 week to 2 years after surgery and is treated with increased doses of immunosuppressive drugs. It is manifested by oliguria or anuria, fever, enlarged tender kidney, fluid retention, increased blood pressure, chronic fatigue, and changes in urinalysis and blood chemistry.
      (3) Chronic rejection signs and symptoms include gradually increasing BUN and serum creatinine levels, fluid retention, and changes in serum electrolyte level.
   b. Acute tubular necrosis (ATN)
      (1) Delay of transplantation after the kidney has been harvested can result in ischemic damage to the kidney resulting in ATN.
      (2) Treat with dialysis until adequate urine output returns and BUN creatinine normalize.
   c. Vascular complications
      (1) Thrombosis of the renal artery
      (2) Vascular leakage or thrombosis

    d. Wound complications, such as hematomas, abscesses, and lymphoceles, which increase the risk for infection

    e. Genitourinary tract complications

        (1) Ureteral leakage, fistula, or obstruction

        (2) Formation of calculi

        (3) Bladder neck contracture

        (4) Graft rupture

7. Provide drug therapy

    a. Immunosuppressives

    b. Corticosteroids

    c. Antilymphocyte preparations

    d. Monoclonal antibodies

    e. Cyclosporine

Community-Based Care

- The case manager helps in planning, coordination, and evaluation of care.

  1. The physical and occupational therapist collaborates with the client and family to evaluate the home environment and to obtain needed equipment prior to discharge.

  2. Refer the client to home health nursing as needed.

- Provide in-depth health teaching about diet and pathophysiology of renal disease and drug therapy.

  1. Provide information and emotional support to assist the client with decisions about treatment course, personal lifestyle, support systems, and coping.

  2. Teach the client about the hemodialysis machine even if it is performed in an outpatient setting.

  3. Teach the client who selects in-home hemodialysis the principles and care of the vascular system and make referrals for the installation of the needed equipment at home.

  4. Provide extensive teaching in the procedures of PD and assist the client to obtain the needed equipment and supplies. Emphasize the importance of strict sterile technique and of reporting manifestations of peritonitis, especially cloud effluent and abdominal pain.

  5. Provide renal transplant clients with detailed instructions about the prescribed immunosuppressive drug therapy.

  6. Assist the client and family to adjust to the diagnosis and treatment regimen.

7. Instruct clients and family members in all aspects of diet therapy, drug therapy, and complications.

8. Teach clients and family members to report complications, such as fluid overload and infection.

9. Stress that although uremic symptoms are reduced as a result of dialysis procedures, the client will not return completely to his or her previous state of well-being.

10. Instruct the family to monitor the client for any behaviors that may contribute to nonadherence to the treatment plan and to report such to the health care provider.

11. Refer the client to a home health nurse and to local and state support groups and agencies.

Respiratory Failure, Acute (ARF)

OVERVIEW

- ARF is classified by blood gas abnormalities with pH less than 7.30, PaO_2 less than 60 mm Hg, SaO_2 less than 90%, or $PaCO_2$ greater than 50 mm Hg.
- Acute respiratory failure can be classified three ways.
  1. *Ventilatory failure* is a ventilation-perfusion mismatch in which perfusion is normal but ventilation is inadequate usually as a result of a mechanical abnormality of the lungs or chest wall, a defect in the respiratory control center of the brain, or impaired ventilatory muscle function, especially the diaphragm. The $PaCO_2$ level is above 45 mm Hg.
  2. *Oxygenation failure* occurs when oxygen is able to reach the alveoli, but is unable to be absorbed or used properly. Causes include impaired diffusion at the alveolar level, right-to-left shunting of blood in the pulmonary vessels, ventilation-perfusion mismatching, breathing air with too low a concentration of oxygen, or abnormal hemoglobin that fails to absorb the oxygen.
  3. *Combined* ventilatory and oxygenation failure involves poor respiratory movements (hypoventilation). The bronchioles and alveoli are diseased, causing oxygen failure

and the work of breathing increases until the respiratory muscles are unable to function effectively, causing ventilatory failure.

COLLABORATIVE MANAGEMENT

Assessment

- Assess for
  1. Dyspnea, the hallmark of respiratory failure
  2. Orthopnea
  3. Change in respiratory rate, pattern, breath sounds
  4. Signs and symptoms of hypoxemia and hypercapnia
  5. Decreased oxygen saturation on pulse oximetry
  6. Abnormal arterial blood gases

Interventions

- Treatment for acute respiratory failure includes
  1. Oxygen therapy to keep the partial pressure of arterial oxygen above 60 mm Hg
  2. Mechanical ventilation, if needed
  3. Assisting the client in finding a position of comfort for easier breathing
  4. Assisting the client with relaxation and diversion techniques to decrease the anxiety typically associated with dyspnea
  5. Energy conservation measures such as minimal self-care and no unnecessary procedures
  6. Pulmonary medications given systemically or by inhaler for bronchodilation
  7. Encouraging deep breathing and other breathing exercises

Restless Leg Syndrome

OVERVIEW

- Restless leg syndrome (RLS) is characterized by leg paresthesia associated with an irresistible urge to move.
- It is associated with peripheral and central nerve damage in the legs and spinal cord.

- RLS is characterized by intense burning or "crawling type" sensations in the limbs and subsequently the client feels the need to move the limbs repeatedly.
- Symptoms are worse in the evening and at night.
- Treatment is symptomatic.
    1. Treat the underlying cause or contributing factor, if known.
    2. Collaborate with the client to develop strategies to minimize insomnia such as limiting caffeine, nicotine, and alcohol; setting a routine bedtime; limiting strenuous exercise 3 hours before bedtime.
    3. Biofeedback, massage, and acupuncture may be effective.
    4. Medications include clonidine hydrochloride (Catapres, Dixarit) and carbamazepine (Tegretol, Mazepine).
    5. Refer the client to the Restless Legs Foundation.

Retinal Holes, Tears, and Detachments

OVERVIEW

- A *retinal hole* is a break in the integrity of the peripheral sensory retina and is frequently associated with trauma and aging.
- A *retinal tear* is a more jagged and irregularly shaped break in the retina that occurs as a result of traction on the retina.
- *Retinal detachment* is the separation of the sensory retina from the pigmented epithelium.
- *Rhegmatogenous detachments* occur after the development of a hole or tear in the retina creates an opening for the vitreous to filter into the subretinal space.
- *Traction detachments* are created when the retina is pulled away from the epithelium by bands of fibrous tissue in the vitreous humor.
- *Exudative detachments* are caused by fluid accumulation in the subretinal space as a result of an inflammatory process.

COLLABORATIVE MANAGEMENT

- Indirect ophthalmoscopic examination reveals gray bulges or folds in the retina that quiver with movement; a hole or tear may be seen.
- Repair of *retinal holes* or *tears* is done by surgery.
- Treatment of *retinal holes* or *tears*, which is directed toward sealing the break by creating an inflammatory response that will bind the retina and choroid together around the break, includes
  1. Cryotherapy
  2. Photocoagulation
  3. Diathermy
- For repair of *retinal detachments,* the treatment is directed toward placing the retina in contact with the underlying structures. The scleral buckling procedure is most often performed. During the scleral buckling procedure, the ophthalmologist repairs wrinkles or folds in the retina so that the retina can assume its normal smooth position.
- Preoperative care for retinal detachments includes
  1. Providing routine preoperative care
  2. Restricting activity
  3. Placing an eye patch over the affected eye to reduce eye movement
  4. Administering topical medications to inhibit accommodation and constriction
- Postoperative care for retinal detachments includes
  1. Providing routine postoperative care
  2. Reporting any drainage to the physician immediately
  3. Not removing the initial eye patch and shield without a specific order
  4. Positioning the client to allow gas that may have been used to promote reattachment to float against the retina
     a. The client lies on the abdomen with the head turned so that the unaffected eye is down.

    b. The client sits on the side of the bed with the head on a bedside stand.

5. Withholding food and fluids until the client is fully awake and nausea has passed. Antiemetics may be given.

6. Administering analgesics for pain. Sudden increase in pain or pain accompanied by nausea is reported to the ophthalmologist.

7. Instructing the client to avoid activities that will increase intraocular pressure, such as sneezing, straining at stool, and bending over from the waist

8. Teaching the client about activity restrictions, including avoidance of reading, writing, and performing close work such as needlepoint

9. Teaching the client about the signs and symptoms of infection and detachment

Rotator Cuff Injuries

- The function of the rotator cuff is to stabilize the head of the humerus in the glenoid cavity during shoulder abduction.
- The rotator cuff undergoes degenerative changes as one ages.
- Older adults tend to have small tears related to aging, repetitive motions, or falls.
- Younger adults usually sustain tears of the cuff by trauma, including falling, throwing a ball, or lifting heavy objects.
- Clinical manifestations include shoulder pain and the inability to initiate or maintain abduction of the arm at the shoulder.
- Treatment involves nonsteroidal anti-inflammatory drugs, physical therapy, sling support, and ice and heat applications.
- Surgery may be required to treat injuries that do not respond to conservative treatment.

R

Sarcoidosis, Pulmonary

- Pulmonary sarcoidosis is a granulomatous disorder of unknown cause that can affect any organ, particularly the lungs.
- The hallmark of sarcoidosis is an autoimmune response in which T-lymphocytes increase and initiate damaging actions in lung tissue.
- Interstitial fibrosis results in a loss of both lung compliance and the ability to exchange gases.
- Cor pulmonale (right-sided heart failure) develops because of the inability of the heart to pump effectively against the stiff, fibrotic lung.
- Clinical manifestations include enlarged lymph nodes in the hilar area of the lungs, cough, dyspnea, lung infiltrates seen on x-ray, skin and eye lesions, hemoptysis, and chest discomfort.
- Indications for treatment vary.
  1. If the client is asymptomatic, with normal pulmonary function tests, there is no treatment.
  2. For reduced pulmonary function, steroids are administered.

Scabies

- Scabies is a contagious skin disease characterized by epidermal curved or linear ridges and follicular papules associated with severe pruritus.
- Hypersensitivity reactions result in excoriated erythematous papules, pustules, and crusted lesions on the palms, wrists, elbows, nipples, lower abdomen, buttocks, thighs, and axillary folds.
- Scabies are transmitted by close and prolonged contact with an infested companion or bedding.
- Scabies mites are carried by pets and occur endemically among schoolchildren, institutionalized older clients, and clients of lower socioeconomic status.

- Treatment consists of chemical disinfection with scabicides such as lindane (Kwell, Hexit ♣) or topical sulfur preparations.
- Clothes and personal items are laundered in hot water.

Sclerosis, Multiple

OVERVIEW

- Multiple sclerosis (MS) is a chronic autoimmune disease that affects the myelin sheath and conduction pathway of the central nervous system.
- MS is one of the leading causes of disability in persons 20 to 40 years of age.
- The major types of MS are
  1. *Relapsing-remitting*, which is characterized by increasingly frequent attacks. Relapses develop over 1 to 2 weeks and resolve over 4 to 8 months, after which the client returns to baseline.
  3. *Progressive-relapsing*, which is characterized by the absence of remission. The client's condition does not return to baseline.
  4. *Primary-progressive*, which involves a steady and gradual neurologic deterioration. There is no remission of symptoms.
  5. *Secondary-progressive*, which begins with a relapsing-remitting course that later becomes steadily progressive. Attacks and partial recoveries may continue to occur.

COLLABORATIVE MANAGEMENT

Assessment

- MS often mimics other neurologic diseases, which makes the diagnosis difficult and prolonged.
- Assess for
  1. Progression of symptoms (Often the client reports having noticed symptoms several years earlier but symptoms disappeared and medical attention was not sought.)

2. Factors that aggravate symptoms
   a. Stress
   b. Fatigue
   c. Overexertion
   d. Temperature extremes
   e. Hot shower or bath
3. Motor function
   a. Fatigue
   b. Stiffness of legs
   c. Flexor spasms
   d. Increased deep tendon reflexes
   e. Clonus
   f. Positive Babinski's reflex
   g. Absent abdominal reflexes
4. Cerebellar function
   a. Ataxic gait
   b. Intention tremor
   c. Dysmetria
   d. Clumsy motor movements
5. Cranial nerve function
   a. Hearing loss
   b. Facial weakness
   c. Swallowing difficulties
   d. Tinnitus
   e. Vertigo
6. Vision
   a. Decreased visual acuity
   b. Blurred vision
   c. Diplopia
   d. Scotoma (changes in peripheral vision)
   e. Nystagmus
7. Sensation
   a. Hypalgesia
   b. Paresthesia
   c. Facial pain
   d. Change in bowel and bladder function
   e. Impotence, difficulty sustaining an erection
   f. Decreased vaginal secretion
8. Cognitive changes seen late in the course of the disease
   a. Memory loss
   b. Decreased ability to perform calculations

        c. Inattention
        d. Impaired judgment
    9. Psychosocial function
        a. Apathy, emotional lability, and depression
        b. Disturbed body image

Interventions

- As a result of weakness and fatigue, the client requires more time to complete activities of daily living (ADLs).
- Collaborate with physical and occupational therapists to teach the client regarding the following:
    1. An exercise program to strengthen and stretch muscles
    2. How to ambulate, as tolerated, with assistive devices as appropriate, such as a cane, walker, or electric (Amigo) cart
    3. How to use assistive-adaptive devices to remain independent in ADLs
    4. The importance of avoiding rigorous activities that lead to an increase in body temperature, which may lead to fatigue, decreased motor ability, and decreased visual acuity
- Drug therapy includes
    1. Steroid therapy
    2. Adjunctive therapy to treat muscle spasticity and paresthesia
    3. Immunosuppressive therapy
    4. Biologic response modifiers
    5. Adjunctive therapy for paresthesia, bladder dysfunction, pain
- Other interventions include
    1. Managing cognitive problems in the areas of attention, memory, problem solving, visual perception, and use of speech
    2. Applying an eye patch to relieve diplopia and switching the eye patch every few hours
    3. Teaching scanning techniques to compensate for peripheral vision deficits
    4. Testing the temperature of the water before bathing (teach the client to do this at home before placing hands in hot water)
    5. Referring the client to a therapist or nurse educated in issues surrounding sexuality

- Clients using complementary therapies, such as nutritional supplements and bee stings, report improvement in their condition, but these modalities have not been scientifically tested.

Community-Based Care

- Home care management includes
  1. Explaining the development of MS and the factors that may exacerbate the symptoms
  2. Stressing the importance of avoiding overexertion, stress, extremes of temperatures (fever, hot baths, overheating, excessive chilling), humidity, and people with upper respiratory tract infections
  3. Providing drug information, as needed
  4. Encouraging the client to follow the exercise program developed by the physical therapist and to remain independent in all activities for as long as possible
  5. Encouraging the client to engage in regular social activities, obtain adequate rest, and avoid stress
  6. Teaching the family strategies to cope with personality changes
  7. Reviewing the established bowel and bladder, skin care, and nutrition program
  8. Referring the client to local and national support groups, as needed

Sclerosis, Progressive Systemic

OVERVIEW

- Progressive systemic sclerosis (PSS), also referred to as *systemic scleroderma*, is a chronic connective tissue disease characterized by inflammation, fibrosis, and sclerosis of skin and vital organs. It is similar to lupus erythematosus.

COLLABORATIVE MANAGEMENT

Assessment

- PSS is manifested by arthralgia; stiffness; painless, symmetric, pitting edema of the hands and fingers, which may progress to include the entire upper or lower extremities and face; and taut and shiny skin that is free from wrinkles.
- In PSS, inflammation is replaced by tightening, hardening, and thickening of skin tissue. The skin loses its elasticity, and range of motion is markedly decreased.
- Joint contractures may develop, and the client is unable to perform activities of daily living (ADLs).
- Major organ involvement is manifested in
  1. Gastrointestinal tract: hiatal hernia, esophageal reflux, dysphagia, reflux of gastric contents that can cause esophagitis, partial bowel obstruction, and malabsorption
  2. Cardiovascular system: Raynaud's phenomenon, digit necrosis, vasculitis, myocardial fibrosis, dysrhythmias, and chest pain
  3. Respiratory system: fibrosis of the alveoli and interstitial tissue, pulmonary hypertension

Interventions

- Treatment of PSS is directed toward forcing the disease into remission and slowing its progress.
  1. Administer drugs such as steroids and immunosuppressants in large doses. Give nonsteroidal anti-inflammatory drugs for joint inflammation and pain.
  2. Protect the client's skin by using mild soap, lotion, and gentle cleaning procedures.
  3. Inspect the skin daily for further changes or open lesions.
  4. Provide a bed cradle and footboard.
  5. Maintain a constant room temperature.
  6. Provide small, frequent meals, minimizing foods that stimulate gastric secretion (e.g., spicy foods, caffeine, alcohol), and have the client sit up for 1 to 2 hours after meals (if there is esophageal involvement).
  7. Joint protection and energy conservation measures are important.
- Refer to Arthritis, Rheumatoid, for care of joint pain.

- Health teaching and discharge planning are similar to those for the client with lupus (see Lupus Erythematosus).

Seizure Disorders

OVERVIEW

- A seizure is an abnormal, sudden, excessive uncontrolled electrical discharge of neurons within the brain that may result in alteration in consciousness, motor or sensory ability, or behavior.
- Epilepsy is a chronic disorder characterized by recurrent seizure activity.
- Three major categories of epilepsy are
  1. *Generalized* seizure
     a. *Tonic-clonic* seizure (formerly called a grand mal seizure) is characterized by stiffening or rigidity of the muscles, followed by rhythmic jerking of the extremities. Immediate unconsciousness occurs, and the client may be incontinent of urine or feces and may bite his or her tongue.
     b. *Tonic* seizures are characterized by an abrupt increase in muscle tone, loss of consciousness, and loss of autonomic signs lasting from 30 seconds to several minutes.
     c. *Clonic* seizures last several minutes and are characterized by muscle contraction and relaxation.
     d. *Absence* seizure (formerly called petit mal seizure) consists of a brief (often seconds) period of loss of consciousness and blank staring, as though the client is daydreaming.
     e. *Myoclonic* seizure is a brief, generalized jerking or stiffening of the extremities, which may occur singly or in groups.
     f. *Atonic* seizures (formerly called "drop attacks") are characterized by sudden loss of muscle tone, which in most cases causes the client to fall.

2. Partial (focal) seizure
   a. *Complex* seizure (often called a *psychomotor* seizure or a *temporal lobe* seizure) causes the client to lose consciousness or black out for 1 to 3 minutes. Characteristic behavior, known as automatism, may occur, such as lip smacking, patting, and picking at clothes.
   b. *Simple* seizure consists of an aura or unusual sensation (déjà vu phenomenon, perception of an offensive smell, or sudden onset of pain) before the seizure takes place. It may be followed by unilateral movement of an extremity, or autonomic or psychic symptoms. Simple seizures do not fit into the generalized or partial classification.
3. *Unclassified* or *idiopathic* seizures occur for no known reason.

■ *Primary* seizures are not associated with any identifiable brain lesions, are usually inherited, and are often age related.
■ *Secondary* seizures often result from underlying brain pathology such as a head injury, vascular disease, brain tumor, aneurysm, opportunistic infections from acquired immunodeficiency syndrome (AIDS), or meningitis. They may also occur in the presence of metabolic and electrolyte disorders, drug withdrawal, acute alcohol intoxication, water intoxication, or kidney and liver failure. Seizures resulting from these disorders are not considered epilepsy.

COLLABORATIVE MANAGEMENT

Assessment

■ Record client information.
1. Complete description of seizure activity that occurs and events surrounding the seizure
2. Current medications, including dosage, frequency of administration, and the time at which the medication was last taken
3. Compliance with the medication schedule and reasons for noncompliance, if appropriate

Interventions

- Care of the client during a tonic-clonic or complete partial seizure includes the following:
  1. Protect from injury.
  2. Do not force anything into the client's mouth.
  3. Turn the client to the side.
  4. Loosen any restrictive clothing.
  5. Maintain the airway and suction as needed.
  6. Do not restrain the client; rather, guide the client's movements.
  7. At the completion of the seizure
     a. Take vital signs.
     b. Perform neurologic checks.
     c. Allow the client to rest.
     d. Document the seizure.
- Nursing observations and documentation of a seizure include
  1. How often the seizures occur; date, time, and duration of the seizures
  2. The type of movement or activity and if more than one type occurs
  3. Sequence of progression
     a. Where the seizure began
     b. Body parts first involved
  4. Observations during the seizure
     a. Changes in pupil size and any eye deviation
     b. Level of consciousness
     c. Presence of apnea, cyanosis, and salivation
     d. Incontinence of bowel or bladder
     e. Eye fluttering
     f. Movement and progression of motor activity
     g. Lip smacking or other automatism
     h. Tongue or lip biting
  5. How long the seizure lasted
  6. Presence and description of aura or precipitating events
  7. Postictal status
  8. Length of time before the client returns to preseizure status
- Drug therapy is the major component of management; the health care provider introduces one anticonvulsant at a time to achieve seizure control.

- Serum drug levels are monitored for the first 3 days after the start of anticonvulsants and thereafter as needed.
- Follow agency policy for the implementation of seizure precautions.
  1. Keep oxygen, suctioning equipment, and an airway available at the bedside.
  2. Maintain a saline lock that may be indicated for clients at risk for tonic-clonic seizures.
  3. Padded tongue blades do *not* belong at the bedside; nothing should be inserted into the client's mouth after a seizure begins.
  4. Use of padded siderails is controversial; siderails are rarely the source of significant injury and the use of padded siderails may embarrass the client and family.
  5. Keep the bed in the low position and siderails up at all times.
- *Status epilepticus* is a seizure that lasts longer than 10 minutes or repeated seizures over the course of 30 minutes. It is a neurologic *emergency* and must be treated promptly or brain damage and possibly death from anoxia, cardiac dysrhythmias, or lactic acidosis may occur. Status epilepticus is usually caused by
  1. Sudden withdrawal from anticonvulsant medications
  2. Acute alcohol withdrawal
  3. Head trauma
  4. Cerebral edema
  5. Metabolic disturbances
- Convulsive status epilepticus is a neurologic emergency and must be treated promptly and aggressively. Notify the health care provider immediately.
- Immediate treatment of status epilepticus includes
  1. Establishing an airway (intubation may be necessary)
  2. Monitoring the client's respiratory status carefully
  3. Administering oxygen
  4. Establishing an intravenous (IV) line and starting 0.9% saline infusion
  5. Drawing blood for arterial blood gas analysis and identifying metabolic, toxic, and other causes of uncontrolled seizures
  6. Administering medications such as IV diazepam (Valium) or lorazepam (Ativan, Apo-Lorazepam ✿) to stop motor

S

movement, followed by phenytoin (Dilantin) or fosphenytoin (Cerebyx) to prevent recurrence. General anesthesia may be used as a last resort to stop the seizure activity.

7. Monitoring vital signs frequently

SURGICAL MANAGEMENT

- Several procedures may be performed when traditional methods fail to maintain seizure control.
  1. *Vagal nerve stimulation* involves surgically implanting a vagal nerve–stimulating device below the left clavicle to control partial seizures.
  2. *Corpuscallostomy* which involves severing the corpus callosum to prevent neuronal discharges from passing through the two hemispheres of the brain. It is used to treat tonic-clonic or atonic seizures.
  3. Other procedures, including *anterior temporal lobe resection* for complex partial seizures of temporal origin, *cortical resection,* and *hemispherectomy,* are procedures in which part or all of a cerebral hemisphere is removed.

Discharge Planning and Health Promotion

- Most clients are treated on an outpatient basis, and little home care preparation is needed.
- Health teaching includes
  1. The importance of taking all medications in the correct dosage, at the right time, by the right route, and not stopping the medications
  2. What to do if a dose is missed or if complications or side effects occur
  3. Precautions to take when ill, under stress, fatigued, or when workload or social activities increase
  4. The importance of not taking any herbal remedies or over-the-counter drugs without notifying the health care provider
  5. Components of a balanced diet and the effects of alcohol (alcohol should be avoided)
  6. The importance of proper rest and stress reduction techniques

7. The importance of keeping a seizure diary to determine whether there are factors that tend to be associated with seizure activity
8. Restrictions, if any, such as driving or operating dangerous equipment and participating in certain physical activities or sports
9. The importance of follow-up visits with physicians
10. The need to wear a medical alert bracelet or necklace

- Inform the client that state laws prohibit discrimination against people who have epilepsy.
- Refer the client to the Epilepsy Foundation of America, National Epilepsy League, or National Association to Control Epilepsy and to local support groups.

Severe Acute Respiratory Syndrome (SARS)

- SARS is an atypical pneumonia caused by a mutated form of the coronavirus and is more virulent than most members of this virus family. The virus infects cells of the respiratory tract, triggering an inflammatory response.
- SARS is easily spread by airborne droplets from infected people through sneezing, coughing, and talking.

S

COLLABORATIVE MANAGEMENT

Assessment

- Clinical manifestations include
  1. Those similar to any respiratory infection
  2. Temperature higher than 100.4° F (38° C)
  3. Runny nose, sore throat, watery eyes
  4. Dry cough
  5. Difficulty breathing
  6. Hypoxia, cyanosis
- Chest x-ray shows a pattern similar to pneumonia or other respiratory distress syndromes.

- Diagnosis is made by documenting manifestations and ruling out other causes.
- Twenty-eight days after infection starts, a blood test for antibodies for the virus or pieces of RNA can confirm the diagnosis.

Interventions

- Use airborne and contact precautions.
- Keep door to client's room closed.
- Adhere to strict handwashing to prevent spread of infection.
- Provide supportive care to allow the client's immune system to fight the infection.
- Give oxygen for hypoxia or dyspnea.
- Provide respiratory treatment to dilate the bronchioles and move respiratory secretions.
- Intubation and mechanical ventilation may be needed.
- Antibiotics and antiviral drugs are not able to kill the virus or prevent its replication.
- Antibiotics are used to treat a bacterial pneumonia that may occur with SARS.

Shock

OVERVIEW

- Shock, the whole-body response to poor tissue perfusion, is a condition rather than a disease process.
- Shock is characterized by generalized abnormal cellular metabolism, which occurs as a direct result of inadequate delivery of oxygen to body tissues or inadequate usage of oxygen by body tissue.
- Stages of uncorrected shock
  1. Initial stage (early shock) occurs when the client's baseline mean arterial pressure (MAP) is decreased less than 10 mm Hg and compensatory mechanisms are effective.
  2. Nonprogressive stage (compensatory stage) occurs when MAP decreases 10 to 15 mm Hg from baseline. Kidney and hormonal mechanisms are activated because cardiovascular

compensation alone is not enough to maintain MAP and supply oxygen to the vital organs.

3. Progressive stage (intermediate) occurs when there is a sustained decrease in MAP of more than 20 mm Hg. Compensatory mechanisms are functioning but no longer deliver sufficient oxygen, even to vital organs.

4. Refractory stage (irreversible) occurs when too much cell death and tissue damage results from too little oxygen reaching the tissue.

- Shock is classified into four types. *More than one type of shock can be present at the same time.*

    1. Hypovolemic shock

        a. Too little circulating blood volume causes a decrease in mean arterial pressure (MAP) so that the body's total need for oxygenation is not met.

        b. Causes include hemorrhage, dehydration, any problem that reduces the levels of clotting factors, and fluid shifts that may occur in trauma, burns, or anaphylaxis.

    2. Cardiogenic shock

        a. The heart muscle is unhealthy and pumping is directly impaired, causing decreased cardiac output and afterload, thus reducing MAP.

        b. Causes include inadequate cardiac output.

            (1) *Direct pump failure* can result from myocardial infarction (MI), cardiac arrest, ventricular dysrhythmias, valvular pathologic changes, and myocardial degeneration associated with inadequate myocardial circulation, systemic infection, and exposure to chemical toxins.

            (2) *Indirect pump failure* can result from cardiac tamponade, electrolyte imbalances (especially hyperkalemia and hypocalcemia), administration of drugs that decrease the rate and vigor of cardiac contractility, and injuries to the cardioregulatory areas of the brain.

    3. Distributive shock

        a. Loss of sympathetic tone, blood vessel dilation, pooling of blood in the venous and capillary beds, and increased blood vessel permeability all contribute to decreased MAP.

S

    b. The origin of this set of reactions may be started by nerve changes (neural induced) or the presence of chemical (chemical induced).

    c. Conditions that cause loss of sympathetic tone include severe pain, anesthesia, stress, spinal cord injury, and head injury.

    d. Chemical-induced shock has the following three common origins:

       (1) Anaphylaxis

       (2) Sepsis

       (3) Capillary leak syndrome

  4. Obstructive shock

    a. The ability of the normal heart muscle to pump effectively is impaired, and conditions outside the heart prevent either adequate filling of the heart or adequate contraction of the healthy heart muscle.

    b. Causes include

       (1) Cardiac tamponade

       (2) Pulmonary embolism

       (3) Pulmonary hypertension

       (4) Arterial stenosis

       (5) Constrictive pericarditis

       (6) Tension pneumothorax

       (7) Thoracic tumors

COLLABORATIVE MANAGEMENT

Assessment

■ Record client information.

  1. Risk factors for shock

  2. Age

  3. History of recent illness, trauma, procedures, or chronic conditions that may lead to shock

  4. Current medications

  5. Allergies

  6. Intake and output for the previous 24 hours

■ Assess for

  1. Cardiovascular manifestations

    a. Decreased cardiac output

    b. Increased pulse rate

c. Thready pulse
   d. Decreased blood pressure (It is important to consider the client's baseline blood pressure when shock is suspected.)
   e. Narrowed pulse pressure
   f. Postural hypotension
   g. Low central venous pressure (CVP)
   h. Flat neck and hand veins in dependent positions
   i. Slow capillary refill in the nail beds
   j. Diminished peripheral pulses; as shock progresses, possible absence of superficial peripheral pulses
2. Respiratory manifestations
   a. Increased respiratory rate
   b. Shallow respirations
   c. Decreased $PaCO_2$ and PaO_2
   d. Cyanosis, especially around the lips and nail beds
3. Neuromuscular manifestations
   a. Anxiety and restlessness
   b. Changes in mental status and behavior
   c. Decreased level of consciousness
   d. Generalized muscle weakness
   e. Diminished or absent deep tendon reflexes
   f. Sluggish pupillary response to light
4. Renal manifestations
   a. Decreased urinary output
   b. Increased specific gravity
   c. Sugar and acetone present in the urine
5. Integumentary manifestations
   a. Color changes
      (1) First evident in mucous membranes and in the skin around the mouth
      (2) As shock progresses, color changes noted in the extremities
   b. Cool to cold
   c. Moist and clammy
   d. Pale to mottled to cyanotic
   e. Mouth dry, pastelike coating present
6. Gastrointestinal manifestations
   a. Decreased motility
   b. Diminished or absent bowel sounds

    c. Nausea and vomiting

    d. Constipation

    e. Increased thirst

■ *Manifestations of the first phase of septic shock are unique and are often different from those seen with other types of shock.*

■ If septic shock is suspected, assesses for the following in addition to the general clinical manifestations:

  1. High output, warm phase (hyperdynamic phase)

    a. Cardiac output is increased, which is reflected by tachycardia, increased stroke volume, and a normal to elevated systolic blood pressure and a normal CVP.

    b. Skin color is normal with pink mucous membrane and warmth.

    c. Respiratory rate and depth are increased.

  2. Progression to hypovolemic stage

    a. Disseminated intravascular coagulation (DIC) occurs. Blood may ooze from gums, other mucous membranes, and venipuncture sites.

    b. Small clots form in tiny capillaries of the liver, kidney, brain, spleen, and heart causing hypoxia and ischemia.

  3. Hypodynamic stage or low-output, cold stage

    a. Acute respiratory distress syndrome (ARDS) occurs.

    b. Skin is cool and clammy, and pallor or cyanosis is present.

    c. There is a change in behavior or verbal response.

Interventions

■ Treat the ABCs of emergency care, that is, airway, breathing, and circulation.

  1. Pulse oximetry values between 90% and 95% occur with the nonprogressive stage of shock.

  2. Pulse oximetry values between 75% and 80% occur with the progressive stage of shock.

  3. Any pulse oximetry value below 70% is considered a life-threatening emergency and may signal the refractory stage of shock.

■ Provide emergency care for the client in *hypovolemic* shock.

  1. Ensure a patent airway.

  2. Insert an intravenous (IV) line and infuse colloids (blood and blood products) to restore plasma volume;

IV crystalloids (Ringer's lactate or normal saline) are given for fluid and electrolyte replacement.

3. Administer oxygen.
4. Assess the client for evidence of injury or apparent bleeding.
5. Cover any wound with a clean cloth or dressing and apply pressure to a wound if bleeding appears to be originating from an artery.
6. Elevate the client's feet, keeping the head flat or elevated 30 degrees.
7. Administer drug therapy, as ordered, to increase venous return and improve myocardial contractility or perfusion.
   a. Vasoconstrictive agents such as dopamine (Intropin, Revimine ✤) and norepinephrine (Levophed)
   b. Agents to increase myocardial contractility such as milrinone (Primacor) and dobutamine (Dobutrex)
   c. Agents to enhance myocardial perfusion such as nitroprusside (Nitropress, Nipride)
8. Monitor vital signs and neurologic signs.
9. Monitor CVP, pulmonary artery pressure, and pulmonary wedge pressure.
10. Monitor coagulation studies, electrolytes.
11. Prepare the client for surgery, if necessary, to treat the underlying cause.

- Provide care for the client in *sepsis*-induced distributive shock.
  1. Ensure a patent airway.
  2. Start and maintains an IV line.
  3. Administer oxygen.
  4. Obtain blood, urine, wound, and sputum specimens for cultures, as indicated.
  5. Examine the client for overt bleeding, especially at the gums or injection or IV sites.
  6. Elevate the client's feet, keeping the head flat.
  7. Frequently take vital signs.
  8. Administer medications.
     a. Drugs to enhance cardiac output and restore vascular volume
     b. Antibiotics to treat infection
     c. Anticoagulants in the early phase when many small clots are forming

d. Clotting factors (cryoprecipitate, plasma, platelets) in the late phase when small clots have formed to such an extent that the client no longer has enough clotting factors to prevent hemorrhage

   e. Synthetic activated protein C, which has been shown to stop the inflammatory responses and small clot formation of septic shock

9. Maintain a safe environment, including strict adherence to aseptic technique during invasive procedures and dressing changes.

Sjögren's Syndrome

- Sjögren's syndrome is a group of problems that often appear with other autoimmune disorders. Inflammatory cells and immune complexes obstruct secretory ducts and glands.
- The disorder is manifested by dry eyes (sicca syndrome), blurred vision, itching of eyes, dry mouth (xerostomia), dry vagina, swelling of the parotid and lacrimal areas, dysphagia, change in taste sensation, and frequent nosebleeds.
- Intensity and progression can be slowed by suppressing immune and inflammatory responses.
- Drug therapy includes
   1. Low-dose chemotherapy with methotrexate (Rheumatrex) or cyclophosphamide (Cytoxan)
   2. Immunosuppressive drugs such as corticosteroids, cyclosporine (Neoral, Sandimmune), or hydroxychloroquine (Plaquenil)
   3. Systemic pilocarpine (Salagen) for dry mouth
- Symptomatic treatment includes meticulous mouth, eye, and perineal care; use of artificial tears and saliva; humidifiers in the home.
- Water-soluble vaginal lubricants and moisturizers can increase client comfort and reduce the incidence of vaginitis.
- Without treatment, the client can lose vision; oral ulceration, dental caries, and difficulty in swallowing or talking may occur.

Sprains

- A sprain is the excessive stretching of a ligament, typically caused by twisting motions from a fall or sports activity.
- Sprains are classified by their severity.
  1. *First-degree* sprain (*mild* sprain) involves the tearing of a few fibers of the ligament; joint function is not impaired.
  2. *Second-degree* sprain (*moderate* sprain) involves many torn fibers of the ligament; the joint is stable.
  3. *Third-degree* sprain (*severe* sprain) involves the tearing of fibers to the point that the joint is unstable.
- Pain and swelling characterize ligament injuries.
- The therapy for mild sprains is minimal. Ice and a compression bandage are used to reduce swelling and provide joint support.
- Clients with second-degree sprains usually require immobilization (elastic bandage, air stirrup ankle brace, splint or cast) and partial weight bearing.
- Clients with third-degree sprains typically require surgery to repair the ligament tear, followed by immobilization for 4 to 6 weeks. Artificial ligament implants may be used, especially for knee ligament injuries.
- Complete healing of knee ligaments can take 6 to 9 months or longer.

Stenosis, Aortic

OVERVIEW

- In aortic stenosis, the aortic valve orifice narrows, obstructing left ventricular outflow during systole.
- Increased resistance to ejection or afterload results in left ventricular hypertrophy.
- As stenosis progresses, cardiac output becomes fixed and unable to meet the demands of the body during exertion and symptoms develop.

- Eventually the left ventricle fails, volume backs up in the left atrium, and the pulmonary system becomes congested.
- Right-sided heart failure can occur late in the disease.

Considerations for Older Adults

- Atherosclerosis and degenerative calcification of the aortic valve are the predominant causative factors in people older than 70 years of age.
- Aortic stenosis has become the most common valvular disorder in countries with an aging population. Of clients with aortic stenosis, 80% are men.

COLLABORATIVE MANAGEMENT

- Assess for
  1. Dyspnea, angina, and syncope on exertion
  2. Fatigue
  3. Debilitation
  4. Peripheral cyanosis
  5. Diamond-shaped systolic crescendo-decrescendo murmur
- Aortic valve surgery is the treatment of choice.
- Balloon valvuloplasty may be performed to repair the valve. A balloon catheter is inserted through the femoral artery and advanced to the aortic valve where the balloon is inflated, enlarging the orifice of the valve.
- In aortic valve replacement surgery, the valve is excised during cardiopulmonary bypass surgery, then replaced with a prosthetic (synthetic) or biologic (tissue) valve.
- The postoperative client requires lifetime anticoagulation therapy to prevent thrombus formation on the valve.
- For preoperative and postoperative care, see Surgical Management under Coronary Artery Disease.

Stenosis, Mitral

OVERVIEW

- Mitral stenosis causes thickening of the mitral valve by fibrosis and calcification.
- Valve leaflets fuse together, becoming stiff; the chordae tendineae contract and shorten; the valve opening narrows, preventing normal blood flow from the left atrium to the left ventricle; and as a result, the left atrial pressure rises, the left ventricle dilates, pulmonary artery pressures increase, and the right ventricle hypertrophies.
- Pulmonary congestion and right-sided heart failure occur; later, preload is decreased and cardiac output declines.
- Rheumatic fever is most often the cause of mitral stenosis.
- Women are most often affected.

COLLABORATIVE MANAGEMENT

- Assess for
    1. Orthopnea
    2. Dyspnea on exertion
    3. Paroxysmal nocturnal dyspnea
    4. Dry cough
    5. Hemoptysis
    6. Pulmonary edema
    7. Hepatomegaly
    8. Neck vein distention
    9. Pitting edema
    10. Atrial fibrillation
    11. Rumbling, apical diastolic murmur
- *Balloon valvuloplasty*, an invasive nonsurgical procedure, involves passing a balloon catheter from the femoral vein, through the atrial septum, to the mitral valve. The balloon is inflated to enlarge the mitral orifice.
    1. After the procedure, observe the client for bleeding from the catheter insertion site and institute postangiogram precautions.

S

2. Observe for signs of a regurgitant valve by closely monitoring heart sounds, cardiac output, and heart rhythm.
   3. Observe for septic emboli.
- *Mitral commissurotomy* is performed during cardiopulmonary bypass surgery. The surgeon removes thrombi from the atria, incises the fused commissures (leaflets), and debrides calcium from the leaflets, thus widening the orifice.
- *Mitral valve replacement* is indicated if the leaflets are calcified and immobile. The valve is excised during cardiopulmonary bypass surgery, and a new valve is sutured into place.
- The postoperative client requires lifetime anticoagulant therapy to prevent thrombus formation on the valve.
- For preoperative and postoperative care, see care of the client undergoing a coronary artery bypass grafting procedure under Coronary Artery Disease.
- Discharge planning includes
   1. Providing health teaching information regarding
      a. Medications
      b. Oral hygiene
      c. Plan of work, activity, and rest to conserve energy
      d. The importance of taking an antibiotic before any procedure (e.g., dental work, surgery)
   2. Referring the client to community resources, such as the American Heart Association

Stenosis, Renal Artery

- Renal artery stenosis involves pathologic processes affecting the renal arteries, resulting in severe narrowing of the lumen and reducing blood flow to the renal parenchyma.
- Uncorrected stenosis leads to ischemia and atrophy of renal tissue.
- Renal artery stenosis is suspected when a sudden onset of hypertension occurs.
- Atherosclerotic changes in the renal artery are associated with corresponding disease of the aorta and other major vessels.

- Fibromuscular changes of the vessel wall occur throughout the length of the renal artery between the aortic junction and branching into the renal segmental arteries.
- The location of the defect, the overall condition of the client, and the size of the atrophied kidney influence the decision for therapeutic intervention.
- Treatment includes
  1. Antihypertensive drugs
  2. Percutaneous transluminal balloon angioplasty
  3. Renal artery bypass surgery

Stomatitis

- Stomatitis is characterized by painful single or multiple ulcerations of the oral mucosa that appear as inflammation and denudation of the oral mucosa, impairing the protective lining of the mouth.
- Common causes include infection, allergy, vitamin deficiency, systemic disease, irritants, chemotherapy, and radiation therapy.
- Primary stomatitis include aphthous stomatitis, herpes simplex infections, and traumatic insults.
- Secondary stomatitis results from infection by opportunistic viruses, fungi, or bacteria in clients who are immuno-compromised.
- The client is instructed to
  1. Brush teeth to stimulate gums and clean the oral cavity.
  2. Rinse the mouth frequently with sodium bicarbonate solution, warm saline or hydrogen peroxide solution (do not use commercial mouthwashes because they have a high alcohol content, causing a burning sensation).
  3. Take medication (antibiotics, antifungals, anti-inflammatory, and immune modulators, symptomatic topical agents) as prescribed.

S

Strains

- A strain, sometimes referred to as a "muscle pull," is an excessive stretching of a muscle or tendon when it is weak or unstable.
- Strains may be caused by falls, lifting heavy items, and exercise.
- Strains are classified according to their severity.
    1. *First-degree* strain (*mild* strain) causes mild inflammation manifested by swelling, ecchymosis (minimal bleeding), and tenderness.
    2. *Second-degree* strain (*moderate* strain) involves tearing of the muscle or tendon, possibly resulting in impaired muscle function.
    3. *Third-degree* strain (*severe* strain) involves a ruptured muscle or tendon and causes severe pain and disability.
- Management usually involves cold and heat applications, activity limitations, progressive exercise, anti-inflammatory drugs, and analgesics.
- Clients with third-degree strains may require surgery to repair the muscle or tendon.

Stroke

OVERVIEW

- Stroke is a disruption in the normal blood supply to the brain.
- Strokes may be classified as
    1. *Ischemic,* caused by the occlusion of a cerebral artery by either a thrombus or embolus
        a. Types of ischemic strokes include
            (1) *Thrombotic,* commonly associated with the development of atherosclerosis of the blood vessel wall. The artery becomes occluded and blood flow to the area is markedly diminished, causing transient

ischemia and then complete ischemia and infarction of brain tissue. Signs and symptoms occur gradually.

    (i) A lacunar stroke is a type of thrombotic stroke that causes a soft area or cavity to develop in the white matter or deep gray matter of the brain.

  (2) *Embolic,* caused by an embolus or group of emboli that travel to the cerebral arteries through the carotid artery and block the artery, causing ischemia. Sudden and rapid development of focal neurologic deficits occurs. Cerebral hemorrhage may result if the vessel wall is damaged.

  b. *Ischemic stroke* may be preceded by warning signs, including

    (1) *Transient ischemic attack (TIA),* a transient focal neurologic deficit such as vertigo or blurred vision that lasts a few minutes to fewer than 24 hours

    (2) *Reversible ischemic neurologic deficit (RIND),* which lasts longer than 24 hours but less than a week

2. *Hemorrhagic,* in which the integrity of the vessel wall is interrupted and bleeding occurs into the brain tissue or spaces surrounding the brain (ventricular, subdural, subarachnoid). Causes include hypertension, ruptured aneurysm, and arteriovenous malformation (AVM).

  a. An *aneurysm* is an abnormal ballooning or blister on the involved artery that may become stretched or thinned and rupture.

  b. *AVM* is a tangled or spaghetti-like mass of malformed, thin-walled, dilated vessels that form an abnormal communication between the arterial and venous systems.

COLLABORATIVE MANAGEMENT

Assessment

- Record client information.
    1. Activity at onset of the stroke
    2. Progression and severity of symptoms, including the presence of a TIA or RIND

3. Level of consciousness, orientation
4. Motor status: gait, balance, reading and writing abilities
5. Sensory status: speech, hearing, vision
6. Medical history
7. Social history, with attention to identifying risk factors such as smoking, diet, and exercise
8. Current medications and nonprescribed drugs, especially anticoagulants, aspirin, vasodilators, and illegal drugs

- Assess for changes in
  1. Level of consciousness, orientation, cognition, memory, judgment, and problem-solving and decision-making abilities
  2. Ability to concentrate and attend to tasks
  3. Motor status (muscle strength, muscle tone, range of motion, proprioception, head and trunk control, balance, gait, coordination, bowel and bladder control)
  4. Sensory status (response to touch and painful stimuli; ability to distinguish between two tactile stimuli presented simultaneously; ability to read, write, and follow verbal directions; ability to name objects and use them correctly)
  5. Speech pattern (rhythm, clarity, aphasia)
  6. Visual system (pupil size and reaction to light, visual field deficits, homonymous hemianopsia, bitemporal hemianopsia, ptosis, amaurosis fugax)
  7. Cranial nerve function, especially nerves V, VII, IX, X, and XII
  8. Cardiac system (hypertension, dysrhythmias, and murmurs)
  9. Disturbed body image and self-concept
  10. Coping mechanisms or personality changes
  11. Emotional lability
  12. Financial status and occupation as a result of hospitalization

- The primary purpose of the initial computed tomography (CT) scan or magnetic resonance imaging (MRI) is to identify the presence of hemorrhage or a cerebral aneurysm. Results also help differentiate stroke from other pathologic changes that mimic a stroke.

Planning and Implementation

NONSURGICAL MANAGEMENT

- Monitor for neurologic changes or complications.
    1. Perform a neurologic assessment at a minimum of every 2 to 4 hours, checking
        a. Verbal response, orientation
        b. Eye opening, pupil size, and reaction to light
        c. Motor response
    2. Monitor vital signs with neurologic checks.
        a. Ask the physician for acceptable limits for blood pressure.
        b. Perform a cardiac assessment.
        c. Monitor the client for dysrhythmias. Auscultate the heart to identify presence of cardiac murmurs or atrial fibrillation.
    3. Elevate the head of the bed per physician order.
    4. Avoid activities that may increase intracranial pressure.
        a. Maintain the client's head in a midline neutral position.
        b. Position the client to avoid extreme hip or neck flexion.
        c. Avoid clustering nursing procedures.
        d. Provide a quiet environment; room lights should be low.
        e. Assess the need for suctioning; hyperoxygenate the client before suctioning.

- Occlusive stroke is treated with anticoagulant therapy (contraindicated in clients with a history of ulcers, uremia, and hepatic failure). Sodium heparin (Hepalean ✖) subcutaneously or by continuous intravenous drip is commonly used.

- Thrombolytic therapy may be used for an acute ischemic stroke.
    1. Recombinant tissue plasminogen activator (rt-PA) may be given within 3 hours of the onset of symptoms.
    2. Clients who have had a stroke or serious head trauma in the past 3 months, a hemorrhagic stroke, recent myocardial infarction, increased partial thromboplastin time (PTT), anticoagulant therapy, or who are pregnant are not candidates for this therapy.

3. Catheter-directed thrombolic therapy may be performed as a first line-treatment or if system therapy was not effective in improving the client's condition.
- Anticoagulant therapy and antiplatelet therapy may be prescribed depending on the health care provider's preference.
    1. Obtain a baseline prothrombin time (for oral anticoagulation therapy) and PTT (for heparin [Hepalean ✚] therapy) before initiating therapy, 6 to 8 hours after the start of the drug, and every morning thereafter. International normalized ratio (INR) is used to monitor warfarin therapy.
    2. Anticoagulation therapy may cause bleeding. Observe for blood in the urine and stool, epistaxis, bleeding gums, and easy bruising.
- Enteric-coated or other forms of aspirin (Ancasal ✚) or dipyridamole (Persantine) may be used to forestall thrombotic and embolic strokes.
- Other medications used to treat a stroke include
    1. Phenytoin (Dilantin) or gabapentin (Neurontin), which may be used to prevent seizures
    2. Calcium channel blockers (nimodipine; Nimotop), which may be administered to treat vasospasm or chronic spasm of the vessel (which inhibits blood flow to the area)
    3. Stool softeners, analgesics for pain, and antianxiety drugs
- Monitor the client for complications such as
    1. Hydrocephalus, enlarged ventricles manifested by change in the level of consciousness (LOC), gait disturbances, and behavior changes
    2. Vasospasm, or narrowing of the cerebral arteries, which leads to cerebral ischemia and infarction and is manifested by a decreased LOC, motor and reflex changes, increased neurologic deficits (cranial nerve deficits, aphasia)
    3. Rebleeding or rupture of an aneurysm
- Carotid artery angioplasty is a nonsurgical intervention to treat certain types of ischemic strokes. A distal protection device may be placed beyond the stenosis to catch any debris that breaks off during the angioplasty or stenting procedure.

SURGICAL MANAGEMENT

- Two surgical procedures that may be used are
    1. *Carotid endarterectomy* to remove atherosclerotic plaque from the inner lining of the carotid artery

2. *Extracranial-intracranial bypass* to bypass the occluded
      area and re-establish blood flow to the affected area
- Surgical procedures to treat *AVM* include
   1. Injecting an embolic agent such as platinum coils, detach-
      able silicone balloons, liquid acrylic, and polyvinyl alcohol
      into the carotid artery, which travel to involved vessels,
      become lodged, and cause the vessels to thrombose
   2. Surgically removing involved vessels
- Surgical procedures to treat *aneurysm* include
   1. Placing a clip or clamp at the base or neck of the
      aneurysm
   2. Wrapping the aneurysm with muscle, muslin, or plastic
      coating
- The nursing care for these procedures is similar to that
  discussed in Surgical Management under Tumors, Brain.

NDx: Impaired Physical Mobility; Self-Care Deficit

- Treatment includes
   1. Performing active and passive range-of-motion exercises
      at least every 2 to 3 hours
   2. Carefully positioning the client in proper body alignment
   3. Maintaining correct use of splints and braces
   4. Using sequential compression devices or pneumatic com-
      pression boots; frequently changing client's position;
      mobilizing the client as soon as possible to prevent deep
      venous thrombosis (DVT) or pneumonia
   5. Monitoring the client for signs of DVT

NDx: Disturbed Sensory Perception

- Nursing interventions include
   1. Providing frequent verbal and tactile cues to help the
      client perform activities of daily living (ADLs)
   2. Breaking down tasks into small steps when cueing
   3. Approaching the client from the nonaffected side
   4. Placing objects within the client's field of vision
   5. Placing a patch over the affected eye if diplopia is
      present
   6. Removing clutter from the room
   7. Orienting the client to time, place, and event
   8. Providing a structured, repetitive, and consistent
      routine or schedule

9. Presenting information in a clear, simple, concise manner
10. Using a step-by-step approach
11. Placing pictures and other familiar objects in the room

◆NDx: Unilateral Neglect

- Interventions include
    1. Teaching the client to use both sides of the body
    2. Teaching the client to scan with eyes and turn the head side to side (when visual impairments occur)

◆NDx: Impaired Verbal Communication

- Interventions to help the client develop communication strategies include
    1. Giving repetitive, simple directions; breaking each task into simple steps
    2. Facing the client and speaking slowly and distinctly
    3. Giving sufficient time for the client to understand the direction
    4. Using pictures or a communication board if necessary
    5. Encouraging the client to communicate and positively reinforcing this behavior
    6. Repeating the names of objects on a routine basis and teaching the family to do the same

◆NDx: Impaired Swallowing

- Nursing interventions include
    1. Before feeding, assessing the client's ability to swallow
        a. Observe for facial drooping and a weak, hoarse voice.
        b. Assess the swallow, gag, and cough reflexes.
        c. Collaborate with the speech-language pathologist to determine the extent of the swallowing problem.
    2. Positioning the client to facilitate swallowing
        a. Place the client in a chair or sitting straight up in bed.
        b. Position the client's head and neck slightly forward and flexed.
    3. Providing soft or semisoft foods and thick fluids (e.g., mechanical soft, dental diet; custards, scrambled eggs)
    4. Maintaining a quiet room with few distractions while the client is eating
    5. Weighing the client twice a week

- Interventions to help the client become continent include
  1. Establishing the type (bowel or bladder) and cause of the problem
     a. Altered level of consciousness
     b. Impaired innervation
     c. Inability to communicate the need to urinate or defecate
  2. Determining the client's usual voiding or bowel movement pattern
  3. Implementing an individualized bladder-training program (see entries on rehabilitation for a thorough discussion)
     a. Use an intermittent catheterization program if urinary incontinence is due to upper motor lesion.
     b. Place the client on a bedpan or commode every 2 hours; encourage fluid intake to 2000 mL daily unless contraindicated.
  4. Implementing an individualized bowel-training program (see entries on rehabilitation for a thorough discussion)
     a. Determine the normal time or routine for bowel elimination.
     b. Place the client on a bedpan or commode at the same time each day; use a suppository or stool softener, if needed.
     c. Provide a diet high in bulk or fiber (may require consultation with a dietitian).

Community-Based Care

S

- Provide a detailed plan of care at the time of discharge for clients to be transferred to a rehabilitation center or long-term care facility (rehabilitation can be a lengthy process; see entries on rehabilitation).
- When possible, a case manager should be assigned to help coordinate plans for the client discharged to the home setting. The case manager should collaborate with the physical and occupational therapists to
  1. Identify and suggest corrections of hazards in the home before discharge.
  2. Ensure that the client and family can correctly use all adaptive devices ordered for home use.
  3. Arrange follow-up appointments, as ordered.

- Discharge teaching includes
    1. Providing drug information as needed
    2. Reinforcing mobility skills (in collaboration with other therapists)
        a. How to safely climb stairs, transfer from bed to chair, and get into and out of a car
        b. How to use adaptive equipment
    3. Teaching the family that depression and emotional lability may occur
        a. Depression is usually self-limiting; antidepressants may be needed.
        b. Advise the family to avoid being overprotective.
        c. Assist the family and client to develop realistic and achievable goals.
- Depending on the location of the lesion, the client may be anxious, slow, cautious, hesitant, or impulsive; may lack initiative; or may be seemingly unaware of the deficit.
- Family members may need a referral for respite care.
- Refer family to a social worker for further support and counseling.
- Provide the family with a variety of publications available from the American Heart Association and National Stroke Association.

Subclavian Steal

- Subclavian steal occurs in the upper extremities from a subclavian artery occlusion or stenosis and results in altered blood flow and ischemia in the arm.
- The disorder occurs at any age but is more common with risk factors for atherosclerosis.
- Assess for
    1. Paresthesias
    2. Light-headedness
    3. Dizziness
    4. Pain and discomfort when the arms are elevated
    5. Difference in blood pressure between arms

6. Subclavian bruit on the occluded side
7. Subclavian pulse decreased on the occluded side
8. Discoloration of the affected arm
- Surgical intervention involves one of three procedures.
    1. Endarterectomy of the subclavian artery
    2. Carotid-subclavian bypass
    3. Dilation of the subclavian artery
- Nursing interventions include
    1. Frequent brachial and radial pulse checks
    2. Observation for ischemic changes of the extremity
    3. Observation for edema and redness

Syndrome of Inappropriate Antidiuretic Hormone

OVERVIEW

- Syndrome of inappropriate antidiuretic hormone (SIADH) occurs when ADH (vasopressin) is secreted even when plasma osmolality is low or normal.
- Water is retained, which results in dilutional hyponatremia and expansion of extracellular fluid volume.
- SIADH is associated with
    1. Small cell carcinoma of the lung
    2. Carcinoma of the pancreas, duodenum, and genitourinary tract
    3. Ewing's sarcoma
    4. Hodgkin's and non-Hodgkin's lymphoma
    5. Viral and bacterial pneumothorax, lung abscess, active tuberculosis, pneumothorax, and chronic lung disease
    6. Central nervous system disorders such as trauma, stroke, infections, tumors, porphyria, and lupus erythematosus
    7. Drugs such as exogenous ADH, chlorpropamide, vincristine, cyclophosphamide, carbamazepine, general anesthetic agents, and tricyclic antidepressants

S

COLLABORATIVE MANAGEMENT

Assessment

- Record the client's medical history and weight, especially a history of weight gain.
- Assess for
  1. Gastrointestinal (GI) disturbances such as loss of appetite, nausea, and vomiting
  2. Water retention
  3. Lethargy, headache, hostility, uncooperativeness, and disorientation
  4. Seizure activity
  5. Decreased or sluggish deep tendon reflexes
  6. Vital sign changes (tachycardia, hypothermia)
  7. Irritability, anxiety
  8. Hyponatremia, decreased serum osmolality

Interventions

- Restrict fluids.
  1. Intake may be as low as 500 to 600 mL daily.
  2. Dilute tube feedings with a solution other than plain water. Use saline to irrigate GI tubes. Mix medications for GI tube administration with saline.
  3. Weigh the client daily (a 1-kg weight increase is equal to a 100 mL of fluid retention).
  4. Monitor strict intake and output.
  5. Provide frequent mouth care.
  6. Suggest hard candy to relieve dryness of the mouth.
- Provide drug therapy, including
  1. Diuretics, particularly if heart failure results from fluid overload
  2. Hypertonic saline, which may be given cautiously because it may add to existing fluid overload and promote heart failure
  3. Routine IV fluids with a saline solution
  4. Demeclocycline (Declomycin)
- Provide a safe environment.
  1. Monitor neurologic status.
  2. Reduce environmental noise and lighting to prevent overstimulation.
  3. Provide basic safety measures.

Syphilis

- Syphilis is a complex sexually transmitted disease that can become systemic and cause serious complications, including death.
- The causative organism is *Treponema pallidum*, a spirochete with a slender, spiral shape.
- In *primary* syphilis, the chancre is the first lesion, which develops at the site of inoculation or entry of the organism.
- During the highly infectious stage, the chancre begins as a small papule; within 3 to 7 days, it breaks down into its characteristic appearance: a painless, indurated, smooth, weeping lesion.
- Without treatment, the chancre disappears within 6 weeks; however, the organism disseminates throughout the bloodstream.
- *Secondary* syphilis, which develops from 6 weeks to 6 months after the onset of primary syphilis, becomes a systemic disease because spirochetes circulate throughout the bloodstream.
  1. Symptoms of secondary syphilis include malaise, low-grade fever, headache, muscular aches and pains, and sore throat.
  2. A generalized rash usually evolves from papules, to squamous papules, to pustules; the lesions are highly contagious.
- *Latent* syphilis is a later stage of the disease.
  1. *Early latent* syphilis occurs during the first year after infection, and infectious lesions can recur.
  2. *Late latent* syphilis is a disease of more than 1 year's duration after infection; it is noninfectious except to the fetus of a pregnant woman.
- *Tertiary* or *late* syphilis develops after a highly variable period, from 4 to 20 years in untreated cases. Manifestations include benign lesions of the skin, mucous membranes, and bones; aortitis and aneurysms; and neurosyphilis.

COLLABORATIVE MANAGEMENT

- Assess for
  1. Sexual history
     a. Type and frequency of sexual activity
     b. Number of contacts
     c. History of sexually transmitted diseases
     d. Potential sites of infection
     e. Sexual preferences
  2. Chief complaint
  3. A chancre lesion on the external genitalia and other physical findings such as enlarged lymph nodes
  4. Positive results from Venereal Disease Research Laboratory (VDRL) and fluorescent treponemal antibody absorption tests
- Management includes antibiotic therapy with benzathine penicillin G. Allergic reactions to the antibiotic occur frequently; monitor for signs and symptoms.
- Client education includes
  1. Treatment and side effects
  2. Complications of untreated syphilis
  3. Follow-up care
  4. Treatment for sexual partners
  5. Disease report to the health department
  6. Contiguousness of the disease
- Refer the client to community agencies as needed for psychological support, self-help groups, and support groups.

Tetanus

- Tetanus, also known as lockjaw, is caused by *Clostridium tetani* and is easily prevented through immunization.
- Tetanus is characterized by muscle rigidity, opisthotonos, cramps, muscle spasms, stiffness, and headache.

- Treatment includes prompt (within 72 hours) intramuscular antitoxin human tetanus immune globulin or hyperimmune equine or bovine serum.
- Antibiotics may be needed for superimposed infections.
- Sedation, antianxiety agents, and muscle relaxants to decrease muscle spasms and increase comfort are provided.
- Propranolol (Inderal) or another antidysrhythmic agent may be given to treat cardiac irregularities, and the client may need aggressive respiratory support.

Thoracic Outlet Syndrome

- Thoracic outlet syndrome is a compression of the subclavian artery at the thoracic outlet by anatomic structures, such as a rib or muscle.
- Damage of the arterial wall produces thrombosis or embolization to distal arteries of the arm.
- The common sites of compression of the thoracic outlet are
  1. The interscalene triangle
  2. Between the coracoid process of the scapula and the pectoralis minor tendon
  3. The costoclavicular space (the most common site)
- Assess for
  1. Neck, shoulder, and arm pain
  2. Numbness of the extremity
  3. Moderate edema of the extremity
  4. Increasing pain and numbness when the arm is held over the head or out to the side
- Conservative treatment includes
  1. Physical therapy
  2. Exercise
  3. Avoidance of aggravating positions
- Surgical treatment involves resection of the anatomic structures compressing the artery.

T

Thrombocytopenic Purpura, Autoimmune

OVERVIEW

- Autoimmune thrombocytopenic purpura was known as idiopathic thrombocytopenic purpura (ITP) before the underlying cause was identified.
- This condition causes the number of circulating platelets to be greatly diminished, although bone marrow platelet production is normal.
- An antiplatelet antibody is created that coats the surface of the platelets, making them more likely to be destroyed by macrophages.
- The spleen is the primary site of platelet destruction.
- When the rate of platelet destruction exceeds the rate of platelet production, the number of circulating platelets decreases, and blood clotting slows.

COLLABORATIVE MANAGEMENT

Assessment

- Assess for
  1. Ecchymoses (bruises)
  2. Petechial rash on the arms, legs, upper chest, and back
  3. Mucosal bleeding
  4. Anemia
  5. Neurologic dysfunction (as a result of an intracranial bleed)
- Interventions include
  1. Administering immunosuppressant drugs to inhibit immune system synthesis of antiplatelet autoantibodies
  2. Using intravenous immunoglobulin and intravenous anti-Rho to prevent the destruction of antibody-coated platelets
  3. Administering more aggressive therapy, which involves low-dose chemotherapy

4. Administering platelet transfusions for acute, life-threatening bleeding (less than 20,000 mm^3)
5. Maintaining a safe environment
- A splenectomy is performed for clients not responding to drug therapy.

Thyroiditis

OVERVIEW

- Thyroiditis is the inflammation of the thyroid gland.
- The three types of thyroiditis are
  1. *Acute suppurative thyroiditis,* caused by bacterial invasion of the thyroid gland and manifested by neck tenderness, pain, fever, malaise, and dysphagia
  2. *Subacute granulomatous thyroiditis,* which results from a viral infection of the thyroid gland and is manifested by fever, chills, dysphagia, and muscle and joint pain; on palpation, the gland feels hard and moderately enlarged
  3. *Chronic thyroiditis* (Hashimoto's thyroiditis), believed to be an autoimmune disease and manifested by dysphagia, painless enlargement of the thyroid gland, low serum thyroid levels, and increased thyroid-stimulating hormone secretion, which causes a euthyroid state for some time, followed by the development of hypothyroidism

COLLABORATIVE MANAGEMENT

- Acute suppurative thyroiditis is treated symptomatically and with antibiotics.
- Subacute granulomatous thyroiditis is treated with rest, fluids, and acetylsalicylic acid (aspirin); severe cases may be treated with corticosteroids.
- Chronic thyroiditis is usually treated with thyroid hormone; a subtotal thyroidectomy may be necessary (see Surgical Management under Hyperthyroidism).

Tonsillitis

- Tonsillitis is an inflammation and infection of the tonsils and lymphatic tissue of the oropharynx.
- Tonsillitis is a contagious airborne infection.
- The acute form lasts 7 to 10 days and is caused by a bacterial organism, usually *Streptococcus,* and viruses.
- Acute symptoms begin with the sudden onset of a mild to severe sore throat, fever, muscle aches, chills, dysphagia, ear pain, headache, anorexia, and malaise.
- The tonsils are swollen and red with pus and covered with white or yellow exudate.
- The uvula may be edematous and inflamed, and the cervical lymph nodes are tender and enlarged.
- Treatment includes
  1. Systemic antibiotics for 7 to 10 days
  2. Warm saline gargles
  3. Analgesics
  4. Antipyretics
  5. Antiseptic anesthetic lozenges
- Tonsillectomy and adenoidectomy are indicated for
  1. Recurrent acute infections or chronic infections unresponsive to antibiotic therapy
  2. Peritonsillar abscess
  3. Hypertrophy of tonsils and adenoids, causing airway obstruction
  4. Repeated group A beta-hemolytic streptococcal infections

Toxic Shock Syndrome (TSS)

- Certain strains of *Staphylococcus aureus* produce a toxin associated with TSS.
- TSS is related to menstruation and tampon use as well as surgical wound infection, nonsurgical focal infections, postpartum conditions, and nonmenstrual vaginal conditions.

- Menstrual-related TSS theories focus on tampon use and conclude that toxins readily cross the vaginal mucosa.
- Highly absorbent tampons rub the vaginal walls and cause ulceration, which allows transport of the toxins. Prolonged or continued tampon use can cause chronic vaginal ulcerations through which *S. aureus* is absorbed; plastic tampon inserters can cause ulceration.
- Diaphragms, cervical caps, and vaginal contraceptives have also been implicated.
- Assess for
  1. Fever (temperature greater than 102° F)
  2. Influenza-type symptoms, including headache, sore throat, vomiting, and diarrhea
  3. Generalized rash
  4. Hypotension
- Primary treatment includes
  1. Fluid replacement for dehydration
  2. Antibiotics (e.g., oxacillin, nafcillin, and cephalosporin)
  3. Administration of platelets, if needed
  4. Corticosteroids for skin changes
- Client education is focused on prevention, including instructions on proper tampon, vaginal sponge, and diaphragm use.

Trachoma

- Trachoma is a chronic, bilateral scarring form of conjunctivitis caused by *Chlamydia trachomatis*.
- Trachoma is the leading cause of blindness in the world. Manifestations include tearing, photophobia, edema of the eyelids, conjunctival edema, profuse drainage, eyelid scars, and eyelids turning inward, leading to corneal abrasion.
- Treatment includes oral tetracycline (Achromycin, Apo-Tetra ✦) or erythromycin (E-Mycin, E.E.S., Apo-Erythro ✦), which may also be used as a topical ointment.
- Teach the client to
  1. Use warm water to clean the face and eye
  2. Not share washcloths for bathing and to launder washcloths separately in hot water

3. Wash the hands before and after touching the eyes
4. Complete the prescribed course of treatment

Transplantation, Liver

- Liver transplantation is performed to treat end-stage liver disease or acute liver failure that has not responded to conventional medical or surgical treatment.
- Extensive physiologic and psychological assessment of the client is required.
- Donors are primarily obtained from trauma victims; living donors may also be used.
- The client is placed on antirejection drugs to prevent organ rejection, which may be acute or chronic.
- Assess for indications of acute rejection, including
  1. Tachycardia
  2. Fever
  3. Right upper quadrant or flank pain
  4. Decreased bile pigment and volume
  5. Increasing jaundice
  6. Elevated serum bilirubin, aminotransferase, prothrombin time, and alkaline phosphatase
- Transplant rejection is treated aggressively with immunosuppressive medications.
- If treatment for regression is not effective, rapid deterioration in liver function occurs, multisystem organ failure including respiratory and renal involvement develops, as do diffuse coagulopathies and portal systemic encephalopathy.
- Immunosuppression increases the client's susceptibility and risk for opportunistic infections.
- In the early transplant period, common infections include pneumonia, wound infection, and urinary tract infections.
- Opportunistic infections such as cytomegalovirus, mycobacterial infections, and parasitic infections may develop after the first postoperative month.
- Other complications include hemorrhage, hepatic artery thrombosis, fluid and electrolyte imbalances, atelectasis,

acute renal failure, chronic graft rejection, and psychological maladjustment.
- Monitor for signs of complications, including
  1. Fever
  2. Increased abdominal pain, distention, and rigidity
  3. Change in neurologic status
  4. Coagulopathy

Trauma, Abdominal

OVERVIEW

- Abdominal trauma is an injury to the structures located between the diaphragm and the pelvis when the abdomen is subjected to blunt or penetrating forces.
- Organs injured include the large or small bowel, liver, spleen, duodenum, pancreas, kidneys, and urinary bladder.
- Two broad categories are
  1. *Blunt trauma,* 50% resulting from automobile accidents and the balance caused by falls, aggravated assaults, and contact sports.
  2. *Penetrating trauma,* most often caused by gunshot wounds and stab wounds.

COLLABORATIVE MANAGEMENT

Assessment

- Assess for airway, breathing, and circulation (ABCs).
- The focus of the assessment is on the risk of hemorrhage, shock, and peritonitis.
  1. In mild shock, the skin is pale, cool, and moist.
  2. In moderate shock, diaphoresis is marked and urine output decreased.
  3. In severe shock, changes in mental status are manifested by agitation, disorientation, and recent memory loss.
- Assess for abdominal trauma by
  1. Asking the client about the presence, location, and quality of pain

2. Inspecting the abdomen, back, flanks, genitalia, and rectum for contusions, abrasions, lacerations, ecchymosis, penetrating injuries, and symmetry. Ecchymosis around the umbilicus (*Cullen's sign*) and ecchymosis in either flank (*Turner's sign*) may indicate retroperitoneal bleeding into the abdominal wall.
3. Auscultating the abdomen for absent or diminished bowel sounds and bruits
4. Percussing for abnormal sounds such as resonance over the liver or dullness over the stomach or intestines (*Ballance's sign*)
5. Lightly palpating the abdomen to identify areas of tenderness, guarding, rigidity, and spasm
6. In splenic injury, looking for Kehr's sign, which is left shoulder pain resulting from diaphragmatic irritation
7. Noting blood in peritoneal lavage

Interventions

NONSURGICAL MANAGEMENT

- Interventions include
  1. Placing two large-bore intravenous catheters
  2. Infusing intravenous fluids at a rapid rate, as ordered
  3. Obtaining blood samples for analysis
  4. Inserting an indwelling Foley catheter
  5. Inserting a nasogastric tube to prevent vomiting
- Physiologic parameters that are measured include
  1. Arterial blood gases (ABGs)
  2. Complete blood count (CBC)
  3. Serum electrolytes, glucose, amylase, and blood urea nitrogen (BUN)
  4. Liver function tests
  5. Clotting studies
  6. Cardiac monitoring
- Analgesics for pain are not given in the initial stage so that clinical manifestations are not masked or overlooked.
- The client who does not have overt signs of bleeding may be admitted to the hospital for observation.
  1. Assess for abdominal or referred pain and nausea.
  2. Monitor mental status, vital signs, bowel signs, urinary

output, and changes in clinical findings every 15 to 30 minutes until stable, then hourly.

3. Report any change immediately to the physician.

4. Analgesics for pain are not prescribed initially so that clinical manifestations are not masked or overlooked.

SURGICAL MANAGEMENT

- For clients with severe abdominal trauma, an exploratory laparotomy with repair of abdominal injuries is performed.
- Most clients with gunshot and stab wounds require an exploratory laparotomy to assess for internal damage.
- A colostomy, either temporary or permanent, may be required. (See the Surgical Management discussion under Cancer, Colorectal.)

Trauma, Bladder

OVERVIEW

- Bladder trauma occurs as a result of blunt or penetrating injury to the lower abdomen.
- The most common cause is a fractured pelvis in which bone fragments puncture the bladder.

COLLABORATIVE MANAGEMENT

- Assess for
  1. Anuria
  2. Hematuria
  3. Bloody urinary meatus
  4. Results of a cystogram and of a voiding cystourethrogram
- Clients with bladder trauma other than a simple contusion require surgical intervention, including closure repair of the anterior or posterior bladder wall and peritoneal membrane.
- Clients with anterior bladder wall injury require a Penrose drain and a Foley catheter.
- Clients with posterior bladder wall injury require a Penrose drain and a Foley or suprapubic catheter.

Trauma, Esophageal

OVERVIEW

- Trauma to the esophagus can occur from blunt injuries, chemical burns from ingestion of caustic substances, surgery or endoscopy, or the stress of protracted, severe vomiting. The incidence is low in adults.

COLLABORATIVE MANAGEMENT

Assessment

- Most clients are initially evaluated and treated in the emergency department.
- Assess for
  1. Airway
  2. Pain
  3. Dysphagia
  4. Vomiting
  5. Bleeding
  6. Results of x-ray examination, computed tomography, and endoscopy

Interventions

- Treatment includes
  1. Maintaining the client on a nothing by mouth status to prevent further leakage of esophageal secretions
  2. Maintaining nasogastric or gastrostomy tube drainage to rest the client's esophagus
  3. Administering total parenteral nutrition during esophageal rest (usually for at least 10 days)
  4. Administering broad-spectrum antibiotics, corticosteroids, and analgesics
- If nonsurgical management is not effective in healing traumatized esophageal tissue, surgery may be needed to remove the tissue. A resection or replacement of the damaged esophageal segment with small bowel tissue may be required (see Surgical Management under Tumors, Esophageal).

Trauma, Facial

OVERVIEW

- Facial trauma is defined by the specific bones (e.g., mandibular, maxillary, zygomatic, orbital, or nasal fracture) and side of the face involved.
- Because the face is very vascular, facial trauma causes a significant amount of bleeding.

COLLABORATIVE MANAGEMENT

Assessment

- The *first* priority in the management of facial trauma is to assess for a patent airway.
- Assess for
  1. Edema of soft tissues
  2. Facial asymmetry
  3. Pain
  4. Leakage of cerebrospinal fluid through the ears or nose (may indicate temporal or basilar skull fracture)
  5. Vision and extraocular movements
  6. Neurologic status
  7. Results of skull and facial x-ray examinations and computed tomography scan

Interventions

- The priority intervention is to establish and maintain a patent airway.
- Other interventions include
  1. Anticipating the need for emergency intubation, tracheotomy, or cricothyroidotomy
  2. Controlling or treating hemorrhage
  3. Assessing for extent of injury
  4. Establishing intravenous access, if not already started
  5. Assisting in stabilization of fractures, if present
  6. Administering antibiotics, as ordered
  7. For mandibular fixation with plates, teaching the client oral care with a water-irrigating device, soft diet restrictions, and the method for cutting wires if emesis occurs

8. Collaborating with the dietitian, as needed, to ensure adequate nutrition

Trauma, Head

OVERVIEW

- Traumatic brain injury (TBI) occurs as a result of an external force applied to the head and brain, causing disruption of physiologic stability locally, at the point of injury as well as globally with elevations in intracranial pressure (ICP) and potentially dramatic changes in blood flow within and to the brain.
- TBI may produce a diminished or altered state of consciousness and changes in cognitive abilities, physical functioning, or behavioral and emotional functioning.
- The damage most frequently occurs to the frontal and temporal lobes and may be either temporary or permanent.
- An *open* head injury occurs when the skull is fractured or penetrated by an object, violating the integrity of brain and dura and exposing them to environmental contaminants.
- Types of cranial fractures include
  1. *Linear,* a simple, clean break
  2. *Depressed,* in which bone is pressed inward into brain tissue to at least the thickness of the skull
  3. *Open,* in which the scalp is lacerated, creating a direct opening to the brain tissue
  4. *Comminuted,* which involves fragmentation of the bone, with depression of bone into the brain tissue
  5. *Basilar,* which occurs at the base of the skull, usually along the paranasal sinus, and results in a cerebrospinal fluid (CSF) leak from the nose or ear, possibly resulting in damage to cranial nerves I, II, VII, and VIII and infection
- *Closed* head injuries are caused by blunt trauma. The integrity of the skull is not violated.
- Damage to brain tissue depends on the degree and mechanism of injury.
  1. A *concussion* is characterized by a brief loss of consciousness.

2. A *contusion* causes bruising of the brain tissue.
3. A *laceration* causes actual tearing of the cortical surface vessels and may lead to secondary hemorrhage.
4. Diffuse axonal injury causes significant damage to the axons in the white matter.

■ Secondary responses include any neurologic damage that occurs after the initial injury and may result in increased morbidity and mortality, including
1. Increased ICP
2. Edema: vasogenic or interstitial
3. Hemorrhage: epidural, subdural, or intracranial
4. Impaired cerebral autoregulation
5. Hydrocephalus
6. Brain herniation

COLLABORATIVE MANAGEMENT

Assessment

■ Record the events surrounding the injury.
1. When, where, and how the injury occurred
2. The client's level of consciousness immediately after the injury and upon admission to the hospital or unit and if there have been any changes or fluctuations
3. Presence of seizure activity

■ Record client information.
1. Age, sex, and race
2. Medical and social history
3. Hand dominance
4. Allergies to medications and foods, especially seafood (clients allergic to seafood are often allergic to the medium used in diagnostic testing)
5. Alcohol and drug use and abuse

■ Assess for
1. Impaired airway or breathing pattern
2. Signs and symptoms of hypovolemic shock or hemorrhage, which may indicate abdominal bleeding or bleeding into soft tissue around major fractures
3. Indications of spinal cord injury
4. Cardiac dysrhythmias from chest trauma, bruising of the heart, or interference with the autonomic nervous system

T

5. Impaired cerebral autoregulation manifested by changes in vital signs
6. Changes in neurologic status and indications of ICP
   a. Decreased level of consciousness (stuporous, comatose)
   b. Inability to follow commands, confused
   c. Behavioral changes
   d. Pupils that are large, pinpoint or ovoid, and nonreactive to light
   e. Cranial nerve dysfunction, especially III, IV, and VII
   f. Decreased or absent motor strength in the extremities; hemiparesis or hemiplegia
   g. Ataxia
   h. Aphasia
   i. Complaints of severe headache, nausea, or vomiting
   j. Seizure activity
   k. Drainage of CSF from the ear or nose ("halo" sign)
7. Indications of post-traumatic sequelae in the client who experienced a minor head injury; symptoms may persist for weeks or months
   a. Persistent headache
   b. Weakness
   c. Dizziness
   d. Loss of memory
   e. Personality and behavioral changes
   e. Problems with perception, reasoning abilities, and concept formation
8. Changes in personality, behavior, and abilities, such as
   a. Increased incidence of temper outbursts, risk-taking behavior, and depression, and denial of disability
   b. Becoming more talkative and developing a very outgoing personality
   c. Decreased ability to learn new information, to concentrate, and to plan
   d. Impaired memory, especially recent or short-term memory; this should not be confused with problems of aphasia

- Assess family dynamics. Family members may be angry at the client for being injured, especially when the client's behavior resulted in an injury that could have been prevented, or they may feel guilty that they could not prevent the injury.

Interventions

NONSURGICAL MANAGEMENT

- Assess vital signs every 1 to 2 hours. Cardiac monitoring to detect cardiac dysrhythmias may be implemented.
- Fever may be a defense mechanism in presence of trauma, sign of infection, or caused by hypothalamic damage.
- Position client to avoid extreme flexion or extension of the neck. Maintain the head in a midline, central position, log roll the client, and elevate the head of the bed 30 degrees unless contraindicated (e.g., in spinal cord injury).
- The client on a respirator may be hyperventilated to maintain an arterial carbon dioxide ($PaCO_2$) level of approximately 35 mm Hg and an arterial oxygen (PaO_2) level of 80 to 100 mm Hg. Monitor arterial blood gases at least twice per day.
- The client may be placed in a barbiturate coma if increased ICP cannot be controlled by other means, using pentobarbital (Nembutal) to decrease the metabolic demands of the brain. This requires sophisticated hemodynamic monitoring techniques, mechanical ventilation, and ICP monitoring. Complications include cardiac dysrhythmias, hypotension, and fluid and electrolyte disturbances. Some facilities use narcotic sedation rather than barbiturates.
- Drug therapy includes
  1. Osmotic diuretics (mannitol) given through or drawn up through a needle with a filter to eliminate microscopic crystals. This is most effective when given as bolus rather than continuous infusion. Insert a Foley catheter and measure output.
  2. Loop diuretics (e.g., furosemide [Furoside ✦]) as adjunctive therapy to reduce the incidence of rebound from mannitol and enhance its therapeutic effect
  3. Codeine or fentanyl (Sublimaze) or paralytic agents (pancuronium), used if the client is mechanically ventilated to control restlessness and agitation in those at risk for increased ICP
  4. Neuromuscular blocking agents for severe agitation or if agitation is causing ICP. These agents must be given with aggressive sedation and analgesia.
  5. Antiepileptic drugs to treat seizure activity

- Fluid and electrolyte management includes
  1. Monitoring electrolytes and serum and urine osmolarity
  2. Measuring intake and output every hour
  3. Measuring urine specific gravity every hour
- Client is at risk for diabetes insipidus and syndrome of inappropriate antidiuretic hormone.
- Sensory and perceptual management includes
  1. Monitoring the client for nutritional deficits that may occur secondary to loss of smell and loss of ability to taste, swallow, or feel food in the oral cavity
     a. Ensure that mealtime is a pleasant experience.
     b. Check the temperature of food and beverages on the tray before serving.
     c. Position the client to maximize swallowing ability.
     d. Collaborate with the speech-language pathologist to develop and implement a swallowing program for the client, as needed.
  2. Keeping the side rails up while the client is in bed and the seat belt on while the client is in a chair
  3. Initiating a sensory stimulation program, such as audiotapes used for no longer than 10 to 15 minutes
  4. Orienting the client to environment, time, place, and the reason for hospitalization
  5. Reassuring the client that family or significant others know where he or she is and explaining when the family will visit
  6. Providing simple, short explanations of procedures and activities immediately before any interventions
  7. Maintaining a normal sleep-wake cycle
  8. Asking the family to bring in familiar objects, such as pictures
  9. Monitoring the client's reaction to television or radio (the client is often unable to differentiate programs from what is happening within his or her own environment)
- Pulmonary management includes
  1. Performing chest physiotherapy and encouraging the client to breathe deeply
  2. Turning and repositioning the client at least once every 2 hours
  3. Suctioning the client as needed

- Behavioral management includes
  1. Orienting the client to the environment
  2. Keeping the bed in the low position
  3. Observing and documenting behavior
- Strategies to prevent complications of immobility are as follows:
  1. Until the client is fully mobile, he or she should wear pneumatic compression boots or sequential compression stockings to prevent venous stasis.
  2. Prophylactic anticoagulants such as heparin, aspirin, or low–molecular weight heparinoids may be ordered.
  3. Perform active and passive range-of-motion exercises at least once every 2 to 3 hours.
  4. Position the client carefully and use splints and braces correctly.
  5. Apply high-top athletic shoes if the client's feet are flaccid. Use these shoes with clients who are spastic only after consultation with physical therapist.
  6. Collaborate with physical and occupational therapists to plan exercise and activities of daily living (ADLs) programs.
- Nutrition management is as follows:
  1. Begin nutritional support as soon as possible with hyperalimentation, tube feedings (nasal or gastrostomy), or oral feedings.
  2. Weigh the client daily.
  3. Monitor the client's serum albumin, prealbumin, and transferrin levels to ensure adequate protein intake.
  4. Check for signs of dehydration.

SURGICAL MANAGEMENT

- A *craniotomy* may be indicated to
  1. Evacuate a subdural or epidural hematoma
  2. Treat uncontrolled increased ICP; remove ischemic tissue or tips of temporal lobe
  3. Treat hydrocephalus
- Surgical insertion of an ICP-monitoring device is often performed. Types of devices include
  1. Intraventricular
  2. Epidural catheter or sensor

T

3. Subarachnoid bolt or screw
4. Fiberoptic transducer-tipped pressure sensor

Community-Based Care

- Discharge planning includes
  1. Providing a detailed plan of care at the time of discharge for clients to be transferred to a rehabilitation or long-term care facility (Rehabilitation may be a lengthy process; see Rehabilitation.)
     a. Medications, including dosage and possible side effects
     b. Current client care plan
     c. Techniques used to motivate or calm the client
     d. Strategies to assist the family to cope with the situation
  2. Referring the client to the National Head Injury Foundation or a local head injury support group
- Health teaching includes
  1. Reviewing seizure precautions
  2. Strategies to adapt to sensory dysfunction and to cope with the personality or behavior problems that may arise
  3. Explaining the purpose, dosage, schedule, and route of administration of medications
  4. Encouraging the client to participate in activities as tolerated
  5. Teaching the client and family measures to treat sensory dysfunctions
     a. The home should have functioning smoke detectors (the client may have loss of sense of smell).
     b. Objects and furniture should be kept in the same place.
     c. The measures described for sensory and perceptual management are relevant here also.
     d. Help the family and client develop a home routine that is structured, repetitious, and consistent.
- For minor head injury, discuss symptoms of post-traumatic syndrome, inform the client that these symptoms are normal, and refer the client and family to a support group if symptoms persist. Symptoms include
  1. Personality changes
  2. Irritability

3. Headaches
4. Dizziness
5. Restlessness
6. Nervousness
7. Insomnia
8. Memory loss
9. Depression

- Respite care may be needed to help the family cope with feelings of isolation, increased responsibility, financial or emotional stressors, or role reversal; refer to support groups.
- The client may experience a sense of isolation and loneliness because personality and behavior changes make it difficult to resume or maintain the social contacts whom he or she had before the injury.
- Refer the client and family to the state and national chapters of the National Head Injury Foundation.

Trauma, Knee

- *Meniscus* injuries are characterized by pain, swelling, and tenderness in the knee and sometimes by a clicking or snapping sound when moving the knee.
- A common diagnostic technique is the *McMurray test.* The examiner flexes and rotates the knee, then presses on the medial aspect while slowly extending the leg. The test result is positive if a clicking sound is palpated or heard, but a negative finding does not rule out a tear.
- Treatment of *locked* knee is manipulation followed by casting for 3 to 6 weeks.
- A *meniscectomy,* or removal of all or part of the meniscus, may be required.
- Postoperative care includes
  1. Monitoring the dressing for drainage and bleeding
  2. Checking circulation: skin temperature and color, movement, sensation, pulses, capillary refill, and pain
  3. Performing leg exercises: quadriceps setting and straight-leg raising

4. Using a knee immobilizer
5. Elevating the leg on pillows; applying ice

- Ligament injuries result in sprains.
- Anterior cruciate ligament (ACL) injuries are characterized by a "snap"; within a few hours, the knee is swollen, stiff, and painful.
- ACL injuries are treated with exercise, bracing, and restriction of activity; surgical repair and casting may be needed.
- For a *rupture* of the *patellar tendon,* the treatment is surgical repair and casting for 6 to 8 weeks or tendon transplant. (For care of the client in a cast, see also Fracture.)

Trauma, Laryngeal

- Laryngeal trauma is the result of a crushing or direct blow injury or fracture, or an intrinsic injury such as prolonged endotracheal intubation.
- Symptoms include hoarseness, dyspnea, aphonia, subcutaneous emphysema, and hemoptysis.
- Respiratory assessment includes assessing pulse oximetry and assessing and frequently monitoring for a patent airway and distress symptoms, which include tachypnea, anxiety, sternal retractions, nasal flaring, decreased oxygen saturation, and stridor.
- Management is cause specific.
- Laceration of the cricoid cartilage requires surgical repair and tracheostomy.

Trauma, Liver

- Liver trauma is the most common organ injury resulting from penetrating abdominal trauma and the second most common organ injury after blunt abdominal trauma.
- Common injuries to the liver include simple lacerations, multiple lacerations, avulsions (tears), and crush injuries.

- Because the liver is a vascular organ, blood loss is massive when trauma occurs.
- Signs of hemorrhagic shock from blood loss include hypotension; tachycardia; tachypnea; pallor; diaphoresis; cool, clammy skin; and confusion.
- Clinical manifestations of liver trauma include right upper quadrant pain with abdominal tenderness, distention, guarding, and rigidity and abdominal pain that is aggravated by deep breathing and is referred to the right shoulder.
- Exploratory laparotomy may be needed with suture placement, wound packing, decompression, or a combination of these procedures; liver lobe resection may be necessary.
- The client requires infusion of multiple blood products, packed red blood cells, fresh frozen plasma, and massive volume to maintain hydration.

Trauma, Peripheral Nerve

- Mechanisms of injury for peripheral nerve trauma include
  1. Partial or complete severance of a nerve
  2. Contusion, stretching, constriction, or compression of a nerve
  3. Ischemia
  4. Electrical, thermal, and radiation sources
- The most commonly affected nerves are the median, ulnar, and radial nerves of the arms and the peroneal, femoral, and sciatic nerves of the legs.
- Regeneration of the damaged nerve may occur.
- Nerve damage is characterized by pain, burning, or other abnormal sensations distal to the trauma; weakness or flaccid paralysis; and change in skin color and temperature (a warm phase and a cold phase).
- Treatment consists of immobilization of the area with a splint, cast, or traction.
- Surgery may include resection and suturing to reapproximate the severed nerve ends, nerve grafts, and nerve and tendon transplants.

- Postoperative nursing care is directed toward frequent skin care and assessment, management of pain, and instructing the client to protect the involved area from trauma.

Trauma, Renal

OVERVIEW

- Renal trauma is injury to one or both kidneys.
- Injuries include
  1. *Minor* injuries: contusion, small lacerations, and tearing of the parenchyma and the calyx; likely to follow falls, contact sports, and blows to the back or torso
  2. *Major* injuries: lacerations to the cortex, medulla, or one of the branches of the renal artery or vein; likely to follow penetrating abdominal, flank, or back wounds
  3. *Pedicle* injuries: a laceration or disruption of the renal artery or vein, resulting in rapid and extensive hemorrhage and death unless diagnosis and intervention are prompt

COLLABORATIVE MANAGEMENT

- Record client information.
  1. History of events surrounding the trauma
  2. History of renal or urologic disease
  3. Previous surgical intervention
  4. History of diabetes or hypertension
- Assess for
  1. Abdominal or flank pain
  2. Presence of flank asymmetry
  3. Presence of flank bruising
  4. Gross bleeding of the urethra
  5. Penetrating injuries of the lower thorax or back
  6. Abdominal ecchymoses
  7. Abdominal distention
  8. Penetrating abdominal wounds
  9. Hemoglobin or red blood cells in the urine
  10. Decreased serum hemoglobin and hematocrit values

- Treatment includes medications for vascular support, fluids to restore volume, and surgery when indicated.
  1. Administer low-dose dobutamine to ensure renal perfusion.
  2. Administer fluids, such as crystalloids and red blood cells, to restore circulatory blood volume; plasma volume expanders may also be given.
  3. Assess the need for clotting factors such as vitamin K and platelets.
- Monitor the client for hemodynamic instability.
- Measure and record urine output hourly.
- Depending on the extent of the injury, *nephrectomy* (the surgical removal of the kidney) may be required.
- For major vascular tearing, the kidney may be surgically removed, repaired through revascularization techniques, and then surgically reimplanted.

Trauma, Spinal Cord

OVERVIEW

- An injury to the vertebral column and spinal cord may be caused by motor vehicle accidents, falls, sports such as diving and football, and penetrating trauma.
- As a result, a loss or decrease in motor function, sensation, reflex activity, and bowel and bladder function may occur.
- The extent of the injury can be classified as
  1. *Complete* when the spinal cord is severed or damaged in a way that eliminates all innervation below the level of injury and total motor and sensory loss occurs
  2. *Incomplete*, the most common, when there is preservation of a mixed pattern of motor, sensory, and reflex function
- Cervical spinal cord injuries may result in specific syndromes.
  1. *Anterior cord injury* is characterized by loss of motor function, pain, and temperature sensation below the level of the injury; sensations of touch, position, and vibration remain intact.

2. *Posterior cord injury* is characterized by intact motor function and loss of vibratory sense, crude touch, and position sense.
3. *Brown-Séquard's paralysis* is characterized by loss of motor function, proprioception, vibration, and deep touch on the same side as the injury; pain, temperature, and light touch are affected on the opposite side of the body.
4. *Central cord injury* is characterized by loss of motor function that is more pronounced in the upper extremities than in the lower extremities.

- Complications of spinal cord injury include heterotrophic ossification manifested by swelling, redness, warmth, and decreased range of motion (ROM) of the involved extremity; pneumonia, urinary tract infection, and pressure ulcers.

COLLABORATIVE MANAGEMENT

Assessment

- Record client information.
  1. Description of how the injury occurred and the probable mechanism of injury
  2. Position immediately after the injury
  3. Symptoms that occurred after the injury and what changes have occurred since
  4. Prehospital rescue personnel are questioned about
     a. Problems encountered during the extrication and transport
     b. Type of immobilization devices used
     c. Medical treatment given at the scene
  5. Medical history, with particular attention to a history of arthritis of the spine, congenital deformities, osteoarthritis or osteomyelitis, cancer, previous back and spinal cord injury, and respiratory problems
- Assess for
  1. Airway, breathing, and circulation (ABCs)
  2. Indication of hemorrhage or bleeding around the fracture sites or in the abdomen
  3. Indications of a head injury such as a change in level of consciousness, abnormal pupil size and reaction to light, and change in orientation

4. Decreased or absent motor strength; the ability to shrug the shoulders, flex and extend the arms, elevate the arms and legs off the bed, extend the wrist, wiggle the toes, and flex and extend the feet and legs; deep tendon reflexes
5. *Spinal shock*, which occurs immediately after the injury and lasts from a few days to several months. Spinal shock is characterized by
   a. Flaccid paralysis
   b. Loss of reflex activity below the level of the lesion
   c. Bradycardia
   d. Paralytic ileus (occasionally)
   e. Hypotension
6. Decreased or absent sensation
7. Cardiovascular dysfunction such as bradycardia, hypotension, hypothermia, and cardiac dysrhythmias
8. Change in thermoregulatory capacity, with the client's body tending to assume the temperature of the environment
10. Paralytic ileus manifested by decreased or absent bowel sounds and distended abdomen
13. Coping strategies used in the past to deal with illness, difficult situations, or disappointments

Planning and Implementation

◆NDx: Ineffective (Spinal Cord) Tissue Perfusion

- Routine care includes
  1. Assessing for changes in respiratory function
  2. Monitoring neurologic signs and vital signs every 2 to 4 hours
  3. Monitoring the client with a cervical cord injury for neurogenic shock manifested by hypotension and bradycardia
  4. Keeping the client in optimal body alignment to prevent further cord injury or irritability
     a. The most commonly used devices for cervical injuries are cervical tongs (Gardner-Wells, Barton, or Crutchfield tongs) and the halo fixation device to immobilize the spine.
     b. Traction is added, with the amount of weight to be used prescribed by the physician.

    c. Weights should hang free at all times; never release the traction.

    d. Monitor insertion sites for infection and clean pins per hospital policy.

    e. Monitor the client's neurologic status for changes in movement or decreased strength.

- The client with thoracic and lumbar or sacral injuries is placed on bedrest; immobilization with a fiberglass or plastic body cast may be done.
- Drug therapy may include
    1. Methylprednisolone (Solu-Medrol) may or may not be given depending on physician preference.
    2. Dextran, a plasma expander, is used to increase capillary blood flow with the spinal cord and to prevent or treat hypotension.
    3. Atropine sulfate is used to treat bradycardia.
    4. Inotropic and sympathomimetic agents treat hypotension.
    5. Dantrolene (Dantrium) or baclofen (Lioresal) is used to treat spasticity.
- Monitor the client for *autonomic dysreflexia (hyperreflexia),* which is generally seen in injuries above the level of the sixth thoracic vertebra and occurs after the period of spinal shock is completed; it is usually caused by a noxious stimulus such as a distended bladder or constipation.
- Key features of autonomic dysreflexia include
    1. Severe, rapidly occurring hypertension
    2. Bradycardia
    3. Flushing above the level of injury
    4. Severe, throbbing headache
    5. Nasal stuffiness
    6. Sweating
    7. Nausea
    8. Blurred vision
- Autonomic dysreflexia treatment includes
    1. Raising the head of the bed to a high Fowler's position
    2. Loosening tight clothing
    3. Checking the Foley catheter tubing (if present) for kinks or obstruction
    4. If a Foley catheter is not present, checking for bladder distention and catheterizing immediately

5. Checking the client for fecal impaction and, if present, disimpacting immediately using anesthetic ointment
6. Checking the room temperature to ensure that it is not too cool or drafty
7. Monitoring blood pressure every 15 minutes; hypertension may be treated with nitrates or hydralazine

SURGICAL MANAGEMENT

- *Decompressive laminectomy* is performed to relieve compression from a hematoma, to remove bone fragments, or to remove a penetrating object such as a bullet.
- *Spinal fusion* or insertion of metal or steel rods to stabilize the vertebral column may be indicated.
- Postoperative care is the same as discussed under Surgical Management under Back Pain or Cervical Spine Pain.

NDx: Ineffective Airway Clearance; Ineffective Breathing Pattern; Impaired Gas Exchange

- Respiratory care includes
  1. Perform a respiratory assessment every 4 hours.
  2. Turn the client at least every 2 hours.
  3. Encourage the client to cough and deep breathe every 1 to 2 hours.
  4. Teach the client to use an incentive spirometer every 2 hours while awake.
  5. Perform tracheal suctioning based on assessment findings.
  6. Use a technique called "quad cough" or "cough assist" to help the quadriplegic client cough: Place your hands on either side of the client's rib cage or upper abdomen below the diaphragm. As the client inhales, push upward to help the client expand the lungs and cough.

NDx: Impaired Physical Mobility; Self-Care Deficit

- To prevent complications of immobility
  1. Reposition the client every 2 hours while the client is in bed and every 30 minutes while in a chair.
  2. Inspect the skin and teach the client to inspect the skin every shift for signs of pressure sores or reddened areas.
  3. Perform ROM exercises to all extremities at least once every 8 hours.

4. Collaborate with physical and occupational therapists to determine positioning and exercise programs; determine the need for splints and a plan to prevent foot drop.
5. Assess for signs of deep venous thrombosis; measure the calf and thigh each day.
6. Apply thigh-high antiembolism stockings; sequential compression devices or pneumatic compression boots may be used.
7. Observe for orthostatic hypotension when raising the head of the bed, dangling the client on the side of the bed, and transferring the client to a chair. Teach the client to change positions slowly.
8. Collaborate with physical and occupational therapists to identify techniques and assistive devices to enable the client to become as independent as possible in activities of daily living (ADLs).

NDx: Impaired Urinary Elimination, Constipation

- Establish an individualized bladder program.
  1. Begin an intermittent catheterization program as soon as possible.
  2. Catheterize the client every 4 hours or more frequently if the urinary output is greater than 500 mL.
  3. Over time, intervals between catheterizations are increased and adjusted to the client's fluid intake and sleep times.
  4. Encourage fluid intake, unless contraindicated, to 2000 to 2500 mL. Clients with lower motor neuron injuries may restrict fluids after 6 or 7 PM.
  5. Teach the client with upper motor injury (spastic bladder problem) to stimulate voiding by stroking the inner thigh, pulling on pubic hair and hair of the upper thigh, pouring warm water over the perineum, or tapping the bladder area to stimulate the detrusor muscle.
  6. Teach the client with a lower motor injury (flaccid bladder problem) to perform the Valsalva maneuver or tighten the abdominal muscles to stimulate emptying the bladder.
  7. Catheterize for residual urine after the client voids to determine the effectiveness of the stimulation techniques.
- Establish an individualized bowel program.
  1. Schedule a consistent time for evacuation.

2. Encourage fluid intake (2000 mL/day) unless contra-indicated.
3. Provide a high-fiber diet.
4. Assess the need for a suppository or stool softener.
5. Place the client on a bedside commode or bedpan at the time determined to be the client's normal time to have a bowel movement; allow for privacy.
6. Teach the client to use the Valsalva maneuver or to massage the abdomen from right to left to stimulate bowel evacuation.

NDx: Impaired Adjustment

- Use the following interventions:
  1. Refer questions about prognosis and potential for complete recovery to the health care provider because the timing and extent of recovery vary greatly.
  2. Invite the client to ask questions; answer questions honestly and openly.
  3. Explore coping strategies with the client.
  4. Redirect socially unacceptable behavior.
  5. Refer the client to clergy, a psychiatric liaison nurse, or a psychologist to help the client adjust to his or her unexpected life change.
  6. Refer the client to social worker or financial counselor for review of insurance and financial status; refer to appropriate social service agencies as needed.

Discharge Planning

- Most clients are discharged to a rehabilitation setting where they learn more about self-care, mobility skills, and bladder and bowel retraining.
  1. Psychosocial adaptation is a crucial factor in determining the success of rehabilitation.
  2. Assist the client to verbalize feeling and fears about body image, self-concept, role performance, and self-esteem.
  3. Talk to the client about the expected reactions of those outside the hospital environment.
- To prepare for discharge to home or for a weekend home visit
  1. Collaborate with the client, family, and rehabilitation professionals to assess the home environment to ensure

that it is free from hazards and can accommodate the client's special needs.

2. Ensure that the client can correctly use all adaptive devices ordered for home use.
3. Ensure that adaptive equipment is installed in the home before discharge.

- Teach the client and family the following in collaboration with other health care team members:
  1. ADL skills
  2. Bowel and bladder training program
  3. Medication regimen
  4. Skin care
  5. Sexual functioning
- Refer the client to local, state, and national support groups.
- Provide the telephone number for the spinal cord injury hotline.

Trauma, Tracheobronchial

- Most tears of the tracheobronchial tree result from severe blunt trauma or rapid deceleration, primarily involving the mainstem bronchi.
- Injuries to the trachea occur at the junction of the trachea and cricoid cartilage.
- Clients with laceration of the trachea develop massive air leaks, which cause air to enter the mediastinum and extensive subcutaneous emphysema.
- Upper airway obstruction may occur, causing severe respiratory distress and inspiratory stridor.
- Large tracheal tears are managed by cricothyroidotomy or tracheostomy below the level of the injury.
- Management includes
  1. Assessing for hypoxemia by arterial blood gas assays
  2. Administering oxygen
  3. Maintaining mechanical ventilation or surgical repair may be needed
  4. Assessing for subcutaneous emphysema
  5. Auscultating the lungs to assess for further complications

6. Providing care to the tracheostomy, if needed
7. Monitoring for hypotension and shock

Tuberculosis, Pulmonary

OVERVIEW

- Pulmonary tuberculosis (TB) is a highly communicable disease caused by *Mycobacterium tuberculosis*.
- The tubercle bacillus is transmitted via aerosolization (airborne route) to a susceptible site in the bronchi or alveoli of the lung and freely multiplies.
- The initial infection is seen most often in the middle or lower lobes, with the upper lobes being the most common sites of reinfection.
- Miliary or hematogenous TB is the spread of TB throughout the body when a large number of organisms enter the blood and infect the brain, meninges, liver, kidney, or bone marrow.
- Foreign immigrants from Mexico, the Philippines, and Vietnam are at high risk for TB.
- People at the greatest risk of developing TB are those in frequent close contact with an untreated individual or with an individual with immune dysfunction or HIV, people who are older and homeless, and people of lower socioeconomic groups as well as those living in crowded conditions such as those in long-term care facilities or prisons.

COLLABORATIVE MANAGEMENT

Assessment

- Record client information.
  1. Past exposure to TB
  2. Country of origin
  3. Travel to foreign countries
  4. Prior TB tests
  5. History of bacille Calmette-Guérin (BCG) vaccination
- Anyone who has received the BCG vaccine in the last 10 years will have a somewhat positive skin test that can complicate interpretation.

- Assess for
    1. Progressive fatigue, lethargy
    2. Anorexia, nausea, weight loss
    3. Irregular menses
    4. Low-grade fever, night sweats
    5. Cough with mucoid, blood-streaked, mucopurulent sputum
    6. Chest tightness; dull, aching chest pain
    7. Dullness with chest percussion
    8. Bronchial breath sounds or rales
    9. Increased transmission of spoken or whispered sounds
    10. Localized wheezing
    11. Positive result on a tuberculin (Mantoux) test
    12. Positive sputum smear for acid-fast bacillus
    13. Positive sputum culture for *M. tuberculosis*
    14. Positive chest x-ray findings
- *TB should be considered for any client with a persistent cough or other symptom such as weight loss, anorexia, night sweats, hemoptysis, shortness of breath, fever, or chills.*
- Management of the client with TB includes
    1. Combination drug therapy, which is the most effective method of treatment
        a. Isoniazid (INH) and rifampin are administered throughout the course of therapy.
        b. Pyrazinamide is administered for the first 2 months of treatment only.
        c. Ethambutol and streptomycin may be given to make a four-drug combination.
    2. Suggesting that the client take medications at bedtime to minimize nausea
    3. Client teaching regarding the importance of strict adherence to medication regimen
    4. Instructing the client to cover the nose and mouth when coughing or sneezing, and instructing the client to place used tissues in plastic bags
    5. Ensuring airborne precautions in a well-ventilated room that exhausts to the outside if the client is hospitalized

6. Wearing an N95 or a high-efficiency particulate air (HEPA) respirator when caring for the client
- Refer clients who do not have money for medications to the appropriate resources to obtain low-cost or no-cost medications.

Community-Based Care

- Client and family education
  1. Airborne precautions are not necessary; the people in the home have already been exposed.
  2. Family members and those in close contact with the client need to be tested for TB.
  3. The client should wear a mask when in contact with crowds until the drug suppresses the infection.
  4. Sputum cultures are needed every 2 to 4 weeks once drug therapy begins; when three cultures are negative, the client is no longer infectious and may return to work or school.
  5. Medication information
     a. The prescribed drug regimen must be adhered to for 6 months or longer.
     b. Emphasize that not taking the drugs as prescribed could lead to an infection that is difficult to treat or has total drug resistance.
     c. Teach side effects and ways to minimize them to ensure compliance.
     d. Directly observed therapy in which a health care provider watches the client swallow the drugs may be indicated in some situations.
  6. Fatigue diminishes as treatment progresses and usual activities should be resumed gradually.
  7. Teach client how to maintain proper nutrition.
  8. Teach client to increase the intake of foods rich in iron, protein, and vitamin C. Refer the client to the American Lung Association and other agencies as needed.

Tuberculosis, Renal

- Renal tuberculosis, or granulomatous nephritis, occurs when the kidney is invaded by *Mycobacterium tuberculosis,* usually by the bloodborne route.
- Normal renal parenchyma is replaced by scar tissue or a granuloma.
- Symptoms include
  1. Urinary frequency
  2. Dysuria
  3. Hypertension
  4. Hematuria
  5. Proteinuria
  6. Renal colic
- Treatment includes
  1. Antitubercular therapy with a 2-month course of rifampin, isoniazid, and pyrazinamide followed by a 4-month course of rifampin and isoniazid. An additional 3 to 6 months of rifampin and isoniazid may be recommended for men who are harboring the organism in the prostate.
  2. Surgical excision of diseased tissue
- Complications include loss of renal function, nephrolithiasis, obstructive uropathy, and bacterial superinfection of the urinary tract.

Tumors, Benign Bone

OVERVIEW

- Benign bone tumors are often asymptomatic and may be discovered on routine radiographic examination or as the cause of pathologic fractures.
- Types of benign tumors include
  1. *Chondrogenic* (from cartilage)
     a. Osteochondroma is the most common and generally involves the femur and tibia. It usually begins in

childhood but may not be diagnosed until adulthood. Males are affected more often than females.

   b. Chondroma, or *endochondroma,* primarily affects the hands, feet, ribs, sternum, spine, and long bones and often causes pathologic fractures after trivial injury. These tumors affect women and men of any age equally.

2. *Osteogenic* (from bone)

   a. *Osteoid osteoma* most often involves the femur and tibia and causes unremitting bone pain. It occurs most often in children and young adults, mostly males.

   b. *Osteoblastoma,* often called the giant osteoid osteoma, affects the vertebrae and long bones. It affects male adolescents and young adults of both sexes.

   c. *Giant cell tumors,* unlike most other benign tumors, affect women older than 20 years of age. These tumors are aggressive and can metastasize to the lung even though the tumors are benign.

COLLABORATIVE MANAGEMENT

Assessment

- Assess for
  1. Severity, nature, and location of pain
  2. Local swelling around the involved area
  3. Muscle spasms or atrophy
  4. Anxiety and fear about diagnosis and surgery

Interventions

- Administer analgesics and nonsteroidal anti-inflammatory drugs (NSAIDs) such as ibuprofen (Motrin).
- Apply heat or cold.
- Curettage, a surgical procedure, is performed to excise the tumor tissue. Bone grafting may be needed.

Tumors, Brain

OVERVIEW

- Brain tumors arise anywhere within the brain structure and are named according to the cell or tissue from which they originate.
- *Primary* tumors originate within the central nervous system (CNS) and occur as a rapid proliferation or abnormal growth of cells normally found within the CNS.
- *Secondary* tumors occur as malignant cells from other tumors outside the CNS, such as the lungs, breast, kidney, or gastrointestinal tract, that metastasize to the brain.
- Complications of brain tumors include cerebral edema, increased intracranial pressure (ICP), focal neurologic deficits, obstruction of the flow of cerebrospinal fluid, and pituitary dysfunction.
- Malignant tumors include
  1. *Gliomas,* which arise from the neuroglial cells and infiltrate and invade surrounding brain tissue. The peak incidence is between 40 and 60 years of age.
     a. *Astrocytoma,* the most common type of glioma, is found anywhere within the cerebral hemispheres.
     b. *Oligodendroglioma,* another type of glioma, is slow growing.
     c. *Glioblastomas* are highly malignant, rapidly growing, invasive astrocytomas.
  2. *Ependymomas,* which arise from the lining of the ventricles and are difficult to treat surgically because of their location
- Benign tumors include
  1. *Meningiomas,* which are highly vascular and arise from the meninges. Although complete removal is possible, they tend to recur.
  2. *Pituitary tumors,* which result in a wide variety of symptoms caused by their effect on the pituitary gland
  3. *Acoustic neuromas,* which arise from the sheath of Schwann cells in the peripheral portion of cranial nerve

VIII. They compress brain tissue and tend to surround adjacent cranial nerves (V, VII, IX, and X).

   a. The remainder of tumors that affect adults are of miscellaneous origin.

   b. Brain tumors in adults are most common in clients between 40 and 60 years of age.

COLLABORATIVE MANAGEMENT

Assessment

- Assess for changes in neurologic status.
   1. Headaches that are usually more severe upon awakening in the morning
   2. Nausea and vomiting
   3. Visual symptoms
   4. Seizures
   5. Changes in mentation or personality
   6. Papilledema (swelling of the optic disk)
- Supratentorial tumors usually result in paralysis, seizures, memory loss, cognitive impairment, language impairment, or visual problems.
- Infratentorial tumors produce ataxia, autonomic nervous system dysfunction, vomiting, drooling, hearing loss, and visual impairment.

Interventions

NONSURGICAL MANAGEMENT

- Treatment depends on tumor size and location, client symptoms and general condition, and whether the tumor is recurrent.
- Drug therapy includes
   1. Analgesic for headache
   2. Dexamethasone (Decadron) to control cerebral edema
   3. Phenytoin (Dilantin) to prevent seizures
   4. Histamine blockers or proton pump inhibitors to prevent stress ulcers
   5. Antiemetics for nausea and vomiting
- Radiation therapy is used alone or in combination with surgery and chemotherapy.

- Chemotherapy may be given alone or in combination with surgery and radiation therapy.
- Chemotherapy may be given intravenously, intra-arterially, or intrathecally.
- Radiosurgical procedures, including the gamma knife, LINAC, and CyberKnife, are alternatives to traditional surgery. The gamma knife employs a single high dose of ionized radiation to destroy intracranial lesions while preserving healthy tissue.

SURGICAL MANAGEMENT

- A craniotomy may be performed, depending on the tumor type, size, and location.
- Provide postoperative care.
    1. Monitor vital signs every 30 to 60 minutes until they are stable.
    2. Monitor neurologic signs every 30 to 60 minutes until they are stable.
    3. Record intake and output every hour; check urine specific gravity every hour or with every voiding.
    4. Implement cardiac monitoring while the client is in the intensive care unit.
    5. Do not position the client on the operative site.
    6. Monitor serum electrolytes, complete blood count (CBC), and osmolarity.
    7. Apply sequential compression stockings or pneumatic compression devices.
    8. Help the client turn, cough, and deep breathe every 2 hours.
    9. Elevate the head of the bed 30 degrees.
    10. Check the head dressing for drainage every 1 to 2 hours.
    11. Measure output from the surgical (Hemovac) drain every 8 hours.
    12. Apply cool compresses to the client's eyes to decrease periorbital edema.
    13. Observe for and report complications of cranial surgery (craniotomy).
        a. ICP: The clinical manifestations include
           (1) Change in level of consciousness, restlessness, or irritability

   (2) Pupils large or pinpoint and nonreactive to light
   (3) Decreased or absent motor movement
   (4) Decerebrate or decorticate posturing
   (5) Seizure activity
   (6) Bradycardia and hypertension with widened pulse pressure
  b. Epidural or subdural hematoma: The clinical manifestations are the same as those for increased ICP, plus
   (1) Severe headache
   (2) Bleeding into the posterior fossa, which may cause cardiac and respiratory arrest
  c. Hydrocephalus: The clinical manifestations are the same as those for increased ICP, plus
   (1) Blurred vision
   (2) Urinary incontinence
  d. Wound infection
   (1) The incision is reddened and puffy.
   (2) The incision may separate.
   (3) The incision is sensitive to touch and feels warm.
   (4) The client may be febrile.
   (5) Treatment is based on the severity of the symptoms.
    (a) Cleanse with alcohol and apply antiseptic ointment.
    (b) Administer systemic antibiotics, as ordered.
  e. Atelectasis, pneumonia
  f. Neurogenic pulmonary edema
  g. Meningitis
  h. Fluid and electrolyte imbalance, including diabetes insipidus and syndrome of inappropriate antidiuretic hormone (SIADH)
   (1) Hypernatremia and increased urinary output are indicative of diabetes insipidus
   (2) Hyponatremia and decreased urinary output are indicative of SIADH

Community-Based Care

- Discharge planning includes
 1. Ensuring that the client understands the importance of follow-up visits

2. Ensuring that the client understands the drug regimen, including the names of medications, dosages, time, route, and side effects
3. Instructing the client to refrain from taking over-the-counter medications unless authorized by the health care provider
4. Ensuring that the client's home is accessible with regard to client's method of mobility
5. Providing a detailed plan of care at the time of discharge for clients to be transferred to a rehabilitation or long-term care facility (rehabilitation may be a lengthy process; see Rehabilitation in Part One)
6. Instructing the client to maintain a program of regular physical exercise within limits of any disabilities
7. Teaching seizure precautions
8. Obtaining a dietary consult to ensure adequate caloric intake for the client receiving radiation or chemotherapy
9. Emphasizing the importance of follow-up visits with the physicians and other therapists
10. Referring the client and family to the American Brain Tumor Association or the National Brain Tumor Association and to the American Cancer Society as a community resource

Tumors, Epithelial Ovarian

- Epithelial ovarian tumors are serous or mucinous cystadenomas that occur in women between 30 and 50 years of age.
- Serous cystadenomas usually occur bilaterally and have greater potential for malignancy than do mucinous cystadenomas.
- Both types of tumors can be irregular and smooth, but mucinous adenomas grow to large sizes (up to 45 kg, or 100 pounds).
- Management includes surgical unilateral salpingo-oophorectomy (surgical removal of a fallopian tube and ovary). Small cystadenomas may be removed by cystectomy.

Tumors, Esophageal

- *Benign* tumors of the esophagus, usually in the form of leiomyomas, are uncommon and usually asymptomatic.
- *Malignant* (cancerous) tumors may develop at any point along the esophagus. They evolve as part of a slow process that begins with benign tissue changes, and they produce widespread disabling effects that are almost always fatal.
- The two types of malignant tumors are
  1. *Squamous epidermoid tumors,* which account for most esophageal cancers and usually develop in the middle third of the esophagus
  2. *Adenocarcinomas,* which develop in the lower third of the esophagus
- Esophageal tumors exhibit rapid local growth and metastatic spread via the lymph nodes.

COLLABORATIVE MANAGEMENT

Assessment

- Record client information.
  1. Alcohol consumption
  2. Tobacco use
  3. History of esophageal disease or problems
  4. Dietary habits and nutritional history
  5. Severe weight loss related to anorexia, dysphagia, or discomfort
  6. Client's racial and cultural background
- Assess for
  1. General physical appearance
  2. Persistent and progressive dysphagia initially associated with swallowing solids, particularly meat, progressing rapidly to difficulty swallowing soft food and liquids
  3. Odynophagia (painful swallowing), reported as a steady, dull, substernal pain, which may radiate
  4. Regurgitation or vomiting
  5. Foul breath

T

6. Chronic hiccups
7. Hoarseness from laryngeal spread
8. Client's response to the diagnosis and prognosis and the client's usual coping strategies
- Assess results of computed tomography scan, barium swallow, and endoscopy, which show the tumor.

Planning and Implementation

◄**NDx:** Imbalanced Nutrition: Less than Body Requirements

NONSURGICAL MANAGEMENT

- Provide nutritional support.
    1. Collaborate with the dietitian to complete a nutritional assessment.
    2. Weigh the client daily at the same time and on the same scale.
    3. Position the client carefully to prevent regurgitation.
    4. Teach the client to remain upright for several hours after meals and to avoid lying flat at any time.
    5. In collaboration with the dietitian, provide soft or semiliquid foods enriched with skim milk powder or commercial protein supplements to maintain adequate nutritional intake.
    6. Monitor ongoing calorie count; provide liquid nutritional supplements as needed.
    7. Provide care for feeding tubes or parenteral nutrition systems that may be required for severe dysphagia.
    8. Consult with the speech-language pathologist to develop an oral exercise program to improve swallowing.
    9. Assist the client to position the head in forward flexion (chin tuck) and place food at the back of the mouth. Check for pocketing of food after the client swallows.
    10. Monitor for signs of aspiration.
- Radiation therapy reduces the size of the tumor and offers consistent short-term relief of symptoms.
- Photodynamic therapy involves the injection of porfimer sodium, a light-sensitive drug that acts to amass cancer cells. Two days after the injection, a fiberoptic probe with a light on the end is threaded into the esophagus. The light activates the photofrin, destroying only the cancer cells.

- Esophageal dilation provides temporary but immediate relief of dysphagia.
- Esophageal dilation may be performed throughout the course of the disease to achieve temporary relief of dysphagia.
- A prosthesis may be inserted to bypass disabling dysphagia and maintain an open esophagus, which preserves the client's ability to take oral nutrition.
- The use of chemotherapy has been only moderately effective and is most often given in combinations with radiation therapy.

SURGICAL MANAGEMENT

- *Esophagectomy* is the removal of all or part of the esophagus.
- *Esophagogastrostomy* involves removal of part of the esophagus and proximal stomach. The remaining stomach may be "pulled up" to take the place of the esophagus, or the jejunum or colon may be used as a conduit.
- Tumors in the upper esophagus may require *radical neck dissection laryngectomy* because of spread to the larynx.
- Tumors that spread to the stomach may require *colon interposition,* which requires removing a section of right or left colon and bringing it up into the thorax to substitute for the esophagus.
- Preoperative care includes
  1. Maintaining nutritional support from 5 days to 2 to 3 weeks before surgery by oral supplements, tube feedings, or parenteral nutrition
  2. Advising the client to quit smoking 2 to 4 weeks before surgery to enhance pulmonary functioning
  3. Monitoring the client's weight, intake and output, and fluid and electrolyte balance
  4. Obtaining a preoperative dental evaluation and any necessary treatment
  5. Teaching the client to perform mouth care four times daily to decrease the risk of postoperative infection
  6. Providing routine preoperative care and teaching
  7. Teaching the client about the incisions, wound drainage tubes, chest tubes, nasogastric (NG) tubes, and intravenous (IV) lines

T

8. Encouraging the client and family to talk about personal feelings and fears
- Postoperative care includes
  1. Assessing the client's respiratory status
  2. Once the client is extubated, implementing deep breathing, turning, and cough routines; implementing chest physiotherapy and incentive spirometer every 4 hours
  3. Maintaining the client in a semi-Fowler's position to support ventilation and prevent reflux
  4. Administering antibiotics as prescribed
  5. Administering supplemental oxygen
  6. Ensuring patency of the chest tube water-seal drainage system
  7. Monitoring for signs of fluid overload, particularly in older clients and those who have undergone lymph node dissection
  8. Providing support of the multiple surgical incisions during turning and activity
  9. Assessing for fever, fluid accumulation, general signs of inflammation, and symptoms of early shock, which could be indicative of anastomosis leakage
  10. Avoiding manipulation and irrigation of the surgically placed NG tube
  11. Providing meticulous mouth care while the NG tube is in place
  12. Maintaining nothing by mouth (NPO) status until gastrointestinal motility is established (usually 3 to 5 days)
  13. Administering IV fluids and parenteral nutrition
  14. Slowly increasing jejunostomy feeding over several days; discontinuing when client is taking adequate oral nutrition
  15. Slowly progressing the client's diet to pureed and semisolid foods
  16. Emphasizing the importance of eating small meals and maintaining an upright position during eating

Community-Based Care

- Provide discharge teaching, including
  1. Instruction on respiratory care, ambulation, splint incisions, incentive spirometer, and reporting symptoms of respiratory infection to the physician immediately

2. Encouraging the client to be as active as possible and to avoid excessive bedrest
3. Inspection of the incision for redness, tenderness, swelling, and drainage
4. The signs of anastomosis leakage and the importance of reporting them immediately to the surgeon
- Reinforce dietary instructions, including
  1. Increasing dietary intake to include high-calorie, high-protein meals that contain soft and easily swallowed foods; small and frequent meals
  2. The importance of eating six to eight small meals per day and to drink fluid between meals rather than with meals to prevent diarrhea
  3. Care for tube feedings and parenteral nutrition, which may be necessary (This requires intensive teaching for the client and caretakers.)
  4. Maintaining an upright position after eating, and elevating the head of the bed
  5. Monitoring weight daily
- Refer the client and family to the appropriate community or home health care organizations, including the American Cancer Society and area hospice services.

Tumors, Spinal Cord

OVERVIEW

- Spinal cord tumors occur most often in the thoracic region, followed by an almost equal distribution in the lumbar and cervical regions.
- Signs and symptoms depend on the location of the tumor and on the speed of growth.
- Primary spinal cord tumors arise from the epidural vessels, spinal meninges, or glial cells of the cord.
- Secondary tumors develop as metastases from the lungs, breasts, kidney, and gastrointestinal tract.

COLLABORATIVE MANAGEMENT

- Assess for
  1. Pain
     a. Quality
     b. Severity
     c. Intensity
     d. Factors that exacerbate and relieve pain
  2. Motor deficits
     a. Weakness or paralysis
     b. Clumsiness
     c. Spasticity
     d. Hyperactive reflexes
  3. Sensory loss
     a. Slowly progressive numbness, tingling, or temperature loss
     b. Decreased appreciation of touch
     c. Inability to sense vibration and loss of position sense
  4. Loss of bowel and bladder control
  5. High cervical manifestation
     a. Respiratory distress
     b. Diaphragm paralysis
     c. Quadriparesis
     d. Stiff neck
     e. Nystagmus
     f. Cranial nerve dysfunction
  6. Abnormal spine x-ray, computed tomography (CT) scan, or magnetic resonance imaging (MRI) results
- Treatment of a spinal cord tumor includes
  1. Surgical removal of as much of the tumor as possible
  2. Radiation therapy
  3. Chemotherapy
- Postoperative care is the same as discussed under back pain surgery, laminectomy.
  1. Vital signs and neurologic checks
  2. Pain control
  3. Prevention of complications of immobility
  4. Development of a bowel and bladder program if necessary

Community-Based Care

- The client may be discharged to a rehabilitation setting or home.
- The teaching plan depends on the level of dysfunction present.
- Refer the client and family to local, state or providence, and national organizations for people with spinal cord injuries that are applicable to spinal cord tumors.
- Refer the client with a malignant tumor to the American Cancer Society.

Ulcers, Peptic

OVERVIEW

- Peptic ulcer disease (PUD) is a mucosal lesion of the stomach or duodenum and results when gastric mucosal defenses become impaired and no longer protect the epithelium from the effects of hydrochloric acid and pepsin.
- Certain drugs, caffeine, smoking, alcohol, radiation, and increased stress contribute to PUD; *Helicobacter pylori* is the most common infectious agent causing PUD.
- Types of peptic ulcers include
  1. *Gastric ulcer,* which occurs when there is a break in the mucosal barrier and hydrochloric acid injures the epithelium. Gastric emptying is delayed, causing regurgitation of duodenal contents. Gastric ulcers are deep and penetrating, and usually occur on the lesser curvature of the stomach near the pylorus.
  2. *Duodenal ulcer,* a chronic break in the duodenal mucosa extending through the muscularis mucosa that leaves a scar with healing. It is characterized by high gastric acid secretion (the most common type of peptic ulcer). Most clients with duodenal ulcers have confirmed *H. pylori* infection.
  3. *Stress ulcer,* which occurs after an acute medical crisis or trauma. Bleeding resulting from gastric erosion is the principal manifestation and multiple lesions occur in the

U

proximal portion of the stomach, beginning with the area of ischemia and evolving into erosions.

- Complications of ulcers include
  1. Hemorrhage
     a. Ulcer bleeding varies from minimal to massive hematemesis, which usually indicates bleeding at the duodenojejunal junction.
     b. Melena is more common in duodenal ulcers than in other types.
     c. Hemorrhage tends to occur most often in clients with gastric ulcers and in older adults.
  2. *Perforation*, with the gastroduodenal contents emptying through the anterior wall of the stomach or duodenum into the peritoneal cavity
     a. A sudden, sharp pain begins in the midepigastric region and spreads over the entire abdomen.
     b. The client may become critically ill in a matter of hours.
  3. Pyloric obstruction
     a. The obstruction occurs at the pylorus.
     b. The cause is scarring, edema, and inflammation, causing abdominal bloating, nausea, and vomiting.
  4. Intractable disease
     a. Pain and discomfort recur.
     b. The client no longer responds to conservative management.
     c. Symptoms interfere with activities of daily living (ADLs).

COLLABORATIVE MANAGEMENT

Assessment

- Record client information.
  1. Tobacco use
  2. Dietary intake, including alcohol, caffeine, other irritants, and patterns of eating
  3. Past medical history focusing on gastrointestinal problems
  4. Prescribed and over-the-counter medication such as corticosteroids and anti-inflammatory agents
  5. Lifestyle, including actual and perceived stress
  6. Symptoms, including epigastric discomfort, abdominal tenderness, cramps, indigestion, nausea, or vomiting and

their onset, duration, location, and frequency, as well as aggravating and alleviating factors
- Assess for
  1. Epigastric tenderness; rigid, boardlike abdomen accompanied by rebound tenderness (if perforation occurred)
  2. Effect of eating on pain. Gastric ulcer pain may be relieved by food; duodenal ulcer pain occurs 90 minutes to 3 hours after eating and often awakens the client at night.
  3. Dyspepsia
  4. Melena, especially in older adults
  5. Vomiting
  6. Orthostatic vital signs
  7. Deficient fluid volume
  8. Dizziness
  9. Low hemoglobin and hematocrit counts
  10. Results of esophagogastroduodenoscopy (EGD), which visualizes the ulcer
  11. Family and individual stressors and the client's usual patterns of coping and problem solving
  12. Impact of chronic disease on the client
  13. Results of esophagogastroduodenoscopy and *H. pylori* testing

 Considerations for Older Adults

- The older adult may use over-the-counter remedies to treat symptoms, often delaying appropriate treatment for PUD.
- Ulcer-producing drugs for chronic illnesses are often consumed by older adults.
- The older adult maybe at increased risk for complications and death following acute peptic ulcer bleeding.

Planning and Implementation

NDx: Acute Pain

- Perform a comprehensive pain assessment. Carefully assess changes in the characteristic of location or peptic ulcer pain because this may indicate the development of complications.
- Drug therapy includes
  1. Triple therapy consisting of bismuth compound or a proton pump inhibitor and a combination of two antibiotics

2. Antisecretory agents, also called proton pump inhibitors
3. H_2-receptor antagonists to inhibit gastric acid secretion
4. Prostaglandin analogues to inhibit acid secretion and contribute to the mucosal barrier
5. Antacids as buffering agents to decrease pain (given 2 hours after meals)
6. Mucosal barrier fortifiers to provide a protective coat, preventing digestive action
7. *H. pylori* infection treatment with "triple therapy" of bismuth compound, metronidazole, and either amoxicillin or tetracycline; some strains of *H. pylori* have demonstrated resistance to metronidazole, raising concerns about long-term treatment with this regimen.

■ There is no evidence that dietary restrictions reduce gastric acid secretion or promote tissue healing. When diet therapy is used, teach the client to
1. Avoid caffeine-containing coffee, tea, and cola and other foods that cause discomfort.
2. Avoid alcohol and tobacco.
3. Eat a bland diet with nonirritating foods during the acute phase.

◆**NDx:** Risk for Deficient Fluid Volume

■ The client is at risk for fluid volume deficit from vomiting and from blood loss due to hemorrhage or perforation.
■ Management of hypovolemia includes
1. Monitoring vital signs
2. Monitoring for fluid loss from bleeding or vomiting
3. Maintaining strict intake and output
4. Monitoring serum electrolytes and hematocrit and hemoglobin
5. Inserting two large-bore peripheral intravenous (IV) catheters
6. Replacing fluids with IV fluids such as normal saline or lactated Ringer's solution
7. Ordering blood products
■ Management of hemorrhage includes
1. Monitoring for sign and symptoms indicating gastrointestinal (GI) bleeding and documenting findings
   a. Observe secretions (emesis, sputum, stool, urine, and nasogastric drainage) for frank or occult blood.

    b. Document color, amount, and character of stools.

    c. Monitor hematocrit, hemoglobin, and coagulation studies for changes from baseline.

2. Inserting a nasogastric (NG) tube to ascertain the presence of blood in the stomach, assess the rate of bleeding, prevent gastric dilation, and provide lavage; irrigating the NG tube to maintain patency and prevent obstruction with blood

3. Instructing the client and family on the need for blood replacement, as necessary. Blood loss of more than 1 L/24 hr may cause signs and symptoms of shock.

    a. Hypotension

    b. Chills, diaphoresis

    c. Palpitations

4. Administering medications such as H_2 blockers, proton pump inhibitors as ordered

- Treatment measures include

  1. Esophagogastroduodenoscopy to identify bleeding sites
  2. Saline lavage
  3. Injection of the bleeding site with diluted epinephrine
  4. Laser photocoagulation
  5. Heater probe therapy
  6. Electrocoagulation through an endoscope

- Treatment of perforation includes the immediate replacement of fluid, blood, and electrolytes.

  1. Maintain nasogastric suction to drain gastric secretions.
  2. Keep the client on nothing by mouth (NPO) status and monitor intake and output carefully.
  3. Check the client's vital signs at least once hourly.
  4. Monitor the client for septic shock.

- Pyloric obstruction is caused by edema, spasm, or scar tissue and is manifested by feelings of fullness, distention, or nausea after eating, as well as vomiting copious amounts of undigested food.

- Treatment of pyloric obstruction is directed toward restoring fluid and electrolyte balance, decompressing the dilated stomach, and, if necessary, surgical interventions.

Surgical Management

- Simple *gastroenterostomy* permits neutralization of gastric acid by regurgitation of alkaline duodenal contents into the stomach. A passageway is created between the body of the stomach and the small bowel, often the jejunum.

- A *vagotomy* eliminates the acid-secreting stimulus to gastric cells and decreases the responsiveness of parietal cells. The three types of vagotomy procedures are

  1. *Truncal,* in which each branch of the vagus nerve may be completely cut and the antrum removed. The remaining stomach is anastomosed to the proximal duodenum.
  2. *Selective,* in which only the branches of the vagus nerve that supply the stomach are cut. The remaining abdominal viscera still has intact vagal innervation.
  3. *Proximal gastric,* which interrupts the nerve supply to only the acid-secreting portion of the stomach. It spares the branches of the vagus nerve that innervate the antrum, making pyloroplasty unnecessary.

- A *vagotomy with pyloroplasty* involves cutting the right and left branches of the vagus nerve and widening the pyloric sphincter to prevent stasis and to enhance emptying of the stomach.

- In clients with *perforation,* surgery entails closure of the perforation after the escaped gastric contents have been evacuated.

- Postoperative care includes

  1. Providing routine postoperative care
  2. Providing pain management
  3. Monitoring the patency of the NG tube and the type of drainage
  4. Not repositioning or irrigating the NG tube
  5. Assessing for fluid and electrolyte imbalances
  6. Assessing for the development of *acute gastric dilation,* in the immediate postoperative period, which is manifested by
     a. Epigastric pain
     b. Tachycardia
     c. Hypotension
     d. Feelings of fullness or hiccups
  7. Assessing for the development of the *dumping syndrome,* which occurs after gastric resection in which the pylorus is bypassed. This postprandial problem is associated with the rapid entry of food into the bowel, which is manifested by

a. Vertigo
b. Tachycardia
c. Syncope
d. Sweating
e. Pallor
f. Palpitations
g. Lightheadedness
h. Epigastric fullness

8. Assisting in the management of the dumping syndrome by
   a. Decreasing the amount of food taken by the client at one time
   b. Providing a high-protein, high-fat, low-carbohydrate diet
   c. Administering pectin in a dry powder form
   d. Placing the client in a recumbent or semirecumbent position during eating
   e. Positioning the client in a flat position after meals
   f. Administering sedatives and antispasmodics, as ordered, to delay gastric emptying

9. Assessing for the occurrence of *alkaline reflux gastritis*, which is the reflux of duodenal contents with bile acids, resulting in injury to the gastric mucosal barrier and manifested by
   a. Abdominal discomfort
   b. Early satiety
   c. Vomiting

10. Assessing for *delayed gastric emptying*, often present after gastric surgery, usually resolving within 1 week, and usually resulting from
    a. Mechanical causes, such as edema at the anastomosis or adhesions obstructing the distal loop
    b. Metabolic causes, such as hypokalemia, hypoproteinemia, or hyponatremia

11. Assessing for development of *afferent loop syndrome*, which occurs when the duodenal loop is partially obstructed after a Billroth II resection, by monitoring for
    a. Painful contractions
    b. Vomiting
    c. Abdominal bloating

U

12. Administering vitamin B_{12}, folic acid, and iron preparations to prevent problems of nutrition that develop from removal of the stomach, including deficiencies of vitamin B_{12}, folic acid, and iron; impaired calcium metabolism; and reduced absorption of calcium and vitamin D

- *Recurrent ulcer* can be due to incomplete vagotomy or persistent *H. pylori* infection.

Community-Based Care

- Discharge planning includes
   1. Collaborating with the client and family to identify gastric irritants and lifestyle stressors and to develop strategies to make lifestyle changes
   2. Instructing the client on symptoms that should be brought to the attention of the health care provider
      a. Abdominal pain
      b. Nausea and vomiting
      c. Black, tarry stools
      d. Weakness and dizziness
   3. Teaching relaxation techniques to increase coping skills and decrease ulcer recurrence
   4. Instructing the client to avoid over-the-counter products containing aspirin or ibuprofen
   5. Teaching dietary management to the postsurgical client, especially the client who had a partial stomach removal. Teach the client to
      a. Eat small, frequent meals.
      b. Avoid drinking liquids with meals.
      c. Abstain from foods that contribute to discomfort.
      d. Eliminate caffeine and alcohol consumption.
      e. Begin a smoking cessation program.
      f. Receive vitamin B_{12} injections as appropriate.

Urethritis

- Urethritis is inflammation of the urethra.
- Symptoms of urethritis in the *male* client are
  1. Burning on urination
  2. Difficult urination
  3. Discharge from the urethral meatus
- Symptoms of urethritis in the *female* client are
  1. Bacterial cystitis (mimics)
  2. Painful urination
  3. Difficulty with urination
  4. Lower abdomen discomfort
  5. Pyuria
- The most common cause of urethritis in males is sexually transmitted disease.
- In postmenopausal women, urethritis is probably caused by tissue changes related to low estrogen and is treated with estrogen vaginal cream.
- Nonspecific urethritis may be caused by *Ureaplasma*, chlamydia, or *Trichomonas vaginalis.*
- Sexually transmitted diseases and infectious processes are treated with appropriate antibiotic therapy.

Urolithiasis

U

OVERVIEW

- Urolithiasis is the presence of calculi (stones) in the urinary tract. The exact mechanism of formation is not known.
- A supersaturation of urinary filtrate with a particular element is believed to be the primary factor contributing to calculi formation.
- Other factors include the acidity or alkalinity of the urine, urinary stasis, and other substances, such as pyrophosphate, magnesium, and citrate.

- Calculi may be formed from calcium, phosphate, oxalate, uric acid, struvite, and cystine crystals, with most stones containing calcium as one component.
- *Nephrolithiasis* refers to calculi formed in the kidney; formation of calculi in the ureter is referred to as *ureterolithiasis.* An enlargement of the ureter is called *hydroureter.*

▐▐▐ Cultural Considerations

- There is an increased incidence of urolithiasis in the southeastern United States and a rising incidence in Japan and Western Europe.
- Urolithiasis is more common in men than in women and tends to occur in young adulthood or early middle adulthood.

COLLABORATIVE MANAGEMENT

Assessment

- Record client information.
  1. History of renal stones
  2. Family history of renal stones
  3. Diet history
  4. Previous interventions to eliminate stones
- Assess for
  1. Renal colic (severe unbearable pain); location and duration of pain
  2. Nausea and vomiting
  3. Hematuria, oliguria, or anuria
  4. Flank pain
  5. Ureteral spasm or colic
  6. Increased turbidity and odor of urine
  7. Bladder distention
  8. Diaphoresis
  9. Pale, ashen skin
  10. Presence of red blood cells, white blood cells, and bacteria in the urine

Planning and Implementation

NDx: Acute Pain

NONSURGICAL MANAGEMENT

- Drug therapy includes

1. Opioid agents, such as morphine sulfate
2. Nonsteroidal anti-inflammatory drugs (NSAIDs) such as ketorolac (Toradol)
3. Spasmolytic agents, such as oxybutynin chloride (Ditropan) and propantheline bromide (Pro-Banthine, Propanthel ✱)

- Assess the client's response to drug interventions.
- Assist the client to find a comfortable position and to use relaxation techniques.
- Relaxation techniques such as hypnosis, imagery, or acupuncture can be used to relieve pain.
- Lithotripsy or extracorporeal shock wave lithotripsy (ESWL) is the application of ultrasound or dry shock wave energies to fragment the calculus. The client receives conscious sedation as the lithotriptor and fluoroscope locate and break up the calculus.

SURGICAL MANAGEMENT

- Stone removal procedures include
    1. *Ureteroscopy,* the use of an endoscope through the urethra to visualize stones and to extract stones with a basket, or the use of a laser to fragment stones. Stents may be used to dilate the ureter and create a passageway for the stone.
    2. *Percutaneous uretero and nephrolithotomy,* the use of an endoscope to visualize the stone with a special attachment to extract the calculus (through a small flank incision)
    3. *Laparoscopic ureterolithotomy,* the use of a laparoscope through the ureter to remove the calculus
    4. *Pyelolithotomy,* direct visualization of the renal pelvis through a large flank incision and removal of the stone
    5. *Nephrolithotomy,* direct visualization of the kidney through a large flank incision and removal of the stone
    6. *Ureterolithotomy,* direct visualization of the ureter through a large flank or lower abdominal incision and removal of the stone
- Preoperative care includes
    1. Providing routine preoperative care
    2. Providing individualized instructions dependent on the procedure to be performed
    3. Preparing bowel per physician preference

U

- Postoperative care includes
  1. Providing routine postoperative care
  2. Monitoring the amount of bleeding from the incisions
  3. Monitoring the client for hematuria
  4. Recording and monitoring urinary output
  5. Straining the client's urine
  6. Encouraging ambulation to promote calculi passage
- Infection prevention includes
  1. Monitoring for signs of infection (fever, chills, altered mental status)
  2. Obtaining urine culture and sensitivity as ordered
  3. Administering antibiotics to eliminate existing infections or prevent new ones
  4. Ensuring adequate nutrition and fluid intake
- Drug therapy includes
  1. Broad-spectrum antibiotics such as aminoglycosides and cephalosporins, and monitoring blood levels depending on antibiotic prescribed
  2. Acetohydroxamic acid (Lithostat) and hydroxyurea (Hydrea) for clients with struvite stones; monitoring serum creatinine (contraindicated for levels above 2 mg/dL)
  3. Thiazide diuretics to treat hypercalciuria (high levels of calcium in the urine)
  4. Allopurinol (Zyloprim) to treat hyperoxaluria (high levels of oxalic acid in the urine) or gout
  5. Alpha-mercaptopropionylglycine (AMPG) and captopril (Capoten) to treat cystinuria (high levels of cystine in the urine)
- Assess for side effects or adverse drug reactions.
- Diet therapy includes
  1. Ensuring adequate caloric intake representing a balance of all food groups
  2. Encouraging fluid intake of 2 to 3 L per day
  3. Limiting calcium intake for calcium stones
  4. Limiting dark green foods such as spinach because oxalate increases as calcium decreases
  5. Reducing purine intake (sources include boned fish and organ meats) for clients with uric acid stones
- Additional diet therapy depends on the type of stone.

- Discharge planning includes
  1. Providing postoperative care instructions, including
     a. Keeping the incision dry
     b. Showering instead of bathing
     c. Monitoring the incision for redness, swelling, and drainage
  2. Informing the client that
     a. Extensive bruising may occur after lithotripsy and may take several weeks to resolve
     b. Urine may be bloody for several days after surgical intervention
  3. Instructing the client on
     a. The importance of finishing all medications
     b. The importance of balancing regular exercise with rest
     c. Diet, depending on stone type
     d. The rationale for preventing dehydration and promoting urine flow; stress the importance of continued adequate fluid intake
     e. The importance of reporting symptoms of recurrent infection or formation of another stone, such as pain, fever, chills, and difficulty with urination
     f. The importance of keeping follow-up appointments to check on infection, have repeat cultures done, and the like

Uveitis

U

OVERVIEW

- *Uveitis* is a general term for inflammatory diseases of the uveal tract of the eye.
- Anterior uveitis
  1. Includes an inflammation of the iris, an inflammation of the ciliary body, or both
  2. Is manifested by moderate periorbital aching, tearing, blurred vision, and photophobia; small, irregularly shaped, nonreactive pupil; purplish discoloration of the cornea;

and an accumulation of purulent material in the anterior chamber
- Posterior uveitis
    1. Includes retinitis, an inflammation of the retina, and chorioretinitis, an inflammation of both the retina and choroid
    2. Is manifested by slow, insidious onset of symptoms, including visual impairment; small, irregularly shaped, nonreactive pupil; and vitreous opacities that are seen as black dots against the background of the fundus

COLLABORATIVE MANAGEMENT

- Treatment is based on symptoms.
    1. Cycloplegic agents to put the ciliary body to rest; instruct the client not to drive or operate machinery because of blurred vision
    2. Steroid drops to decrease inflammation
    3. Analgesics for pain
    4. Antibiotics for posterior uveitis
    5. Warm or cool compresses
    6. Darkened room, sunglasses
- Teach the client the signs and symptoms of increased intraocular pressure.

Vaginitis

OVERVIEW

- Vaginitis is an inflammation of the lower genital tract.
- Vaginitis develops when there is a disturbance of hormone balance and bacterial interaction in the vagina as a result of menopause, sexually transmitted diseases, fungal (yeast) infections, changes in normal flora, an alkaline pH level, insertion of foreign objects such as tampons or condoms, use of chemical irritants such as douches or sprays, use of medications, especially antibiotics; and health problems such as diabetes.

- Record client information.
  1. Onset of symptoms
  2. Characteristics and color of discharge
  3. Odor of discharge
  4. Associated symptoms such as itching and dysuria
  5. Type of contraceptive used
  6. Recent antibiotic use
  7. Sexual activity
  8. History of previous vaginal infections
  9. Hygiene practices, such as douching and tampon use
- Physical examination includes
  1. Abdominal palpation for tenderness and pain
  2. External genitalia inspection for erythema, edema, excoriation, odor, and discharge
  3. Vaginal examination to note the source of the discharge and inflammation
- Interventions include special hygiene practices, including
  1. Cleaning the perineum from front to back after urination and defecation
  2. Wearing cotton underwear
  3. Avoiding strong douches and feminine hygiene sprays
  4. Avoiding tight-fitting pants
  5. Using estrogen creams as prescribed
- Health teaching focuses on preventive measures and information on infection transmission.

Veins, Varicose

V

OVERVIEW

- Varicose veins are distended, protruding veins that appear darkened or tortuous.
- The vein walls weaken and dilate. Venous pressure increases, and the valves become incompetent.
- Incompetent valves enhance vessel dilation, and veins become tortuous and distended.

- Varicose veins occur primarily in clients subjected to prolonged standing. They also occur in pregnant women and in clients with systemic problems such as heart disease, obesity, and a family history of varicose veins.

COLLABORATIVE MANAGEMENT

- Assess for
  1. Pain after standing
  2. Fullness in the legs
  3. Distended, protruding veins
- The Trendelenburg test assists in diagnosis. As the client sits up from a supine position with legs elevated, varicose veins fill from the proximal end rather than from the normal distal end.
- Conservative treatment measures include
  1. Wearing elastic stockings
  2. Elevating the extremities as often as possible
  3. Sclerotherapy, in which the physician injects a chemical to sclerose the vein, performed on small or a limited number of varicosities
- Surgical intervention entails *ligation* (tying) and *stripping* (removal) of the affected veins under general anesthesia.
- Postoperative care includes
  1. Assessing the groin and entire leg through the elastic (Ace) bandage dressing for bleeding
  2. Instructing the client to keep the legs elevated and to perform range-of-motion (ROM) exercises
  3. Discharging the client to the home, as ordered, by the first postoperative day and instructing the client to
     a. Continue wearing elastic stockings.
     b. Exercise by walking.
     c. Limit sitting for long intervals, and keep the legs elevated when seated.
     d. Avoid standing in one place.
- RF (radio frequency) energy involves heating the vein from the inside by the RF energy and shrinking the vein. Collateral veins take over.
- EndoVenous Laser treatment uses a laser fiber to heat and close the main vessel that is contributing to the varicosity.

Venous Disease, Peripheral

OVERVIEW

- Peripheral venous disease (PVD) is a group of diseases that alter the natural flow of blood through the veins of the peripheral circulation.
- Veins must be patent and have functioning valves.
- Venous blood flow may be altered by thrombus formation and defective valves.
- *Venous thromboembolism* includes both thrombus and embolus complications.
- Thrombus formation has been associated with stasis of blood flow, endothelial injury, and hypercoagulability (Virchow's triad).
- A *thrombus* (blood clot) results from an endothelial injury, venous stasis, or hypercoagulability.
- *Thrombophlebitis* occurs when a thrombus is associated with inflammation in superficial veins.
- *Phlebothrombosis* is the presence of a thrombus without inflammation.
- *Deep venous* thrombophlebitis, commonly referred to as *deep vein thrombosis* (DVT), usually occurs in the deep veins of the lower extremities and presents a major risk for pulmonary embolism. Risk factors include hip or open prostate surgeries. Other conditions that seem to promote thrombus formation are heart failure, immobility, pregnancy, and ulcerative colitis.
- *Phlebitis*, vein inflammation, is associated with invasive procedures such as intravenous (IV) therapy and can predispose clients to thrombosis.
- *Venous insufficiency* occurs from prolonged venous hypertension, which stretches the veins and damages valves, resulting in venous stasis ulcers with swelling and cellulitis.

COLLABORATIVE MANAGEMENT

Assessment

- For the client with DVT, assess for
  1. Calf or groin tenderness and pain

2. Unilateral swelling of the leg
3. Warmth and edema of the extremity
4. Induration along the blood vessel
5. Size comparison with the contralateral limb
6. Localized pitting edema
- For the client with venous insufficiency, assess for
  1. Discoloration along the ankles, extending up to the calf
  2. Ulcer formation
     a. Arterial ulcers develop on the toes, between the toes, or on the upper aspect of the foot; they are painful.
     b. Diabetic ulcers develop on the plantar surface of the foot, over metatarsal heads, or on the heel and pressure areas; they may not be painful.
     c. Venous stasis ulcers occur at the ankles; minimal pain is present.
- Diagnostic test for DVT include
  1. Contrast venography
  2. Duplex ultrasonography
  3. Doppler flow studies
  4. Impedance plethysmography

Interventions

- For DVT, interventions include
  1. Preventing pulmonary emboli and an increase in the size of the thrombus
  2. Bedrest and elevation of the extremity
  3. Applying warm, moist soaks to the affected area
  4. Administering anticoagulants such as heparin and warfarin (Coumadin), unfractionated heparin therapy, or low–molecular weight heparin
- Thrombolytic therapy may be effective for dissolving the thrombus.
- To prevent DVT, the following actions may be taken:
  1. Low–molecular weight heparin (enoxaparin), dextran, dihydroergotamine (DHE), or aspirin may be prescribed.
  2. Client may be ambulated and mobilized early, and a thigh-high graduated compression elastic stocking and external intermittent or sequential compression devices may be used.
- Elevate the client's legs when in bed or in a chair to prevent peripheral edema.

- For venous insufficiency, interventions include
    1. Having the client wear elastic or compression stockings during the day and evening
    2. Teaching the client to elevate his or her legs for 20 minutes four or five times a day and to avoid long periods of sitting or standing in place
    3. Teaching the client to use a sequential gradient compression device, if ordered
    4. Treating open venous ulcers with occlusive dressings and topical agents, with or without antibiotics to chemically debride the ulcer
    5. If the client is ambulatory, using an Unna boot
- Surgical management of DVT includes a thrombectomy, inferior vena caval interruption or ligation, and insertion of external clips in the inferior vena cava.

Community-Based Care

- Clients recovering from venous disease are usually discharged from the hospital on a regimen of warfarin.

Considerations for Older Adults

- Warfarin is used with caution in older or debilitated clients to prevent bleeding.
- A reduced dose may be used to prevent spontaneous intracranial bleeding or excessive bleeding related to trauma.
- Older adults may have reduced liver or kidney function and a decreased ability to metabolize and excrete warfarin.

- Teach anticoagulation instructions to the client and family.
    1. Avoid potential trauma.
    2. Observe and report signs and symptoms of bleeding.
        a. Hematuria
        b. Frank or occult blood in the stool
        c. Ecchymoses
        d. Petechiae
        e. Altered level of consciousness
        f. Pain
    3. Apply direct pressure to bleeding sites.
    4. Seek medical assistance immediately if bleeding occurs.
    5. Wear a medical alert bracelet or necklace and carry a medical alert card at all times.

V

6. Inform other health care providers, such as dentists, about the therapy.
7. Avoid other medications unless prescribed by the same physician.
8. Avoid high-fat and vitamin K–rich foods.
9. Have routine monitoring of prothrombin time or international normalized ratio (INR) levels.

- Teach the client with chronic venous status to
  1. Avoid standing still or sitting for long periods.
  2. Avoid crossing the legs when sitting.
  3. Avoid constrictive garments.
  4. Wear support hose or antiembolism stockings, if prescribed.
  5. Follow the prescribed exercise program.
  6. Follow the prescribed weight reduction plan, if needed.
  7. Follow written and oral foot care instructions (see Continuing Care under Arterial Disease, Peripheral).

- The client may need referral to other health care providers for emotional support and to cope with necessary lifestyle adjustments.

Vulvitis

OVERVIEW

- Vulvitis is an inflammatory condition of the vulva associated with pruritus (itching) and a burning sensation.
- The vulvar skin is sensitive to hormonal, metabolic, and allergic influences. Symptoms can be caused by systemic conditions, by direct contact with an irritant, or by extension of infections from the vagina.
- The most common skin disease affecting the vulva is contact dermatitis caused by irritants such as feminine hygiene sprays, fabric dyes, soaps and detergents, and allergens.
- Primary infections affecting the vulva include herpes genitalis and condyloma acuminatum (venereal warts).
- Secondary infections are caused by organisms responsible for vaginitis, including candidiasis.
- Common parasitic infections include pediculosis pubis (crab lice) and scabies (itch mites).

- Other causes include atrophic vaginitis, vulvar kraurosis (a postmenopausal disorder causing dryness and atrophy), vulvar leukoplakia (postmenopausal atrophy and thickening of vulvar tissue), cancer, and urinary incontinence.

COLLABORATIVE MANAGEMENT

- Assess for
  1. Itching
  2. Burning sensation
  3. Erythema, edema, and superficial skin ulcerations
  4. White and thickened vulvar tissue
  5. Dry and scaly skin
- Treatment depends on the cause and includes
  1. Antibiotics
  2. Removal of irritants or allergens
  3. Treatment for pediculosis and scabies
  4. Interventions to relieve itching, such as warm compresses, sitz baths, and topical steroids
  5. If vulvitis is chronic or severe, laser therapy or "skinning vulvectomy"
- Health teaching focuses on preventive measures.

Warts

- Warts, or verrucae, are small tumors caused by infection of the keratinocytes with papillomavirus.
- Warts occur singly or in groups.
- *Common warts* are raised, flesh-colored papules with a rough, hyperkeratotic surface, commonly occurring on the hands and fingers.
- *Flat warts* appear as elevated reddish-brown or flesh-colored papules with flat tops and minimal scale.
- *Plantar warts* are painful warts occurring on the bottom of the foot and are usually covered with thick callus.
- Wart treatment, aimed at destroying keratinocytes containing the virus, includes
  1. Cryosurgery (preferred)

W

2. Surgical excision
3. Electrodesiccation and curettage
4. Topical caustic agents

West Nile Virus

- West Nile virus is an arbovirus that typically affects animals, especially birds.
- The incubation period is 3-12 days after being bitten by an infected mosquito. Other sources of transmission include blood products, breast milk, or transplanted organs.
- The virus primarily affects older adults and those with weakened immune systems and can result in long-term residual fatigue and weakness, as well as death.
- Symptoms are mild and include fever, headache, body aches, skin rash, and swollen lymph glands.
- Severe symptoms include severe headache, high fever, stiff neck, stupor, disorientation, convulsions, and paralysis.
- Immediate medical attention is needed.
- Treatment is symptomatic.
- Prevention measures include
  1. Repairing or replacing screens in home
  2. Removing all sources of standing water outdoors
  3. Wearing long-sleeved shirts and long pants when outdoors; spraying clothing with insect repellent
  4. Staying indoors at dawn and dusk, when mosquitos are most active

APPENDIXES

Guide to Head-to-Toe Physical Assessment of Adults

GUIDE TO HEAD-TO-TOE PHYSICAL ASSESSMENT OF ADULTS*

Nursing Activity	Typical Finding	Changes Associated with Aging
NEUROLOGIC SYSTEM		
1. Determine level of consciousness.	1. Alert	1. None
2. Test for orientation.	2. Oriented	2. None
SKIN		
1. Inspect skin during each part of assessment.	1. Intact, warm, dry, elastic skin	1. Excessive dryness; presence of wrinkles; presence of "age spots" and hemangiomas; inelastic, sagging skin
2. Test for orientation.	2. No lesions	2. Presence of ecchymotic areas as a result of increased capillary fragility
HEAD AND FACE		
1. Inspect and palpate the scalp, hair, and skull.	1. No lesions, shiny hair	1. Thinning and dullness of hair
2. Inspect face for symmetry of expression.	2. Symmetric expression	2. None
3. Palpate the temporal arteries.	3. Faint pulsation	3. None
4. Palpate TMJs.	4. No tenderness	4. Possible tenderness or crepitus

EYE

1. Inspect the external eye structures.	1. No structural abnormalities	1. Presence of an entropion (inverted eyelid) or ectropion (everted eyelid)
2. Inspect the conjunctivae, sclerae, corneas, and irides.	2. No abnormalities; round irides	2. None
3. Use a penlight to test pupillary response (direct and consensual).	3. Pupils are equal and round and react to light and accommodation	3. None
4. Test vision by asking the client to read (if able). NOTE: Be sure that glasses or contact lenses are in place, if used.	4. No vision impairment	4. Presence of presbyopia (farsightedness)

ICS, intercostal space; *JVD*, jugular venous distention; *MCL*, midclavicular line; *PMI*, point of maximal impulse; *ROM*, range of motion; *TMJ*, temporomandibular joint.

*Additional assessments may be needed, depending on the client's concerns and the medical diagnoses. For more information on physical assessment, see Ignatavicius DD, Workman ML. (2005). *Medical-surgical nursing: critical thinking for collaborative care*, 5th ed., Philadelphia: W.B. Saunders.

Continued

GUIDE TO HEAD-TO-TOE PHYSICAL ASSESSMENT OF ADULTS—cont'd

Nursing Activity	Typical Finding	Changes Associated with Aging
EAR		
1. Inspect the external structure.	1. No structural abnormalities	1. No major change
2. Inspect the auditory meatus for drainage.	2. No drainage; small amount of cerumen may be present	2. None
3. Test hearing by whispering to the client while turning head away. NOTE: Be sure that hearing aid, if used, is in place.	3. No difficulty in hearing	3. Presence of presbycusis
MOUTH		
1. Use a penlight to inspect mouth, teeth, and gums.	1. No lesions, extensive dental caries, or gum disease	1. None
NECK		
1. Inspect for symmetry, lesions, pulsations, and JVD.	1. Symmetric, without lesions or JVD	1. None
2. Palpate the carotid pulse, one side at a time; check for bruits.	2. No bruits; pulses equal	2. None
3. Palpate the cervical lymph nodes.	3. Unable to palpate	3. None
4. Test ROM.	4. No limitations	4. Slight decreased; possible crepitus

CHEST (POSTERIOR, ANTERIOR, AND LATERAL)

1. Inspect the chest for deformity, symmetry, expansion, and lesions; note pulsations or heaves (lifts).

   1. Symmetric; without lesions; anteroposterior/lateral ratio of 1:2; no heaves
   1. Slight change in anteroposterior/lateral ratio (1:1.5)

2. Palpate any chest lesions.

   2. No lesions
   2. None

3. Locate the PMI.

   3. PMI at the left MCL, fifth ICS
   3. None

4. Palpate each vertebra of the spine.

   4. No tenderness or bony spurs
   4. Thoracic kyphosis

5. Auscultate breath sounds throughout all lung fields.

   5. Unlabored excursion of air; no adventitious sounds
   5. Shallow respirations

6. Auscultate apical rate and rhythm; auscultate heart sounds.

   6. Presence of S_1 and S_2 heart sounds
   6. Possible S_4 heart sound

ICS, intercostal space; *JVD*, jugular venous distention; *MCL*, midclavicular line; *PMI*, point of maximal impulse; *ROM*, range of motion; *TMJ*, temporomandibular joint.

Continued

GUIDE TO HEAD-TO-TOE PHYSICAL ASSESSMENT OF ADULTS—cont'd

Nursing Activity	Typical Finding	Changes Associated with Aging
UPPER EXTREMITIES		
1. Inspect and palpate joints for swelling, tenderness, and deformity.	1. No swelling, tenderness, or deformity	1. Tenderness of 1 or more joints
2. Palpate brachial and radial arteries; assess for pulse deficit.	2. Pulses equal and within normal limits	2. None
3. Test ROM in all joints and sensation.	3. No restriction	3. Slight decrease in ROM; possible crepitus
4. Test muscle strength of arms, hands, and shoulders.	4. 5/5 movement against resistance	4. Slight decrease (4+/5 or 4/5)
5. Palpate axillary nodes.	5. Nodes not palpable	5. None
ABDOMEN		
1. Inspect for contour, symmetry, lesions, and pulsations.	1. Symmetric; without lesions or pulsations	1. None
2. Auscultate bowel sounds in all 4 quadrants.	2. 5–15 sounds/min in each quadrant	2. May be slightly decreased [hypoactive]
3. Auscultate over abdominal aorta for bruit.	3. No bruit	3. None
4. Palpate for liver enlargement.	4. Liver not below costal margin	4. None

LOWER EXTREMITIES

1. Inspect and palpate for swelling, tenderness, and deformity.
2. Test ROM and sensation.

3. Test muscle strength.

4. Palpate femoral, popliteal, and pedal pulses.
5. Palpate inguinal nodes.

1. No swelling, tenderness, or deformity
2. No limitation

3. 5/5 movement against resistance fifth ICS
4. Pulses equal and within normal range
5. Nodes not palpable

1. Tenderness of 1 or more joints
2. Slight decrease in ROM; possible crepitus
3. Slight decrease (4+/5 or 4/5)

4. Pedal pulses may be weak or not palpable
5. None

GENITALIA

1. Inspect external genitalia for lesions or drainage.

1. No lesions or drainage

1. None

ICS, intercostal space; *JVD,* jugular venous distention; *MCL,* midclavicular line; *PMI,* point of maximal impulse; *ROM,* range of motion; *TMJ,* temporomandibular joint.

Laboratory Values

Terminology Associated with Fluid and Electrolyte Balance

active transport Assisted movement of a substance through a permeable membrane between two fluid compartments; occurs against a concentration, electrical, or pressure gradient; requires the expenditure of chemical energy

adenosine triphosphate (ATP) A substance that is generated by the metabolism of glucose or fat within cells and releases chemical energy for physiologic function when a high-energy phosphate bond ($\sim$P) is broken

aldosterone A hormone secreted by the adrenal cortex that stimulates the renal reabsorption of sodium and water and the renal excretion of potassium

anion A molecule (electrolyte) that carries an overall negative charge when dissolved in water

antidiuretic hormone (ADH) A hormone secreted from the posterior pituitary gland that increases the renal reabsorption of pure water and decreases urine output

atrial natriuretic peptide (ANP) A hormone secreted by cardiac atrial cells that increases the renal excretion of sodium and water

brownian motion Inherent molecular motion

capillary (plasma) hydrostatic pressure The force generated by fluid within a capillary that tends to move fluid out from the capillary and into the interstitial space

capillary (plasma) osmotic pressure The force generated by the concentration of plasma solutes (osmotic and oncotic pressures) that tends to retain fluid within the capillary or move fluid from the interstitial space into the capillary

cation A molecule (electrolyte) that carries an overall positive charge when dissolved in water

cofactor A substance required to enhance the activity of an enzyme or a physiologic reaction

colloidal oncotic pressure The osmotic pressure exerted by the concentration of colloids (proteins) within a solution

diffusion Unimpeded movement of a substance through a permeable membrane between two fluid compartments; occurs down a concentration gradient; does not require the expenditure of chemical energy

disequilibrium A state in which two fluid compartments are unequal in at least one characteristic

electrolytes Substances that carry an electrical charge when dissolved in water

electroneutrality A state in which a body fluid has an equal number of cations and anions so that the fluid does not express an electrical charge

equilibrium A state in which two fluid compartments are equal in one or more characteristics

extracellular fluid (ECF) Body fluid present outside of cells: includes plasma, interstitial fluid, and transcellular fluid

facilitated diffusion Assisted movement of a substance through a permeable membrane between two fluid compartments; occurs down a concentration gradient; does not require the expenditure of chemical energy

filtration The movement of fluid through a biologic membrane as a result of hydrostatic pressure differences on the two sides of the membrane

gradient A graded difference in some characteristic between two fluid compartments

hydrostatic pressure The force of pressure exerted by static water in a confined space—"water-pushing" pressure

hypertonic (hyperosmotic) Any solution with a solute concentration (osmolarity) greater than that of normal body fluids (>310 mOsm/L)

hypotonic (hyposmotic) Any solution with a solute concentration (osmolarity) less than that of normal body fluids (<270 mOsm/L)

impermeable membrane A membrane separating two fluid compartments that does not permit the movement of one or more substances through the membrane (by diffusion) from one compartment to the other

insensible fluid loss Unregulated fluid losses from the skin, gastrointestinal tract, wounds, and pulmonary epithelium

interstitial fluid Fluid present in tissues between cells

intracellular fluid (ICF) Fluid found inside cells

isotonic (isosmotic) Any solution with a solute concentration equal to the osmolarity of normal body fluids or normal saline (0.9% NaCl), ~300 mOsm/L

obligatory urine output The minimal amount of urine output necessary to ensure the excretion of metabolic wastes (~400 mL/day)

osmolality The concentration of solute within a solution as measured by the amount of solute osmoles per kilogram of solvent

osmolarity The concentration of solute within a solution as measured by the amount of solute osmoles per liter of solution

Continued

osmoreceptor Specialized sensory nerve cells in the thalamus or hypothalamus that are sensitive to changes in the osmolarity of extracellular fluid

osmosis Diffusion of water (no other substance) through a selectively permeable membrane from an area of lower osmotic pressure to an area of greater osmotic pressure

osmotic pressure The pressure exerted by a solution that contains a relatively high concentration of solute; this pressure draws water from areas or compartments with lower concentrations of solute into the areas or compartments with higher concentrations of solute—"water-pulling" pressure

permeable membrane A membrane separating two fluid compartments that permits the movement of one or more substances through the membrane (by diffusion) from one compartment to the other

solubility The degree to which any given solute completely dissolves (dissociates) in water

solute The solid particles dissolved in a solution

solvent The fluid (water) portion of a solution

tissue hydrostatic pressure (THP) The force generated by fluid within the interstitial spaces that tends to move fluid into the capillary from the interstitial space

tissue osmotic pressure (TOP) The force generated by the concentration of interstitial fluid solutes that tend to retain fluid in the interstitial space or move fluid from the capillary into the interstitial space

transcellular fluid Extracellular fluid confined to a specific area or region of the body (cerebrospinal fluid, pericardial fluid, visceral fluid, aqueous humor, peritoneal fluid, and pleural fluid)

viscosity Gumminess or thickness of the molecules in a solution, causing friction within that solution

Major Serum Electrolyte Concentrations and Functions

Electrolyte	Reference Range	International Recommended Units	Functions
Sodium (Na$^+$)	136–145 mEq/L	136–145 mmol/L	Maintenance of plasma and interstitial osmolarity Generation and transmission of action potentials Maintenance of acid-base balance Maintenance of electroneutrality
Potassium (K$^+$)	3.5–5.0 mEq/L	3.5–5.0 mmol/L	Regulation of intracellular osmolarity Maintenance of electrical membrane excitability Maintenance of plasma acid-base balance
Calcium (Ca^{2+})	9.0–10.5 mg/dL	2.25–2.75 mmol/L	Cofactor in blood-clotting cascade Excitable membrane stabilizer Adds strength/density to bones and teeth Essential element in cardiac, skeletal, and smooth muscle contraction
Chloride (Cl$^-$)	98–106 mEq/L	98–106 mmol/L	Maintenance of plasma acid-base balance Maintenance of plasma electroneutrality Formation of hydrochloric acid

Data from Pagana, K. & Pagana, T. (2002). *Mosby's manual of diagnostic and laboratory tests* (2nd ed). St. Louis: C.V. Mosby.

Continued

Major Serum Electrolyte Concentrations and Functions—cont'd

Electrolyte	Reference Range	International Recommended Units	Functions
Magnesium (Mg^{2+})	1.3–2.1 mEq/L	0.66–1.07 mmol/L	Excitable membrane stabilizer Essential element in cardiac, skeletal, and smooth muscle contraction Cofactor in blood-clotting cascade Cofactor in carbohydrate metabolism Cofactor in DNA and protein synthesis Activation of B-complex vitamins
Phosphorus (Pi)	3.0–4.5 mg/dL	0.97–1.45 mmol/L	Formation of adenosine triphosphate and other high-energy substances Cofactor in carbohydrate, protein, and lipid metabolism

Data from Pagana, K. & Pagana, T. (2002). *Mosby's manual of diagnostic and laboratory tests* (2nd ed). St. Louis: C.V. Mosby.

Normal Urine Electrolyte Values

Electrolyte/Characteristics	Normal Value*	Significance of Abnormal Value†
Calcium	2.5–7.5 mmol/day	Increased: Malignancy, thyrotoxicosis, hyperparathyroidism, osteoporosis, vitamin D intoxication Decreased: Hypoparathyroidism, rickets, kidney disease, hypothyroidism
Chloride	110–250 mEq/day 110–250 mmol/day	Increased: Increased salt intake, drug-induced diuresis, adrenocortical insufficiency Decreased: Reduced salt intake, water retention, vomiting, cerebral edema, adrenocortical hyperfunction
Magnesium	3.0–5.0 mmol/day	Increased: Alcohol intake, diuretics, corticosteroid therapy, cisplatin therapy Decreased: Dietary insufficiency

Data from Tietz, N. (Ed.). (1995). *Clinical guide to laboratory tests* (3rd ed.). Philadelphia: W.B. Saunders; and Pagana, K., & Pagana, T. (2002). *Mosby's manual of diagnostic and laboratory tests* (2nd ed.). St. Louis: C.V. Mosby.

SIADH, Syndrome of inappropriate antidiuretic hormone.

*Based on a 24-hour total volume urine sample.

†Common conditions associated with abnormal values.

Continued

Normal Urine Electrolyte Values—cont'd

Electrolyte/Characteristics	Normal Value*	Significance of Abnormal Value[†]
Phosphorus	12.9–42.0 mmol/day	Increased: Hyperparathyroidism, renal tubular damage, immobility, nonrenal acidosis Decreased: Hypoparathyroidism
Potassium	25–100 mmol/day (varies with diet)	Increased: Early starvation, hyperaldosteronism, metabolic acidosis Decreased: Addison's disease, renal disease
Sodium	40–220 mEq/day 40–220 mmol/day	Increased: Increased dietary intake, adrenal failure, diuretic therapy Decreased: Low sodium intake, sodium and water retention, adrenocortical hyperfunction, excessive diaphoresis, diarrhea
Osmolarity (osmolality) random	50–1200 mOsm/kg water	Increased: Dehydration, SIADH Decreased: Diabetes insipidus, primary polydipsia
Specific gravity	1.015–1.025	Increased: Dehydration, SIADH, diabetes mellitus, toxemia of pregnancy Decreased: Chronic renal insufficiency, diabetes insipidus, lithium toxicity, early renal disease

Data from Tietz, N. (Ed.). (1995). *Clinical guide to laboratory tests* (3rd ed.). Philadelphia: W.B. Saunders; and Pagana, K., & Pagana, T. (2002). *Mosby's manual of diagnostic and laboratory Tests* (2nd ed.). St. Louis: C.V. Mosby.
SIADH, Syndrome of inappropriate antidiuretic hormone.
*Based on a 24-hour total volume urine sample.
[†]Common conditions associated with abnormal values.

Interventions for Common Environmental Emergencies

	Clinical Manifestations	Collaborative Management
HEAT-RELATED ILLNESS		

Heat exhaustion	Client complains of flu-like symptoms
	  Headache
	  Fatigue
	  Anorexia
	  Nausea
	  Vomiting
	  Hypotension
	  Tachycardia
	May have normal temperature
		Home care
		  Move to cool environment
		  Remove constrictive clothing
		  Provide an oral rehydrating solution such as a sports drink or intravenous fluids (9% saline solution)
		  Place cool/cold packs on neck, chest, abdomen and groin
		  Soak in cool water
		  Fan while spraying water on the skin
		Hospital care (if necessary)
		  Monitor vital signs
		  Rehydrate with oral or IV fluids

Heat stroke: elevated temperature (>105° F or 40.5° C)	Hot, dry skin
	Mental status changes
	  Anxiety
	  Confusion
	  Bizarre behavior
	  Loss of coordination
	  Hallucinations
	  Agitation
	  Seizures
		Prehospital care
		  Call for emergency help
		  Rapid cooling
		  Remove clothes
		  Place ice packs on neck, axillae, chest and groin
		  Immerse in cold water
		  Wet the body with tepid water and fan rapidly to aid in cooling by evaporation

Coma
Hypotension
Tachycardia
Tachypnea

Hospital care
ABCs of airway, breathing, and circulation
    are a priority
Oxygen
Intravenous fluids with 9% saline solution
Aggressive methods to decrease
    temperature (continuously monitor
    temperature)
        Cooling blanket
        Iced lavage
        Peritoneal lavage
Monitor neurologic status
        Seizure precautions

Continued

	Clinical Manifestations	Collaborative Management
COLD-RELATED INJURIES		
Hypothermia: core body temperature below 95° F (35° C)	**Mild**	**Mild**
Mild: 32–35° C	Shivering	Shelter from cold environment
Moderate: 28–32° C	Dysarthria	Remove wet clothes and apply warm clothes or blankets, warm packs, warm room
Severe: <28° C	Muscular incoordination, impaired cognitive abilities and diuresis	Provide warm high-carbonate liquids that do not contain alcohol or caffeine
	Tachycardia	**Moderate and severe**
	Increased respiratory rate	Hospital care required
	Moderate	Do *not* use external rewarming methods. This promotes "after drop," a *continued* decrease in core body temperature after the victim is removed from the cold environment. Applying external heat may produce peripheral vasodilation, which stimulates return of cold blood from periphery to warmer core.
	Obvious motor impairment such as stumbling, falling	
	Weakness	
	Confusion, apathy	
	Irrational, incoherent	
	Stupor and coma	
	Shivering stops	
	Client may perceive warmth and undress	Standard resuscitation measure, if needed
	Bradycardia and hypotension	Handle gently to prevent ventricular defibrillation
	Decreased respiratory rate and cardiac output	Place client in horizontal position
	Dysrhythmias	Core rewarming methods include administration of warm IV fluids, heated oxygen, or inspired gas
	Coagulopathy	
	Thrombocytopenia	

Severe	Absent neurologic reflexes; no response to pain Hypotension Acid-base abnormalities Ventricular fibrillation, asystole Coagulopathy Thrombocytopenia	Extracorporeal rewarming methods used for severe hypothermia such as cardiopulmonary bypass, hemodialysis, or continuous arteriovenous rewarming Administer medications cautiously: Metabolism is unpredictable and can accumulate without obvious therapeutic effect while client is cold, but will become active and may lead to drug toxicity as effective rewarming is under way.

Frostbite	Frostnip
	  Pain, numbness, pallor of affected area (white or waxy appearance)
	First-degree frostbite
	  Hyperemia and edema
	Second-degree frostbite
	  Large, fluid-filled blisters with partial thickness skin necrosis
	Third-degree frostbite
	  Small blisters that contain dark fluid
	  Affected area cool, numb, blue or red that does not blanch
	  Full thickness and subcutaneous necrosis
		Frostnip
		  Use body heat to warm affected area. For example, place warm hands over cold ears or cold hands under axillary region
		Frostbite
		  Hospital care required
		  Rapid rewarming in a water bath at temperature of 38° C–41° C
		  Premedicate for pain before rewarming
		  Do *not* apply dry heat or rub affected area
		  After rewarming, elevate an involved extremity above the heart to decrease tissue edema
		  Administer tetanus prophylaxis, if needed

Continued

	Clinical Manifestations	Collaborative Management
COLD-RELATED INJURIES—cont'd		
Frostbite—cont'd	Fourth-degree frostbite No blisters or edema Affected area is numb, cold, and bloodless Full-thickness necrosis extends into muscle and bone	Surgical management for deep wounds Amputation may be necessary
SNAKE BITES		
North American pit viper Rattlesnake Copperhead Water moccasin (cottonmouth)	One or more puncture wounds Severe pain Swelling Redness or ecchymosis Later: vesicles or hemorrhagic bullae Minty, rubbery, or metallic taste in mouth Tingling or paresthesias of scalp, face, and lips Muscle fasciculations and weakness Nausea, vomiting Hypotension Seizures Coagulopathy Disseminated intravascular coagulation	Prehospital care Move client to safe location Encourage client to rest to decrease venom circulation Remove constrictive clothing and jewelry If extremity is affected, immobilize and keep below level of heart Keep client warm Provide reassurance If hospital care and definitive treatment will be delayed, a constricting band may be applied proximal to an extremity wound to impede venom circulation via lymphatic flow but *not* tight enough to impair venous drainage or arterial flow. Loosen band if it becomes too tight due to edema

Hospital care
  ABCs of airway, breathing, and circulation
  Assess distal circulation frequently
  Insert two large-bore IV catheters and begin
    fluids
  Continuous cardiac and blood pressure
    monitoring
  Pain management
  Tetanus prophylaxis
  Broad-spectrum antibiotic to reduce risk of
    wound infection
  Laboratory studies
    CBC, electrolytes
    Coagulation studies
    Creatinine kinase
    Type and crossmatch
    Urinalysis
  Electrocardiogram
  Measure and record circumference of bite
    site every 15–30 minutes if possible
  Monitor for bleeding due to potential of
    coagulopathy
  Contact the poison control center
  Administer antivenom if ordered and monitor
    for adverse reactions and anaphylaxis

Continued

	Clinical Manifestations	Collaborative Management
SNAKE BITES—cont'd		

Coral snake	Pain may be only mild and transient
	Fang marks difficult to visualize
	Coagulopathy does not occur
	Toxic effect may be delayed
	  12–13 hours
	Nausea, vomiting
	Headache
	Pallor
	Abdominal pain
	Neurologic manifestations
	  Paresthesias
	  Numbness
	  Mental status changes
	  Cranial and peripheral nerve
	    involvement
	Later may see total flaccid paralysis
	Difficulty speaking, swallowing,
	  and breathing
	Cardiovascular collapse
		Continuous cardiac, blood pressure, and pulse
		  oximetry monitoring
		Aggressive airway management
		Monitor and initiate interventions to prevent
		  aspiration
		Contact the poison control center
		Administer antivenom if ordered and monitor
		  for side effects

ARTHROPOD (spider) BITES

Brown recluse spider

Bite is painless, stinging, sharp, or painful
Intense local aching and pruritus
Central bite site appears as a bleb or vesicle surrounded by edema and erythema, which may expand
Over 1–3 days, central lesion becomes dark and necrotic; eschar forms. When the eschar sloughs, an open would or ulcer can remain for weeks to months
Surgical intervention may be needed
Systemic toxicity manifested by
Fever, chills
Nausea and vomiting
Malaise, joint pain
Petechiae
Hemolytic reactions, renal failure, and death may occur

Home care
Cold compresses—never use heat
Rest, elevate an extremity if affected
Hospital care
Wound care includes antibiotics, antiseptic cream, and a sterile dressing to cover the bite area
Surgical evaluation to determine the need for debridement and skin grafting

Continued

Clinical Manifestations	Collaborative Management

ARTHROPOD (spider) BITES—cont'd

Clinical Manifestations	Collaborative Management
Black widow spider	Home care
Little to severe pain	Apply ice pack
Tiny papule or small red punctuate mark	Hospital care
Systemic signs and symptoms	ABCs of airway, breathing, and circulation
Severe abdominal pain	Pain medication
Muscle rigidity/spasm	Muscle relaxants
Hypertension	Calcium gluconate may be used for muscle spasms, rigidity, and pain
Nausea and vomiting	Institute seizure precautions
Facial edema	Medications include
Ptosis	Tetanus prophylaxis
Diaphoresis	Antihypertensive agents
Weakness	Monitor for pulmonary edema and shock
Increased salivation	Hospital admission is recommended for pregnant women and clients with hypertension
Priapism	
Respiratory difficulty	
Increased respiratory secretions	
Fasciculations	
Paresthesias	

Tarantula	Pain at bite site	Supportive management
	Swelling	Analgesics
	Redness	Elevate and immobilize an extremity if affected
	Numbness	
	Lymphangitis	
Scorpions	Pain and inflammation	Analgesics, supportive management
	Mild systemic symptoms	Basic wound care
Bark scorpion	Severe pain	Vital signs
	Systemic manifestations	Continuous cardiac monitoring
	Respiratory failure	Monitor for respiratory failure
	Pancreatitis	IV fluids
	Musculoskeletal dysfunction	Analgesics
	Cranial nerve dysfunction	Tetanus prophylaxis
		Atropine is used if hypersalivation occurs
		Antivenom if ordered

Continued

Interventions for Common Environmental Emergencies   **719**

	Clinical Manifestations	Collaborative Management
LIGHTNING INJURIES		

	Cardiovascular
	  Asystole or ventricular fibrillation
	  Mottled skin
	  Absent peripheral pulses
	Respiratory
	  Arrest, hypoxia
	Central nervous system
	  Temporary paralysis lasting from
	    minutes to hours
	  Loss of consciousness
	  Amnesia
	  Confusion, disorientation
	  Photophobia
	  Seizures
	  Hemorrhage
	  Cerebellar dysfunction
	  Spinal cord injury
	Integumentary
	  Burns (superficial to full thickness)
		ABCs of airway, breathing, and circulation
		Follow advanced life support guidelines
		Cardiac monitoring
		Immobilize for spinal cord injury
		Vital signs
		Burn care if needed
		Laboratory studies such as creatinine kinase
		Tetanus prophylaxis if needed
		Monitor for rhabdomyolysis and kidney failure

ALTITUDE–RELATED ILLNESSES

High altitude is an elevation above 5000 feet

Acute mountain sickness (AMS)	Throbbing headache
	Anorexia
	Nausea and vomiting
	Irritability, apathy
	Variable vital signs
	Dyspnea on exertion, at rest
		Rest, allow time to acclimate to altitude
		Remove to lower altitude
		Administer oxygen if available
		Medications
		  Acetazolamide (Diamox) to prevent and treat AMS
		  Dexamethasone (Decadron) may be given while client moves to lower altitude

High altitude cerebral edema (HACE)	Unable to perform activities of daily living
	Extreme apathy
	Confusion, lack of judgment
	Cranial nerve dysfunction
	Seizures
	Stupor, coma, death
		Rapid descent to lower altitude
		Supplemental oxygen
		Keep client warm
		Medications if available during descent
		  Dexamethasone
		  Loop diuretics
		Hospital care required
		ABCs of airway, breathing, and circulation
		Symptom management

Continued

Clinical Manifestations	Collaborative Management
ALTITUDE-RELATED ILLNESSES—cont'd	
High altitude pulmonary edema (HAPE)	Poor exercise tolerance Dyspnea on exertion Dry cough Cyanosis of nails and lips Tachycardia, tachypnea Rales, pink frothy sputum	As above

Chemical and Biological Agents of Terrorism

The Centers for Disease Control and Prevention list the following indications of intentional release of a biologic agents:

1. An unusual clustering of illness (e.g., persons who attended the same public event or gathering) or patients presenting with clinical signs and symptoms that suggest an infectious disease outbreak
2. An unusual age distribution for common diseases (e.g., an increase in what appears to be a chickenpox-like illness among adult patients, but which might be smallpox)
3. A large number of cases of acute flaccid paralysis with prominent bulbar palsies, suggestive of a release of *Botulinum* toxin

Information for this Appendix is taken from the Centers for Disease Control and Prevention website *www.bt.cdc.gov/*.

Chemical and Biological Agents of Terrorism

Agent	Clinical Manifestations	Mode of Transmission	Collaborative Management
Anthrax, cutaneous A bacterial infection caused by the gram-positive, rod-shaped organism, *Bacillus anthracis*, which lives as a spore in contaminated soil	Raised vesicle that may itch and resemble an insect bite; Center of the vesicle becomes hemorrhagic and sinks inward An area of necrosis and ulceration begins; the tissue around the wound swells and becomes edematous. It is distinguished from insect bites or other skin lesion in that it is painless and that eschar forms regardless of treatment	Incubation period of 3–5 days after exposure Direct contact	Treatment includes ciprofloxacin (Cipro) or doxycycline (Doryx, Vibramycin) Vaccine is not available to the general public

| Anthrax, inhalation | Prodromal stage (early) fever
Fatigue
Mild chest pain
Dry cough
No manifestations of upper respiratory infection of rhinitis, headache, watery eyes, or sore throat
Fulminant stage (late)
Sudden onset of breathlessness, progressing to severe respiratory distress
Diaphoresis
Stridor on inhalation and exhalation
Hypoxia
High fever
Mediastinitis and pleural effusion
Hypotension
Septic shock, meningitis | Incubation period of 1 day–6 weeks
Spread through direct contact
It is *not* spread by person-to-person contact | Combination therapy with ciprofloxacin, doxycycline, and amoxicillin
These same drugs are used individually in oral form for prophylaxis when people have been exposed to inhalation anthrax
Death within 24–36 hours after the onset of breathlessness, even if antibiotic is started at this stage |

Continued

Agent	Clinical Manifestations	Mode of Transmission	Collaborative Management
Botulism A muscle-paralyzing disease caused by a toxin made by a bacterium called *Clostridium botulinum*	Foodborne botulism Abdominal cramps Nausea, vomiting, diarrhea Drooping eyelids Blurred or double vision Dysphagia Dry mouth Slurred speech Descending muscle weakness Inhalation botulism includes all of the above except the GI symptoms plus dyspnea, decreasing respirations that may lead to apnea, and respiratory arrest	Incubation period is 12–72 hours Airborne or foodborne illness	Antitoxin Intravenous fluids

Chemical and Biological Agents of Terrorism—cont'd

Smallpox

An acute, contagious, and sometimes fatal disease caused by the variola virus

Initial symptoms:

Fever, malaise, vomiting

Head and body aches

Fever is usually high

Small red spots on the tongue and in the mouth

Rash that starts on the face and spreads to the arms and legs, hands, and feet

After 3 days, rash becomes raised bumps, which fill with a thick, opaque fluid and often have a depression in the center that looks like a bellybutton (This is a major distinguishing characteristic of smallpox.)

Bumps become pustules

Pustules begin to form a crust and then scab

By the end of the second week after the rash appears, most of the sores have scabbed over

Incubation period of 7–17 days

Prolonged face-to-face contact with someone who has smallpox (usually someone who already has a smallpox rash)

Direct contact with infected bodily fluids or an object such as bedding or clothing that has the virus on it

Exposure to an aerosol release of smallpox

The person is contagious to others until all of the scabs have fallen off

No proven treatment

Intravenous fluids

Medication to control fever or pain, and antibiotics for any secondary bacterial infections that may occur

Smallpox vaccination is not available to the general public

Continued

Chemical and Biological Agents of Terrorism—cont'd

Agent	Clinical Manifestations	Mode of Transmission	Collaborative Management
Plague A disease caused by *Yersinia pestis* (*Y. pestis*), a bacterium found in rodents and their fleas	Fever, weakness Rapidly developing pneumonia Dyspnea chest pain Cough, bloody or watery sputum Nausea, vomiting, and abdominal pain May lead to respiratory failure, shock, and rapid death	Incubation period 2–4 days Respiratory droplets Intentional aerosol release	Tetracycline (e.g., doxycycline) Fluoroquinolone (e.g., ciprofloxacin) For injection or intravenous use, streptomycin or gentamicin antibiotics are used
Tularemia Inhalational *Francisella tularensis*	Resembles the flu Fever, fatigue Swollen glands Sore throat Pneumonia	Incubation period of 3–7 days	

| Hemorrhagic fever (Ebola, Marburg, Lassa, and Crimean-Congo hemorrhagic fever viruses) Viral illness caused by several viruses, resulting in multisystem organ failure syndrome | Specific signs and symptoms vary by the type of VHF (viral hemorrhagic fever) Marked fever, fatigue Dizziness Muscle aches Loss of strength Bleeding under the skin, in internal organs, or from body orifices like the mouth, eyes, or ears Signs of shock Nervous system malfunction, coma, delirium, and seizures Renal failure | Carried by rodents and mosquitoes, tics Incubation period 5–10 days May spread from one person to another, once an initial person has become infected Secondary transmission of the virus can occur directly, through close contact with infected people or their body fluids It can also occur indirectly, through contact with objects contaminated with infected body fluids | Supportive therapy There is no other treatment or established cure for VHFs Ribavirin, an antiviral drug, has been effective in treating some individuals with Lassa fever Treatment with convalescent-phase plasma has been used with success in some patients with Argentine hemorrhagic fever |

Chemical Agents

Agent	Clinical Manifestations	Mode of Transmission	Collaborative Management
Ricin A toxic protein made from castor beans. The toxin (poison) can be extracted from the beans, purified, and treated to form a powder that can be inhaled.	**Inhalation:** Respiratory distress (difficulty breathing), tightness in the chest Fever, cough, nausea Heavy sweating Pulmonary edema Hypotension and respiratory failure, leading to death **Ingestion:** Vomiting and diarrhea that may be bloody Severe dehydration may result Hypotension Hallucinations Seizures Blood in the urine **Skin and eye exposure:** Redness and pain of the skin and the eyes	Symptoms within 8 hours of inhalation	No antidote exists Supportive care Death could take place within 36–72 hours of exposure, depending on the route of exposure and the dose received. If death has not occurred in 3–5 days, the victim usually recovers

Sarin (GB) and Soman (GD) Both are human-made chemical warfare agents classified as nerve agents. They can evaporate into a vapor (gas) and spread into the environment.	Runny nose Watery eyes Small, pinpoint pupils Eye pain Blurred vision Drooling and excessive sweating Cough Chest tightness Rapid breathing Diarrhea Increased urination Confusion Drowsiness Weakness Headache Nausea, vomiting, abdominal pain Slow or fast heart rate Low or high blood pressure Loss of consciousness Convulsions Paralysis Respiratory failure possibly leading to death	Incubation is from a few minutes to several hours Clothing can give off vapors for up to 30 minutes after exposure The client can be exposed through skin or eye contact, breathing air that contains the agents; touching or drinking water, eating contaminated food, or touching contaminated clothes	Full protective gear for emergency responders and emergency department personnel Remove client's clothing Rapidly wash the client's entire body with soap and water Give antidote as ordered Provide airway, breathing, and circulatory support Supportive care based on client's signs and symptoms

Continued

Chemical Agents—cont'd

Agent	Clinical Manifestations	Mode of Transmission	Collaborative Management
Tabun Tabun is a manmade chemical warfare agent classified as a nerve agent	Same as sarin and soman	Tabun is an immediate but short-lived threat and does not last a long time in the environment Tabun is more volatile than VX, it will remain on exposed surfaces for a shorter period of time compared with VX Tabun is less volatile than sarin, it will remain on exposed surfaces for a longer period of time compared with sarin	

VX
VX is a human-made
chemical warfare
agent classified as a
nerve agent
VX is the most potent
of all nerve agents affecting
breathing function.

As above

Symptoms will appear
within a few seconds
after exposure to the
vapor form of VX, and
within a few minutes to
up to 18 hours after

form
Under average weather
conditions, VX can last
for days on objects that
it has come in contact
with. Under very cold
conditions, VX can last
for months. It
evaporates slowly and
can be a long-term
threat as well as a
short-term threat.
Surfaces contaminated
with VX should
therefore be considered
a long-term hazard

Recovery from VX exposure
is possible with treatment,
but the antidotes available
must be used quickly to be
effective

exposure to the liquid

Chemical and Biological Agents of Terrorism **733**

Discharge Planning

- Discharge planning begins on admission.
- Information to ask the client to assist with discharge planning:
  - Where do you live?
  - How will you get home?
  - Do you live in a house, apartment, condominium?
  - How many stairs must you climb to get into your house?
  - Is your bedroom, bathroom, and kitchen on the same floor or will you need to use steps?
  - Do you live alone or does someone live with you?
    - Who lives with you?
    - Will they be able to help you after your discharge?
    - Is there a neighbor or church member who can help you when you are discharged?
  - Is anyone available to help you with grocery shopping or driving to doctors' appointments?
- Collaborate with social worker, case manager or discharge planner to identify client needs related to care after hospitalization including meal preparation, dressing changes, activities of daily living, and personal hygiene.
- If equipment or supplies are needed for use at home, make sure they are ordered and delivered before the client is discharged.
- Ensure that the client and family knows how to use the specific type of supplies and equipment that are to be used at home.
- Refer to rehabilitation (physical, occupational, or speech therapy), community, and health care agencies as appropriate.
- Client may need referrals or help in planning housing, finances, insurance, legal services, funeral arrangements, and spiritual counseling.
- Support the client and family as they make discharge arrangements.

- Provide client and family education:
  - Provide information about the disease process, how to recognize complications (if appropriate), and how to manage the disease at home.
  - Medications:
    - Name of medications
    - Purpose
    - Dosage
    - Side effects
    - Interactions, if any, with foods or other drugs
    - Importance of taking medications as prescribed
- Teach the patient and family members how to perform any dressing changes, suctioning, tube feeding, or other special care that may be required at home.
- Signs and symptoms should be reported to the health care provider. Focus on information that must be reported immediately.
- Collaborate with the registered dietitian to provide dietary information.
- Stress the importance of follow-up care with the health care provider.

Electrocardiographic Complexes, Segments, and Intervals

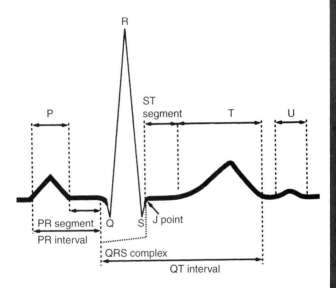

The first step in reading an electrocardiogram is to analyze the aspects of the heart rhythm.

P wave: represents atrial depolarization.

PR segment: represents the time required for the impulse to travel through the atrioventricular (AV) node (where it is delayed) and through the bundle of His, bundle branches, and Purkinje fiber network, just before ventricular depolarization.

PR interval: represents the time required for atrial depolarization and impulse travel through the conduction system and Purkinje fiber network, inclusive of the P wave and PR segment. Measured from the beginning of the P wave to the end of the PR segment. Normally measures 0.12–0.2 second.

QRS complex: represents depolarization of both ventricles and is measured from the beginning of the Q (or R) wave to the end of the S wave. Measured from the end of the PR interval to the J point. Normally measures 0.014–0.1 second.

J point: represents the junction where the QRS complex ends and the ST segment begin.

ST segment: represents early ventricular repolarization. Measured from the J point to the beginning of the T wave.

T wave: represents ventricular repolarization.

U wave: represents late ventricular repolarization. Not normally seen in all leads.

QT interval: represents the total time required for ventricular depolarization and repolarization. Measured from the beginning of the QRS complex to the end of the T wave. Normally measures 0.32–0.4 second.

Next, estimate the heart rate by counting the number of P-P or R-R intervals that occur in 6 seconds and multiply that number by 10. Finally, interpret the rhythm.

NORMAL SINUS RHYTHM

Refer to the figure on page 739. Note both atrial and ventricular rhythms are essentially regular (a slight variation in rhythm is normal). Atrial and ventricular rates are both 92/minute. One P wave occurs before each QRS complex, and all P waves are of a consistent morphology (shape). The PR interval measures 0.14 second and is constant; the QRS complex measures 0.08 second and is constant. The T waves vary in amplitude, from flat to positive, because of respirations (flat with inspiration, positive with expiration).

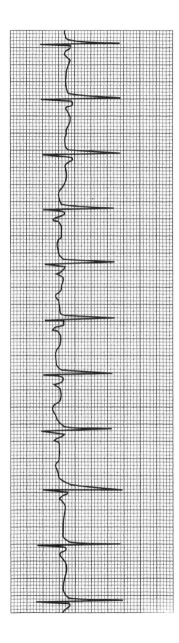

Electrocardiographic Complexes, Segments, and Intervals **739**

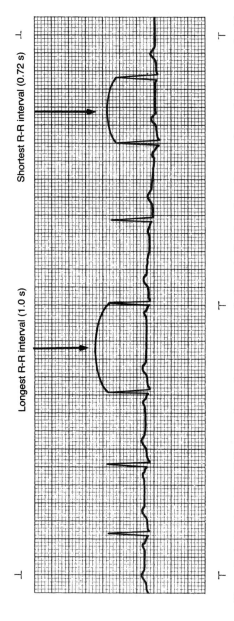

Shortest R-R interval (0.72 s)

Longest R-R interval (1.0 s)

Sinus Arrhythmia ■ All P waves have the same morphology, indicating that they are from the sinus node. The rhythm is irregular, with the shortest R-R interval (0.72 second) varying more than 0.12 second from the longest R-R interval (1 second).

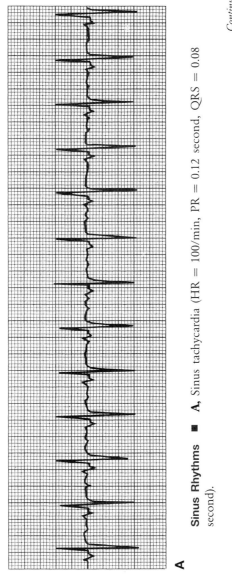

Sinus Rhythms ■ **A,** Sinus tachycardia (HR = 100/min, PR = 0.12 second, QRS = 0.08 second).

Continued

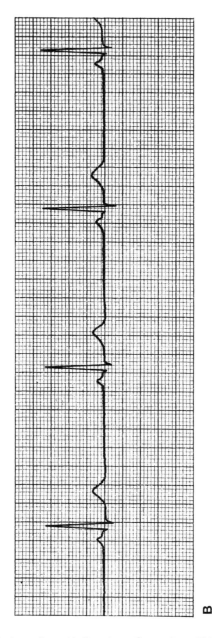

B

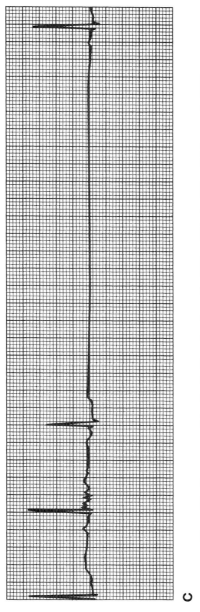

Sinus Rhythms—cont'd ■ **B,** Sinus bradycardia (HR = 35/min, PR = 0.16 second, QRS = 0.10 second). **C,** Sinus pause (underlying HR = 60/min, PR = 0.20 second, QRS 5 0.08 second, with just under a 5-second pause).

C

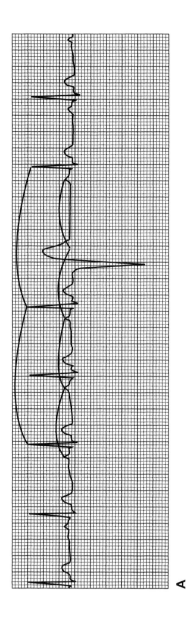

A

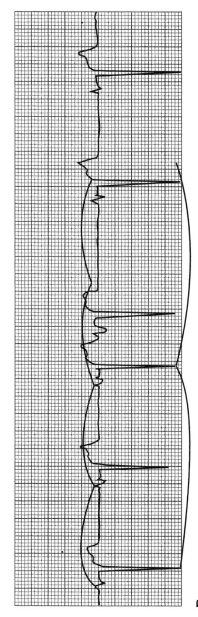

B

Normal Sinus Rhythm with a Premature Contraction ■ **A,** Normal sinus rhythm with a premature ventricular contraction (PVC). A complete compensatory pause follows the PVC, indicated by the fact that the sinus P wave following the pause comes exactly when it was due to occur. The P wave can also be determined by the R-R intervals, measuring between two complete intervals, with the R wave following the pause coming exactly when it was due to occur. **B,** Normal sinus rhythm with a premature atrial contraction (PAC). An incomplete or noncompensatory pause follows the PAC, indicated by the sinus P wave following the pause coming before it was originally due to occur. The QRS complex also comes before it would have been due.

Electrocardiographic Complexes, Segments, and Intervals   **745**

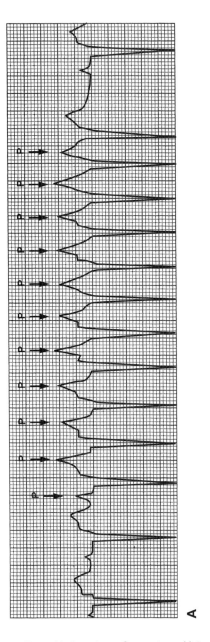

A

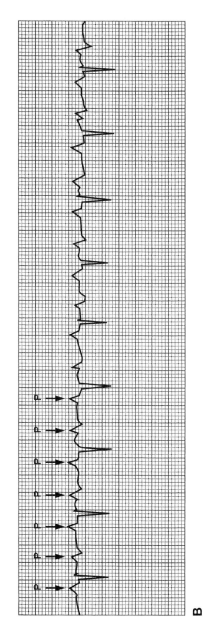

Atrial Dysrhythmias ■ **A,** Normal sinus rhythm with an 11-beat run of paroxysmal atrial tachycardia (PAT) with 1:1 conduction. **B,** Atrial tachycardia with a 2:1 block. The atrial rate is 164/min; the ventricular rate is 82/min.

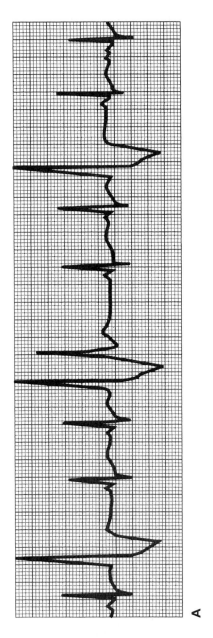

A

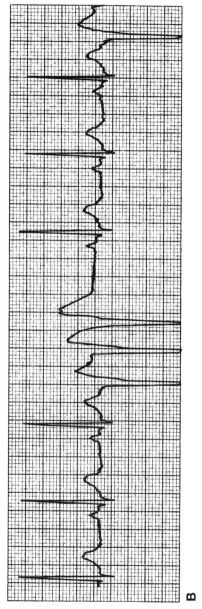

Ventricular Dysrhythmias ■ **A,** Normal sinus rhythm with unifocal premature ventricular complexes (PVCs). Note the pair of PVCs. **B,** Normal sinus rhythm with a three-beat run of ventricular tachycardia (three consecutive PVCs) and another unifocal PVC.

Continued

B

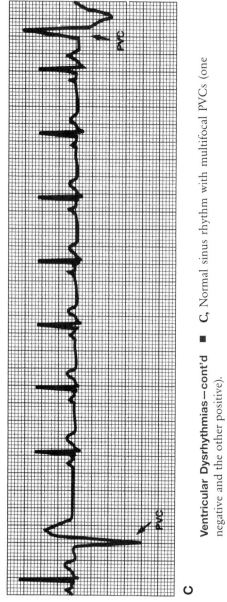

Ventricular Dysrhythmias—cont'd ■ **C,** Normal sinus rhythm with multifocal PVCs (one negative and the other positive).

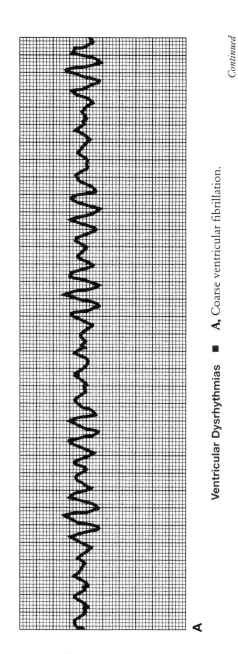

Ventricular Dysrhythmias ▪ **A,** Coarse ventricular fibrillation.

Continued

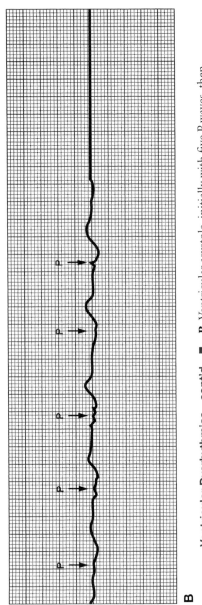

Ventricular Dysrhythmias—cont'd ■ **B,** Ventricular asystole, initially with five P waves, then no P waves (arterial and ventricular standstill).

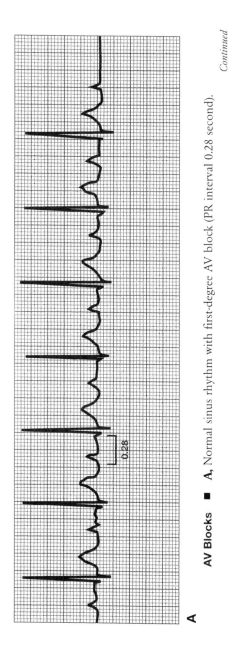

0.28

AV Blocks ■ **A,** Normal sinus rhythm with first-degree AV block (PR interval 0.28 second).

Continued

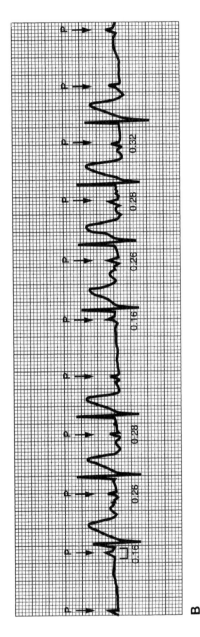

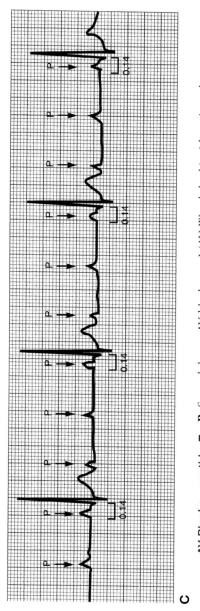

AV Blocks—cont'd ■ **B,** Second-degree AV block type I (AV Wenckebach) with an irregular rhythm, grouped beating, and progressive prolongation of the PR interval until a P wave is completely blocked and not followed by a QRS complex. **C,** Second-degree AV block type II (Mobitz II) with 3:1 conduction and a constant PR interval.

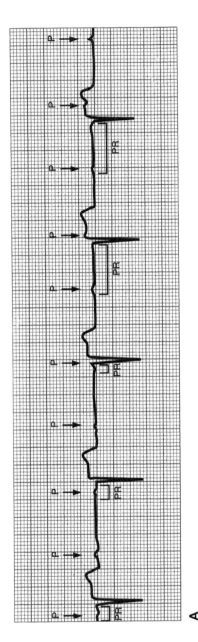

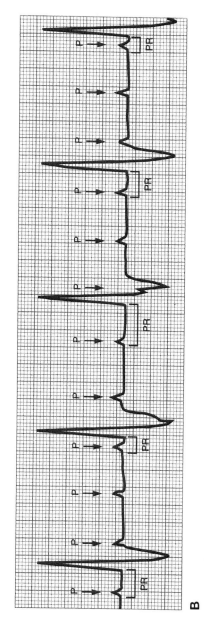

AV Blocks ■ **A,** Third-degree AV block (complete heart block) with regular atrial and ventricular rhythms, inconsistent PR intervals (AV dissociation), and a junctional escape focus (normal QRS complexes) pacing the ventricles at a rate of 38/min. **B,** Third-degree AV block with regular atrial and ventricular rhythms, inconsistent PR intervals (AV dissociation), and a ventricular escape focus pacing the ventricles at a rate of 35/min, with wide QRS complexes.

Continued

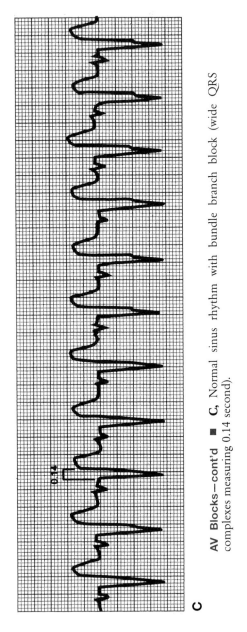

AV Blocks—cont'd ■ **C,** Normal sinus rhythm with bundle branch block (wide QRS complexes measuring 0.14 second).

0.14

C

The Client Requiring Intubation and Mechanical Ventilation

OVERVIEW

- Mechanical ventilation is usually a temporary life support technique, although it may be lifelong, especially for clients with chronic, progressive neuromuscular diseases that reduce effective ventilation.

INTUBATION

- The goals of *intubation* are to maintain a patent airway, provide a means to remove secretions, and provide ventilation and oxygen.
- Endotracheal tube (ET)
  1. Most often, the ET tube is passed through the mouth into the trachea. The nasal route is reserved for facial or oral trauma.
  2. When properly positioned the ET tube rests about 0.8 to 1.2 inches (2 to 3 cm) above the carina.
- Preparing for emergency intubation
  1. Follow institutional procedure for summoning intubation personnel to the bedside.
  2. Bring the code (or crash) care, airway equipment, and suction equipment to the bedside.
  3. Maintain a patent airway through positioning; insert an oral airway until the client is intubated.
  4. During intubation, continuously monitor for changes in vital signs, signs of hypoxia or hypoxemia, dysrhythmias, and aspiration.
  5. Ensure each intubation attempt lasts no longer than 30 seconds. After 30 seconds, provide oxygen by means of a mask and Ambu bag to prevent hypoxia and cardiac arrest.
  6. Stabilize the tube per institution policy; mark the tube where it touches the incisor tooth or naris.
  7. An oral airway may be inserted to keep the client from biting an oral tube.

- Verifying tube placement
  1. The most accurate method is to check end-tidal carbon dioxide.
  2. Assess for bilateral breath sound and chest movement and for air emerging from the ET tube.
  3. Auscultate over the stomach to rule out esophageal intubation.
  4. Continuously monitor chest wall movement and breath sounds until tube placement is verified by chest x-ray.
- Nursing care
  1. Assess tube placement, breath sounds, and chest wall movement.
  2. Prevent pulling or tugging on the tube by the client to prevent dislodgement or slipping of the tube.
     a. Sedation may be needed.
     b. As a last resort, obtain an order for soft wrist restraints per institutional policy.
  3. Check the pilot balloon to ensure that the cuff is inflated.
  4. To prevent accidental tube dislodgement or slipping:
     a. Prevent neck flexion that moves the tube away from the carina.
     b. Prevent neck extension that moves the tube closer to the carina.
     c. Minimize rotation of the head, which causes the tube to move.
     d. Suction the client's mouth as needed to prevent the tape from loosening and the tube from moving.

MECHANICAL VENTILATION

- The goals of *mechanical ventilation* are to improve oxygenation and ventilation and decrease the work needed for an effective breathing pattern.
- Positive pressure ventilators
  1. Generate pressure during inspiration that pushes air into the lungs and expands the chest. An ET tube or tracheostomy is needed.
  2. Inspiration is terminated or cycled in the following three major ways:
     a. Timed cycle ventilators push air into the lungs until a preset time has elapsed. Tidal volume and pressure vary.

b. Volume cycled ventilators push gas into the lungs until a preset volume is delivered. A constant tidal volume is delivered regardless of the pressure needed to deliver the tidal volume.

c. Microprocessor ventilators are computer-managed positive pressure ventilators used for clients with severe lung disease and those who need prolonged weaning trials.

3. Modes of ventilation

a. In assist-control (AC) ventilation, the ventilator takes over the work of breathing for the client. The tidal volume and ventilatory rate are preset. If the client does not trigger spontaneous breaths, a minimal ventilatory pattern is established.

b. Synchronized intermittent mandatory ventilation (SIMV), similar to AC ventilation, allows spontaneous breathing at the client's own rate and tidal volume between ventilator breaths.

c. Bi-level positive airway pressure (BiPAP) provides noninvasive pressure support ventilation by nasal or facemask used most often for clients with sleep apnea.

d. Other modes of ventilation include pressure support and continuous flow, maximum mandatory ventilation (MMV), inverse inspiration-expiration (I/E), ratio permissive hypercapnia, jet ventilation, and high-frequency oscillation.

4. Ventilator controls and settings

a. Tidal volume (TV) is the volume of air that the client receives with each breath. TV can be measured on either inspiration or expiration.

b. Rate or breaths per minute is the number of ventilator breaths delivered per minute.

c. Fraction of inspired oxygen (FIO_2) is the oxygen level delivered to the client. The oxygen is warmed and humidified.

d. Sighs are volumes of air that are 1.5 to 2 times the set tidal volume. Sighs are delivered 6 to 10 times per hour, but are rarely used because they can cause barotrauma.

e. Peak airway (inspiratory) pressure (PIP) indicates the pressure needed by the ventilator to deliver a set tidal volume at a given dynamic compliance. It is the highest pressure reached during inspiration.

    f. Continuous positive airway pressure (CPAP), used most often to help in the weaning process, applies positive airway pressure throughout the entire respiratory cycle for spontaneously breathing clients, keeping the alveoli open during inspiration and preventing alveolar collapse during expiration.

    g. Positive end-expiratory pressure (PEEP) is positive pressure exerted during the expiratory phase of ventilation. PEEP improves oxygenation by enhancing gas exchange and preventing atelectasis.

    h. Flow is how fast the ventilator delivers each breath. It is usually set at 40 L/min.

5. Nursing care

    a. The nursing goals are to monitor and evaluate the client's response to the ventilator, manage the ventilator system safely, and prevent complications.

    b. Explain the purpose of the ventilator and acknowledge that the client might feel some different sensations.

    c. Provide frequent, repeated explanations and reassurances.

    d. Assess vital signs and listen to breath sounds.

    e. Monitor respiratory parameters and check arterial blood gasses and other laboratory values.

    f. Assess breathing pattern in relation to the ventilatory cycle to determine whether the client is tolerating or fighting the ventilator.

    g. Assess and record equal breath sounds to ensure proper ET tube placement.

    h. To determine the need for suctioning, observe secretion type, color, and amount.

    i. Assess the area around the ET tube or tracheostomy site every 4 hours for color, tenderness, skin irritation, and drainage.

    j. Position the ventilator tubing in such a way that the client can move without pulling on the ET or tracheostomy tube.

    k. Pace activities so that oxygenations and ventilation are adequate.

l. Provide for the psychological needs of the client and family.

m. Plan methods of communication to meet the client's needs.

n. Try to anticipate the client's needs and provide access to frequently used belongings.

o. Keep the call light within easy reach of the client.

p. Perform and document ventilator checks according to institution policy.

q. Respond to alarms promptly; ensure they are activated and functional at all times.

    (1) Increased PIP means increased airway resistance in the client or the ventilator tube (bronchospasm, pinched tubing), increased amount of secretions, pulmonary edema, or decreased pulmonary compliance.

    (2) Monitor the client for agitation, restlessness, and other signs of air hunger, which may indicate that the flow rate is set too low.

    (3) Low exhaled volume alarm sounds when there is a disconnection or leak in the ventilator circuit or a leak in the client's artificial airway cuff.

r. Indications that the client needs suctioning include

    (1) Presence of secretions

    (2) Increased PIP

    (3) Presence of rhonchi (wheezes)

    (4) Decreased breath sounds

s. Document the client's response to mechanical ventilation and the ventilator setting according to institution policy.

6. Most complications are due to positive pressure from the ventilator and include

a. Cardiac problems such as hypotension and fluid retention

b. Lung complications such as barotraumas, volutrauma, and acid-base imbalance

c. Stress ulcers

d. Malnutrition

e. Infection

f. Aspiration

g. Muscular complications from immobility

h. Ventilator dependence

7. Extubation (removal of the ET tube)
   a. Explain the procedure to the client.
   b. Set up the prescribed oxygen delivery system.
   c. Have equipment ready if reintubation is necessary.
   d. Ensure that the balloon is completely deflated.
   e. Suction the client when the ET tube is removed.
   f. Monitor vital signs including pulse oximetry every 2 hours and assess ventilatory pattern.
   g. Encourage the client to cough and deep breathe and use the incentive spirometer.
   h. Document the client's response after extubation.

Health Care Organizations and Resources

NURSING ORGANIZATIONS

Academy of Medical-Surgical Nurses
E. Holly Avenue, Box 56
Pitman, NJ 08071-0056
(856) 256-2323
www.medsurgnurse.org

American Academy of Ambulatory Care Nursing
E. Holly Avenue, Box 56
Pitman, NJ 08071-0056
(856) 256-2350
www.aaacn.org

American Academy of Nurse Practitioners
PO Box 12846
Austin, TX 78711
(512) 442-4262
www.aanp.org

American Association of Critical-Care Nurses
101 Columbia
Aliso Viejo, CA 92656-4109
(800) 899-2226
www.aacn.org

American Association of Diabetes Educators
100 W. Monroe, Suite 400
Chicago, IL 60603
(800) 338-3633
www.aadenet.org

American Association of Legal Nurse Consultants
4700 W. Lake Avenue
Glenview, IL 60025-1485
(877) 402-2562
www.aalnc.org

American Association of Managed Care Nurses, Inc.
4435 Waterfront Drive, Suite 101
Glen Allen, VA 23060
(804) 747-9698
www.aamcn.org

American Association of Neuroscience Nurses
4700 W. Lake Avenue
Glenview, IL 60025-1485
(888) 557-2266
www.aann.org

American Association of Nurse Anesthetists
222 South Prospect Avenue
Park Ridge, IL 60068-4001
(847) 692-7050
www.aana.com

American Association of Nurse Attorneys
7794 Grow Drive
Pensacola, FL 32514
(877) 538-2262
www.taana.org

American Association of Occupational Health Nurses, Inc.
2920 Brandywine Road, Suite 100
Atlanta, GA 30341
(770) 455-7757
www.aaohn.org

American Association of Office Nurses
109 Kinderkamack Road
Montvale, NJ 07645
(800) 457-7504
www.aaon.org

American Association of Spinal Cord Injury Nurses
75-20 Astoria Boulevard
Jackson Heights, NY 11370
(718) 803-3782
www.aascin.org

American College of Nurse-Midwives
818 Connecticut Avenue, Suite 900
Washington, DC 20006
(202) 728-9860
www.acnm.org

American College of Nurse Practitioners
1111 19th Street NW, Suite 404
Washington, DC 20036
(202) 659-2190
www.nurse.org/acnp

American Forensic Nurses
255 N El Cielo, Suite 195
Palm Springs, CA 92262
(760) 322-9925
www.amrn.com

American Holistic Nurses Association
PO Box 2130
Flagstaff, AZ 86003-2130
(800) 278-2462
www.ahna.org

American Nephrology Nurses Association
E. Holly Avenue, Box 56
Pitman, NJ 08071-0056
(888) 600-2662
www.annanurse.org

American Nurses Association
600 Maryland Avenue SW, Suite 100 W
Washington, DC 20024-2571
(800) 274-4262
www.ana.org

American Radiological Nurses Association
820 Jorie Boulevard
Oak Brook, IL 60523-2251
(630) 571-9072
www.arna.net

American Society of Ophthalmic Registered Nurses
PO Box 193030
San Francisco, CA 94119
(415) 561-8513
http://webeye.ophth.uiowa.edu/asorn

American Society of Pain Management Nurses
7794 Grow Drive
Pensacola, FL 32514
(888) 342-7766
www.aspmn.org

American Society of Perianesthesia Nurses
10 Melrose Avenue, Suite 110
Cherry Hill, NJ 08003-3696
(877) 737-9696
www.aspan.org

American Society of Plastic and Reconstructive Surgical Nurses
E. Holly Avenue, Box 56
Pitman, NJ 08071-0056
(856) 256-2340
http://asprsn.inurse.com

Association of Nurses in AIDS Care
80 S. Summit Street
500 Courtyard Square
Akron, OH 44308
(800) 260-6780
www.anacnet.org

Association of Occupational Health Professionals
11250 Roger Bacon Drive, Suite 8
Reston, VA 20190-5202
(800) 362-4347
www.podi.com/aohp

Association of Perioperative Registered Nurses (AORN)
2170 South Parker Road, Suite 300
Denver, CO 80231-5711
(800) 755-2676
www.aorn.org

Association for Professionals in Infection Control and Epidemiology, Inc.
1275 K Street NW, Suite 1000
Washington, DC 20005-4006
(202) 789-1890
www.apic.org

Association of Women's Health, Obstetric, and Neonatal Nurses
2000 L Street NW, Suite 740
Washington, DC 20036
(800) 673-8499
www.awhonn.org

Canadian Association of Critical Care Nurses
PO Box 25322
London, ON
Canada N6C 6B1
(519) 652-1989
www.caccn.ca

Case Management Society of America
8201 Cantrell, Suite 230
Little Rock, AR 72227
(501) 225-2229
www.cmsa.org

Dermatology Nurses' Association
E. Holly Avenue, Box 56
Pitman, NJ 08071-0056
(856) 256-2330
http://dna.inurse.com

Emergency Nurses Association
915 Lee Street
Des Plaines, IL 60016-6569
(800) 243-8362
www.ena.org

Home Healthcare Nurses Association
228 7th Street SE
Washington, DC 20003
(202) 546-4754
www.hhna.org

Hospice and Palliative Nurses Association
Penn Center West One, Suite 229
Pittsburgh, PA 15276
(412) 787-9301
www.hpna.org

Infusion Nurses Society
220 Norwood Park S
Norwood, MA 02062
(781) 440-9408
www.ins1.org

International Society of Caring
1770 E Lancaster Avenue, Suite 1B
Paoli, PA 19301-1575
(610) 640-5755

International Society of Nurses in Genetics
Seven Haskins Road
Hanover, NH 03755
(601) 643-5706
http://nursing.creighton.edu/isong

International Transplant Nurses Society
1739 E Carson Street, Box 351
Pittsburgh, PA 15203-1700
(412) 488-0240
www.itns.org

National Association of Clinical Nurse Specialists
3969 Green Street
Harrisburg, PA 17110
(717) 234-6799
www.nacns.org

National Association of Orthopaedic Nurses
E. Holly Avenue, Box 56
Pitman, NJ 08071-0056
(856) 256-2310
http://naon.inurse.com

National Association of School Nurses
PO Box 1300
Scarborough, ME 04070-1300
(877) 627-6476
www.nasn.org

National Black Nurses Association
8630 Fenton Street, Suite 330
Silver Spring, MD 20910-3803
(301) 589-3200
www.nbna.org

National Gerontological Nursing Association
7794 Grow Drive
Pensacola, FL 32514
(800) 723-0560
www.ngna.org

National League for Nursing
61 Broadway
New York, NY 10006
(800) 669-1656
www.nln.org

National Nursing Staff Development Organization
7794 Grow Drive
Pensacola, FL 32514
(800) 489-1995
www.nnsdo.org

National Student Nurses' Association
555 W. 57th Street, Suite 1327
New York, NY 10019
(212) 581-2211
www.nsna.org

Oncology Nursing Society
501 Holiday Drive
Pittsburgh, PA 15220-2749
(412) 921-7373
www.ons.org

Sigma Theta Tau International
550 W. North Street
Indianapolis, IN 46202
(888) 634-7575
www.nursingsociety.org

Society of Gastroenterology Nurses and Associates, Inc.
401 N. Michigan Avenue
Chicago, IL 60611-4267
(800) 245-7462
www.sgna.org

Society of Otorhinolaryngology and Head-Neck Nurses
116 Canal Street, Suite A
New Smyrna Beach, FL 32168
(386) 428-1695
www.sohnnurse.com

Society of Urologic Nurses and Associates
E. Holly Avenue, Box 56
Pitman, NJ 08071-0056
(888) 827-7862
http://suna.inurse.com

Society for Vascular Nursing
7794 Grow Drive
Pensacola, FL 32514
(888) 536-4786
www.svnnet.org

Wound, Ostomy and Continence Nurses Society
1550 S. Coast Highway, Suite 201
Laguna Beach, CA 92651
(888) 224-9626
www.wocn.org

COMMUNITY ORGANIZATIONS AND OTHER RESOURCES

Alternative and Complementary Therapies
American Holistic Nurses' Association
PO Box 2130
Flagstaff, AZ 86003-2130
(800) 278-2462
www.ahna.org

American Massage Therapy Association
820 Davis Street, Suite 100
Evanston, IL 60201-4444
(847) 864-0123
www.amtamassage.org

Healing Touch International, Inc.
12477 W. Cedar Drive, Suite 202
Lakewood, CO 80228
(303) 989-7982
www.healingtouch.net

HealthAtoZ.com
www.healthatoz.com/atoz/centers/alternative/altindex.html

Nurses Certification Program in Imagery
PO Box 8177
Foster City, CA 94404
(650) 570-6157
www.imageryrn.com

The Wellness Center
(704) 683-3369

Whole Nurse
www.wholenurse.com

CANCER/DEATH AND DYING

American Brain Tumor Association
2720 River Road, Suite 146
Des Plaines, IL 60018
(847) 827-9910
www.abta.org

American Cancer Society
1599 Clifton Road NE
Atlanta, GA 30329
(404) 320-3333
www.cancer.org

Breast Care Helpline
(800) 462-9273
Canadian Cancer Society, National Office
10 Alcorn Avenue, Suite 200
Toronto, ON
Canada M4V 3B1
(416) 961-7223
www.cancer.ca

Cancer Information Services Hotline
(800) 4-CANCER

Cancer411.org
12411 Ventura Boulevard
Studio City, CA 91604-2407
(877) CANCR411
www.cancer411.org

CDC Tobacco Information and Prevention Source Page
www.cdc.gov/nccdphp/osh/tobacco.htm

Funeral Consumers Alliance
PO Box 10
Hinesburg, VT 05461
(802) 482-3437
www.funerals.org

Hospice Association of America
228 Seventh Street SE
Washington, DC 20003
(202) 546-4759
www.hospice-america.org

Leukemia & Lymphoma Society
1311 Mamaroneck Avenue
White Plains, NY 10605
(914) 949-5213
www.leukemia.org

National Cancer Institute
Building 31, Room 10A31
31 Center Drive, MSC 2580
Bethesda, MD 20892-2580
(800) 422-6237
www.nci.nih.gov

National Hospice and Palliative Care Organization
1700 Diagonal Road, Suite 300
Alexandria, VA 22314
(703) 837-1500
www.nhpco.org

National Ovarian Cancer Coalition
500 NE Spanish River Boulevard, Suite 14
Boca Raton, FL 33431
(561) 393-0005
www.ovarian.org

Partnership for Caring, National Office
1620 Eye Street NW, Suite 202
Washington, DC 20007
(202) 296-8071
www.partnershipforcaring.org

QuitNet (smoking cessation)
www.quitnet.com

Susan G. Komen Breast Cancer Foundation
5005 LBJ Freeway, Suite 250
Dallas, TX 75244
(972) 855-1600
www.komen.org

Y-ME National Breast Cancer Organization
212 W. Van Buren, Suite 500
Chicago, IL 60607
(312) 986-8338
www.y-me.org

CARDIOVASCULAR AND HEMATOLOGIC PROBLEMS

American Association of Blood Banks
117 N. 19th Street, Suite 600
Arlington, VA 22209
(703) 528-8200
www.aabb.org

American Heart Association, National Center
7272 Greenville Avenue
Dallas, TX 75231
(800) AHA-USA1
www.americanheart.org

American Heart Association—Take Wellness to Heart
7272 Greenville Avenue
Dallas, TX 75231
(888) MY HEART
www.women.americanheart.org

Heart Information Network
www.heartinfo.org

Mended Hearts, Inc.
7272 Greenville Avenue
Dallas, TX 75231
(800) AHA-USA1
www.mendedhearts.org

National Hemophilia Foundation
116 W. 32nd Street, 11th Floor
New York, NY 10001
(800) 424-2634
www.hemophilia.org

Sickle Cell Disease Association of America, Inc.
200 Corporate Point, Suite 495
Culver City, CA 90230-8727
(800) 421-8453
www.sicklecelldisease.org

DIABETES MELLITUS

American Diabetes Association
1701 N. Beauregard Street
Alexandria, VA 22311
(800) 342-2383
www.diabetes.org

American Dietetic Association
216 W. Jackson Boulevard, Suite 800
Chicago, IL 60606-6995
(312) 899-0040
www.eatright.org

CDC Diabetes Home Page
www.cdc.gov/nccdphp/ddt/ddthome.htm

National Institute of Diabetes & Digestive & Kidney Diseases (NIDDK)
31 Center Drive, MSC 2560
Bethesda, MD 20892-2560
www.niddk.nih.gov

EYE AND EAR PROBLEMS

American Foundation for the Blind
11 Penn Plaza, Suite 300
New York, NY 10001
(800) 232-5463
www.afb.org

American Speech-Language-Hearing Association
10801 Rockville Pike, Department AP
Rockville, MD 20852
(800) 638-8255
www.asha.org

Deafness Research Foundation
1050 17th Street NW, Suite 701
Washington, DC 20036
www.drf.org

The Ear Foundation
1817 Patterson Street
Nashville, TN 37203
(800) 545-4327
www.theearfound.org

Eye Bank Association of America
1015 18th Street NW, Suite 1010
Washington, DC 20036
(202) 775-4999
www.restoresight.org

Self-Help for Hard of Hearing People, Inc.
7910 Woodmont Avenue, Suite 1200
Bethesda, MD 20814
(301) 657-2248
www.shhh.org

GASTROINTESTINAL PROBLEMS

American Anorexia Bulimia Association, Inc.
165 W. 46th Street, Suite 1108
New York, NY 10036
(212) 575-6200
www.aabainc.org

Crohn's and Colitis Foundation of America
386 Park Avenue S., 17th Floor
New York, NY 10016-8804
(800) 932-2423
www.ccfa.org

IMMUNOLOGIC PROBLEMS/INFECTION CONTROL AND PREVENTION

AIDS Treatment Data Network
www.aidsinfonyc.org

Allergy, Asthma & Immunology Online
http://allergy.mcg.edu

American Academy of Allergy, Asthma & Immunology
611 E. Wells Street
Milwaukee, WI 53202
(414) 272-6071
www.aaaai.org

Centers for Disease Control and Prevention
1600 Clifton Road NE
Atlanta, GA 30333
(404) 639-3311
www.cdc.gov

HIV/AIDS Surveillance Report
Centers for Disease Control and Prevention
1600 Clifton Road NE
Atlanta, GA 30333
(404) 639-3311
www.cdc.gov/hav/stats/hasrlinc.htm

Immune Deficiency Foundation
40 W. Chesapeake Avenue, Suite 308
Towson, MD 21204
(800) 296-4433
www.primaryimmune.org

Latex Allergy Home Page
http://allergy.mcg.edu/physicians/ltxhome.html

National AIDS Treatment Advocacy Project
580 Broadway, Suite 1010
New York, NY 10012
(212) 219-0106
www.natap.org

Safer Sex Institute
www.safersex.org

MUSCULOSKELETAL PROBLEMS

Arthritis Foundation
1330 W. Peachtree Street
Atlanta, GA 30309
(404) 872-7100
www.arthritis.org

Back Pain Hotline
Texas Back Institute
3801 W 15th Street
Plano, TX 75075
(800) 247-2225
www.texasback.com

**National Institute of Arthritis and Musculoskeletal
and Skin Diseases**
One AMS Circle
Bethesda, MD 20892-3675
(877) 226-2467
www.naims.nih.gov

**Osteoporosis and Related Bone Diseases–National Resource
Center**
1232 22nd Street NW
Washington, DC 20037-1292
(800) 624-BONE
www.osteo.org

Spondylitis Association of America
14827 Ventura Boulevard, Suite 22
Sherman Oaks, CA 91403
(800) 777-8189
www.spondylitis.org

NEUROLOGIC PROBLEMS AND REHABILITATION

The ALS Association
27001 Agoura Road, Suite 150
Calabasas Hills, CA 91301-5104
(800) 782-4747
www.alsa.org

Christopher Reeve Paralysis Foundation
500 Morris Avenue
Springfield, NJ 07081
(800) 225-0292
www.apacure.com

The Epilepsy Foundation
4351 Garden City Drive, Suite 406
Landover, MD 20785-7223
(800) 332-1000
www.efa.org

Epilepsy Ontario
One Promenade Circle, Suite 338
Thornhill, ON
Canada L4J 4P8
(416) 229-2291
www.epilepsyontario.org

Huntington's Disease Society of America
158 W. 29th Street, 7th floor
New York, NY 10001-5300
(800) 345-HDSA
www.hdsa.org

Michael J. Fox Foundation for Parkinson's Research
Grand Central Station
PO Box 4777
New York, NY 10163
www.michaeljfox.org

The Migraine Relief Center
www.migrainehelp.com

National Headache Foundation
428 W. St. James Place, 2nd Floor
Chicago, IL 60614-2750
(888) 643-5552
www.headaches.org

National Multiple Sclerosis Society
733 Third Avenue, 6th Floor
New York, NY 10017
(800) 344-4867
www.nmss.org

National Parkinson's Foundation, Inc.
1501 NW Ninth Avenue
Miami, FL 33136-1494
(800) 327-4545
www.parkinson.org

National Stroke Association
9707 E. Easter Lane
Englewood, CO 80112-3747
(800) 787-6537
www.stroke.org

Neurosciences on the Internet
www.neuroguide.com
Parkinson's Society of Canada
4211 Yonge Street, Suite 316
Toronto, ON
Canada M2P 2A9
www.parkinson.ca

OLDER ADULTS/GERONTOLOGY

Alzheimer's Association
919 N. Michigan Avenue, Suite 1100
Chicago, IL 60611-1676
(800) 272-3900
www.alz.org

American Association of Retired Persons
601 E. Street NW
Washington, DC 20049
(800) 424-3410
www.aarp.org

American Federation for Aging Research
1414 Avenue of the Americas, 18th Floor
New York, NY 10019
(212) 752-2327
www.afar.org

National Institute on Aging
Building 31, Room 5C27
31 Center Drive, MSC 2292
Bethesda, MD 20892
(301) 496-1752
www.nih.gov/nia/

REPRODUCTIVE HEALTH PROBLEMS

Bair PMS Home Page
www.bairpms.com

Center for Human Reproduction
www.centerforhumanreprod.com

Endometriosis Association, International Headquarters
8585 N 76th Place
Milwaukee, WI 53223
(800) 992-3636
www.endometriosisassn.org

Georgia Reproductive Specialists
www.ivf.com/endohtml.html

North American Menopause Society
PO Box 94527
Cleveland, OH 44101-4527
(440) 442-7550
www.menopause.org

Planned Parenthood Federation of America, Inc.
810 Seventh Avenue
New York, NY 10019
(212) 541-7800
www.ppfa.org

Sexual Health InfoCenter
www.sexhealth.org

RESPIRATORY PROBLEMS

American Lung Association
1740 Broadway
New York, NY 10019-4374
(212) 315-8700
www.lungusa.org

Cystic Fibrosis Foundation
6931 Arlington Road
Bethesda, MD 20814
(800) 344-4823
www.cff.org

URINARY AND RENAL PROBLEMS

American Urogynecologic Society
2025 M. Street NW, Suite 800
Washington, DC 20036
(202) 367-1167
www.augs.org

National Association for Continence
PO Box 8310
Spartanburg, SC 29305-8310
(864) 579-8310
www.nafc.org

National Kidney Foundation
30 E. 33rd Street
New York, NY 10016
(800) 622-9010
www.kidney.org

The Simon Foundation for Continence
PO Box 815
Wilmette, IL 60091
(800) 23-SIMON
www.simonfoundation.org

WOMEN'S HEALTH CONSIDERATIONS

Breast Care Helpline
(800) 462-9273

Endometriosis Association
8585 N. 76th Place
Milwaukee, WI 53223
(414) 355-2200
www.endometriosisassn.org

Estronaut: A Forum for Women's Health
www.womenshealth.org

Healthy Weight
www.healthyweight.com

National Ovarian Cancer Coalition, Inc.
500 NE Spanish River Boulevard, Suite 14
Boca Raton, FL 33431
(888) OVARIAN
www.ovarian.org

Osteoporosis and Related Bone Diseases–National Resource Center
1150 17th Street NW, Suite 500
Washington, DC 20036-4603
(800) 624-BONE

MISCELLANEOUS RESOURCES

Agency for Health Care Research and Quality (AHRQ)
2101 E. Jefferson Street, Suite 501
Rockville, MD 20852
(301) 594-1364
www.ahcpr.gov

American Academy of Dermatology
930 N. Meacham Road
PO Box 4014
Schaumburg, IL 60168-4014
(847) 330-0230
www.aad.org

American Academy of Pain Management
13947 Mono Way, Suite A
Sonora, CA 95370
(209) 533-9744
www.aapainmanage.org

American Council on Alcoholism
3900 North Fairfax Drive, Suite 401
Arlington, VA 22203
(703) 248-9005
www.aca-usa.org

American Hospital Association
One N. Franklin
Chicago, IL 60606-3421
(312) 422-3000
www.aha.org

American Red Cross
430 17th Street
Washington, DC 20006
(202) 737-8300
www.redcross.org

American Thyroid Association, Inc.
PO Box 1836
Falls Church, VA 22041-1836
Fax (703) 998-8893
www.thyroid.org

Lupus Foundation of America, Inc.
1300 Piccard Drive, Suite 200
Rockville, MD 20850-4303
(800) 558-0121
www.lupus.org

MedicAlert Foundation
2323 Colorado Avenue
Turlock, CA 95382
(800) 633-4298
www.medicalert.org

Medicare
(800) 633-4227
www.medicare.gov

National Graves' Disease Foundation
PO Box 1969
Brevard, NC 28712
(828) 877-5251
www.ngdf.org

National Institutes of Health (NIH)
Bethesda, MD 20892
www.nih.gov

National Institute of Nursing Research (NINR)
Bethesda, MD 20892-2178
(301) 496-0207
www.nih.gov/ninr

National Psoriasis Foundation
6600 SW 92nd Avenue, Suite 300
Portland, OR 97223-7195
(800) 723-9166
www.psoriasis.org

Transplant Recipients of America
1000 16th Street NW, Suite 602
Washington, DC 20036-5705
(800) 874-6386

United Network for Organ Sharing
1100 Boulders Parkway, Suite 500
PO Box 13770
Richmond, VA 23225-8770
(804) 330-8576
www.unos.org

US Department of Health and Human Services (DHHS)
200 Independence Avenue SW
Washington, DC 20201
(877) 696-6775
www.hhs.gov

U.S. Food and Drug Administration (FDA)
5600 Fishers Lane
Rockville, MD 20857-0001
(888) 463-6332
www.fda.gov

World Health Organization, Regional Office
525 23rd Street NW
Washington, DC 20037
(202) 974-3000
www.who.org

Communication Quick Reference for Spanish-Speaking Clients

The Body • El Cuerpo (ehl KWEHR-poh)

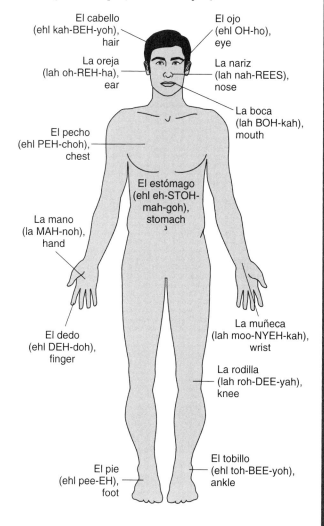

El cabello
(ehl kah-BEH-yoh),
hair

El ojo
(ehl OH-ho),
eye

La oreja
(lah oh-REH-ha),
ear

La nariz
(lah nah-REES),
nose

La boca
(lah BOH-kah),
mouth

El pecho
(ehl PEH-choh),
chest

El estómago
(ehl eh-STOH-mah-goh),
stomach

La mano
(la MAH-noh),
hand

La muñeca
(lah moo-NYEH-kah),
wrist

El dedo
(ehl DEH-doh),
finger

La rodilla
(lah roh-DEE-yah),
knee

El pie
(ehl pee-EH),
foot

El tobillo
(ehl toh-BEE-yoh),
ankle

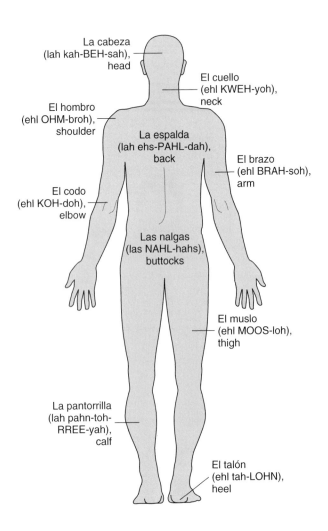

La cabeza
(lah kah-BEH-sah),
head

El cuello
(ehl KWEH-yoh),
neck

El hombro
(ehl OHM-broh),
shoulder

La espalda
(lah ehs-PAHL-dah),
back

El brazo
(ehl BRAH-soh),
arm

El codo
(ehl KOH-doh),
elbow

Las nalgas
(las NAHL-hahs),
buttocks

El muslo
(ehl MOOS-loh),
thigh

La pantorrilla
(lah pahn-toh-
RREE-yah),
calf

El talón
(ehl tah-LOHN),
heel

COMMON INSTRUCTIONS TO BE USED WITH BODY PARTS

Move the, Mueva *(moob-EH-bab)*
Touch the, Toque *(TOH-keb)*
Point to the, Señale *(seb-NYAH-leb)*

MORE PARTS OF THE BODY

Armpit, la axila *(lah ahk-SEE-lah)*
Breasts, los senos *(lohs SEH-nohs)*
Collarbone, la clavícula *(lah klah-BEE-koo-lah)*
Diaphragm, el diafragma *(ehl dee-ah-FRAH-mah)*
Forearm, el antebrazo *(ehl ahn-teh-BRAH-soh)*
Groin, la ingle *(lah EEN-gleh)*
Hip, la cadera *(lah kah-DEH-rah)*
Kneecap, la rótula *(lah ROH-too-lah)*
Nail, la uña *(lah OON-yah)*
Pelvis, la pelvis *(lah PEHL-beece)*
Rectum, el recto *(ehl REHK-toh)*
Rib, la costilla *(lah koh-STEE-yah)*
Spine, el espinazo *(ehl ehs-pee-NAH-soh)*
Throat, la garganta *(lah gahr-GAHN-tah)*
Tongue, le lengua *(lah LEHN-gwah)*

ORGANS

Appendix, el apéndice *(ehl ah-PEHN-dee-seh)*
Bladder, la vejiga *(lah beh-HEE-gah)*
Brain, el cerebro *(ehl seh-REH-broh)*
Colon, el colon *(ehl KOH-lohn)*
Esophagus, el esófago *(ehl eh-SOH-fah-goh)*
Gallbladder, la vesícula biliar *(lah beh-SEE-koo-lah bee-lee-AHR)*
Genitals, los genitales *(lohs heh-nee-TAH-lehs)*
Heart, el corazón *(ehl koh-rah-SOHN)*
Kidney, el riñón *(ehl ree-NYOHN)*
Large intestine, el intestino grueso *(ehl een-tehs-TEE-noh groo-EH-so)*
Liver, el hígado *(ehl EE-gah-doh)*
Lungs, los pulmones *(lohs pool-MOH-nehs)*
Pancreas, el páncreas *(ehl PAHN-kreh-ahs)*
Small intestine, el intestino delgado *(ehl een-tehs-TEE-noh dehl-GAH-doh)*
Spleen, el bazo *(ehl BAH-soh)*
Thyroid gland, la tiroides *(lah tee-ROH-ee-dehs)*
Tonsils, las amígdalas *(lahs ah-MEEG-dah-lahs)*
Uterus, el útero *(ehl OO-teh-roh)*

Good ... morning.	Buenos(as) ... días.	BWEH-nohs (nahs) ... DEE-ahs.
afternoon.	tardes.	TAHR-dehs.
night.	noches.	NOH-chehs.
Hello.	Hola.	OH-lah.
How are you?	¿Cómo está?	¿Koh-moh ehs-TAH?
Good (Fine)	Bien	Byehn.
Bad, Better, Worse.	Mal, Mejor, Peor.	Mahl, Meh-HOHR, Peh-OHR.
The same.	Igual.	Ee-GWAHL.
Do you speak English?	¿Habla inglés?	¿Ah-blah een-GLEHS?
I don't understand.	No comprendo.	Noh kom-PREHN-doh.
Excuse me.	Discúlpeme.	Dees-KOOL-peh-meh.
Please speak slowly.	Por favor, hable más lento.	Pohr fah-VOHR, AH-bleh MAHS LEHN-toh.
Are you in pain?	¿Está adolorido(a)?	¿Ehs-TAH ah-doh-loh-REE-doh(dah)?
Yes, No.	Sí, No.	SEE, Noh.
Tell me where it hurts.	Dígame donde le duele.	DEE-gah-meh DOHN-deh leh DWEH-leh.
Here, There.	Aquí, Ahi.	Ah-KEE, Ah-EE.

Is your pain ... burning?	Tiene un dolor ... ¿quemante?	Tee-EH-neh oon doh-LOHR ...¿keh-MANH-teh?
constant?	¿constante?	¿kohn-STAHN-teh?
dull?	¿sordo?	¿SOHR-doh?
intermittent?	¿intermitente?	¿een-tehr-mee-TEHN-teh?
mild?	¿moderado?	¿moh-deh-RAH-doh?
severe?	¿muy fuerte?	¿MOO-ee FWEHR-teh?
Is your pain ... sharp?	Tiene un dolor ... ¿agudo?	Tee-EH-neh oon doh-LOHR ... ¿ah-GOO-doh?
throbbing?	¿pulsante?	¿pool-SAHN-teh?
worse?	¿peor?	¿peh-OHR?

Are you allergic to any medication?	¿Es usted alérgico(a) a alguna medicación?	¿Ehs oos-TEHD ah-LEHR-hee-koh(kah) ah ahl-GOO-nah meh-dee-kah-SYOHN?
I'm here to help you.	Estoy aquí para ayudarle.	Ehs-TOY ah-KEE pah-rah ah-yoo-DAHR-leh.
Calm down.	Cálmese.	KAHL-meh-seh.
Please.	Por favor.	Pohr fah-VOHR.
Thank you.	Gracias.	GRAH-syahs.
You're welcome.	De nada.	Deh NAH-dah.
May I?	¿Puedo?	¿PWEH-doh?
Who, What, When, Where?	¿Quién, Qué, Cuándo, Dónde?	¿Kyehn, Keh, KWAHN-doh, DOHN-deh?
Zero, One, Two, Three, Four	Cero, Uno, Dos, Tres, Cuatro	SEH-roh, OO-noh, dohs, trehs, KWAH-troh
Five, Six, Seven, Eight, Nine, Ten	Cinco, Seis, Siete, Ocho, Nueve, Diez	SEEN-koh, sehs, SYEH-teh, OH-choh, NWEH-beh, dee-EHS

PRELIMINARY EXAMINATION

My name is— —, and I am your nurse.	Me llamo— —, y soy su enfermera(o).	Meh YAH-moh — —, ee SOY soo ehn-fehr-MEH-rah(roh).
I'm going to ... take your vital signs.	Le voy a ... tomar los signos vitales.	Leh voy ah ... toh-MAHR lohs SEEG-nohs vee-TAH-lehs.
I'm going to ... weigh you.	Le voy a ... pesarle.	Leh voy ah ... peh-SAHR-leh.
take your blood pressure.	tomar la presion.	toh-MAHR lah preh-SYOHN.
Extend your arm and relax.	Extienda su brazo y de-scánselo.	Ehks-TYEHN-dah soo BRAH-soh ee dehs-KAHN-seh-loh.
I'm going to take your ... pulse.	Le voy a tomar ... el pulso.	Leh voy ah toh-MAHR ... ehl POOL-soh.
temperature.	su temperatura.	soo tehm-peh-rah-TOO-rah.
I'm going to count your respirations.	Voy a contar sus respiraciones.	Voy ah kohn-TAHR soos rehs-pee-rah-SYOH-nehs.

Communication Quick Reference for Spanish-Speaking Clients **793**

OBTAINING A BLOOD SAMPLE

I need to draw a blood sample.	Necesito tomar una muestra de la sangre.	*Neh-seh-SEE-toh toh-MAHR OO-nah MWEHS-trah deh lah SAHN-greh.*
Please give me your arm.	Por favor, déme el brazo.	*Pohr fah-VOHR, DEH-meh ehl BRAH-soh.*
It may cause a little discomfort.	Le puede causar alguna molestia.	*Leh PWEH-deh kahw-SAHR ahl-GOO-nah moh-LEHS-tyah.*
I am going to put a tourniquet around your arm.	Le voy a poner una liga alrededor del brazo.	*Leh voy ah poh-NEHR OO-nah LEE-gah ahl-reh-deh-DOHR dehl BRAH-soh.*
I am going to draw blood from this vein.	Voy a sacar la sangre de esta vena.	*Voy ah sah-KAHR lah SAHN-greh deh EHS-tah VEH-nah.*

OBTAINING BLOOD FROM A FINGER STICK

I need to take a few drops of blood from your finger.	Necesito sacarle unas gotas de sangre de uno de sus dedos.	*Neh-seh-SEE-toh sah-KAHR-leh OO-nahs GOH-tahs deh SAHN-greh deh OO-noh deh soos DEH-dohs.*

OBTAINING A URINE SAMPLE

We also need a urine sample.	También necesitamos una muestra de la orina.	*Tahm-BYEHN neh-seh-see-TAH-mohs OO-nah MWEHS-trah deh lah oh-REE-nah.*
It has to be from the middle of the stream.	Tiene que ser de la mitad del chorro.	*TYEH-neh keh sehr deh lah mee-TAHD dehl CHOH-rroh.*
Put the urine in this cup.	Ponga la orina en este vaso.	*POHN-gah lah oh-REE-nah ehn EHS-teh VAH-soh.*

OBTAINING A STOOL SPECIMEN

I need a sample of your stool.	Necesito una muestra de su excremento.	*Neh-seh-SEE-toh OO-nah MWEHS-trah deh soo ehks-kreh-MEN-toh.*
Please put a small amount in this cup.	Por favor ponga un poco en este vaso.	*Pohr fa-VOHR POHN-gah oon POH-koh ehn EHS-teh VAH-soh.*

OBTAINING A SPUTUM SPECIMEN

I need a sample of your sputum.	Necesito una muestra de su esputo.	*Neh-seh-SEE-toh OO-nah MWEHS-trah deh soo ehs-POO-toh.*
Please spit in this cup.	Por favor, escupa en este vaso.	*Pohr fah-VOHR, ehs-KOO-pah ehn EHS-teh VAH-soh.*

ORDERS

You need ... a bandage.	Necesita ... un vendaje.	*Neh-seh-see-TAH ... oon behn-DAH-heh.*
a blood transfusion.	una transfusión de sangre.	*OO-nah trahns-foo-SEE-ohn deh SAHN-greh.*
a cast.	una armadura de yeso.	*OO-nah ahr-mah-DOO-rah deh YEH-soh.*
gauze.	la gasa.	*lah GAH-sah.*
intensive care.	el cuidado intensivo.	*ehl kwee-DAH-doh een-tehn-SEE-boh.*
intravenous fluids.	los líquidos intravenosos.	*lohs LEE-kee-dohs een-trah-beh-NOH-sohs.*
an operation.	una operación.	*OO-nah oh-peh-rah-see-OHN.*
physical therapy.	la terapia física	*lah teh-RAH-pee-ah FEE-see-kah.*
a shot.	una inyección.	*OO-nah een-yehk-see-OHN.*
x-rays.	los rayos equis.	*lohs RAH-yohs EH-kees.*

We're going to ... change the bandage.	Vamos a ... cambiarle el vendaje.	*VAH-mohs ah ... kahm-bee-AHR-leh ehl behn-DAH-heh.*
give you a bath.	darle un baño.	*DAHR-leh oon BAH-nyoh.*
take out the I.V.	sacarle el tubo intravenoso.	*sah-KAHR-leh ehl TOO-boh een-trah-beh-NOH-soh.*

DESCRIPTION OF TUBES

The tube in your ... arm is for I.V. fluids.	El tubo en su ... brazo está para los líquidos intravenosos.	*Ehl TOO-boh ehn soo ... BRAH-soh ehs-TAH PAH-rah LEE-kee-dohs een-trah-beh-NOH-sohs.*
bladder is for urinating.	vejiga es para orinar.	*beh-HEE-gah ehs PAH-rah oh-ree-NAHR.*
stomach is for the food.	estómago es para la comida.	*ehs-TOH-mah-goh ehs PAH-rah lah koh-MEE-dah.*
throat is for breathing.	garganta es para respirar.	*gahr-GAHN-tah ehs PAH-rah rehs-pee-RAHR.*

Index

Genitalia, assessment of, 699
Genitourinary system assessment
  in infection, 452
  postoperative, 28
  in renal failure
    acute, 568
    chronic, 573
GERD. See Gastroesophageal reflux
  disease.
Germinal testicular tumor, 198
Gerontology, organizations and
  resources for, 781–782. See also
  Older adults.
Gestational diabetes mellitus,
  276–277
GHB. See Gamma hydroxybutyrate
  abuse.
GI system. See Gastrointestinal
  system.
Giant cell tumor, 657
Gigantism, 408
Glaucoma, 343–344
Glioblastoma, 658
Glioma, 658
Glomerulonephritis
  acute, 345–347
  chronic, 347–348
  rapidly progressive, 349
Glucophage. See Metformin.
Glucose
  in diabetic ketoacidosis, 277
  exercise and, 284
  in hyperglycemic hyperosmolar
    nonketotic coma, 277
  self-monitoring of, 282
Glycoprotein 11a/111b inhibitors,
  250
Goiter, 437
Gold therapy for rheumatoid
  arthritis, 125
Gonorrhea, 349–350
Gout, 351–352
Gradient, defined, 703
Grading of tumor, 147
Graft
  for burn injury, 142
  coronary artery bypass
    minimally invasive direct,
      256–257
    for recurrent chest pain, 255
Grand mal seizure, 592
Granulomatous thyroiditis, subacute,
  625
Graves' disease, 415
Grieving in colorectal cancer,
  168–169

Group A beta-hemolytic
    Streptococcus
  in peritonsillar abscess, 63
  rheumatic endocarditis and, 208
Group D streptococci in prostatitis,
  554
Guillain-Barré syndrome, 352–357
Guillotine amputation, 93
Gynecomastia, 357

H

HAART. See Highly active
  antiretroviral therapy.
HACE. See High altitude cerebral
  edema.
Haemophilus ducreyi, 216
Haemophilus influenzae, 243
Hair loss. See Alopecia.
Hallucinogens abuse, 45–48
Hand fracture, 333
Handicap, defined, 33
HAPE. See High altitude pulmonary
  edema.
Hashimoto's thyroiditis, 625
HAV. See Hepatitis A virus.
hBNP. See Human B-type natriuretic
  peptides.
HbS. See Hemoglobin S.
HBV. See Hepatitis B virus.
HCM. See Hypertrophic
  cardiomyopathy.
HCV. See Hepatitis C virus.
HDV. See Hepatitis delta virus.
Head
  assessment of, 694
  trauma to, 634–641
    assessment of, 635–636
    community-based care in,
      640–641
    interventions for, 637–640
    overview of, 634–635
Head lice, 532
Headache
  cluster, 358
  migraine, 359–360
  tension, 360
Head-to-toe physical assessment of
  adults, 693–699
Health care organizations and
  resources, 765–787
  cancer/death and dying, 773–775
  cardiovascular and hematologic,
    775–776
  community, 772–773
  diabetes mellitus, 776–777
  eye and ear problems, 777

Monoclonal antibodies for bronchial asthma, 129
Morbid obesity, 489
Morphine
in care of dying client, 13, 14
for sickle cell anemia-associated pain, 103
Morphine sulfate
for chest pain, 249
for heart failure, 372
Motor function
in cancer, 148
in multiple sclerosis, 588
in Parkinson's disease, 529
in spinal cord tumors, 668
in stroke, 612
Motor neuron disease, bowel program for, 42
Mountain sickness, acute, 721
Mouth
assessment of, 696
stomatitis of, 609
MRSA. *See* Methicillin-resistant *Staphylococcus aureus.*
MS. *See* Multiple sclerosis.
MTT. *See* Myoblast transfer therapy.
Mucositis due to chemotherapy, 152
for lung cancer, 177
Mucous membrane, impaired oral
in dehydration, 272
in oropharyngeal cancer, 183–184
Multiple sclerosis, 587–590
Muscle relaxants for osteoarthritis, 498
Muscle weakness in myasthenia gravis, 482, 483
Muscular dystrophy, 303–304
Musculoskeletal system
assessment of
in hypokalemia, 427
in hypothyroidism, 438
in leukemia, 469
in preoperative nursing care, 19
in rehabilitation, 36
organizations and resources for problems with, 779–780
Myasthenia gravis, 482–487
Myasthenic crisis, 484
Mycobacterium avium-intracellulare complex infection in AIDS, 76
Mycobacterium tuberculosis
in pulmonary tuberculosis, 653
in renal tuberculosis, 656
Myelocytic leukemia, 468
Myoblast transfer therapy, 304
Myocardial hypertrophy related to heart failure, 366

Myocardial infarction, 247–258
Myoclonic seizure, 592
Myoma, uterine, 464–468
Myomectomy, 466
Myopia, 563
Myotonic muscular dystrophy, 304
Myringoplasty, 222
Myringotomy, 510
Myxedema coma, 437–438

N

Nasal cancer, 180–181
Nasal fracture, 321–322
Nasogastric intubation
in intestinal obstruction, 493
in peptic ulcer disease, 673
Nasointestinal intubation, 493
Native American population
care of dying client and, 13
diabetes mellitus in, 279
Natrecor. *See* Nesiritide.
Natriuretic peptides, human B-type, 370
Nausea
due to chemotherapy, 151
for lung cancer, 177
in intestinal obstruction, 492
Nearsightedness, 563
Neck, assessment of, 696
Necrosis
acute tubular following renal transplantation, 579
avascular as complication of fracture, 323
in peripheral arterial disease, 114
Needle bladder neck suspension, 446
Neglect, unilateral, in stroke, 616
Neisseria gonorrhoeae
in gonorrhea, 349
in pelvic inflammatory disease, 532
Neomycin sulfate, 236
Neoplasia, 146. *See also* Cancer.
cervical intraepithelial, 164
Nephrectomy before renal transplantation, 578
Nephritic syndrome
acute, 345–347
chronic, 347–348
Nephrogenic diabetes insipidus, 273
Nephrolithiasis, 678
Nephrolithotomy, 679
Nephropathy, diabetic, 278
Nephrosclerosis, 487
Nephrotic syndrome, 488
Nerve agents, 731–733

Testes—cont'd
  hydrocele of, 390–391
Testosterone for hypopituitarism, 436–437
Tetanus, 143, 622–623
Thalamotomy, unilateral, 531
Theca-lutein cyst, 266–267
Thermal injury, 137
Thiazide diuretics
  in heart failure treatment, 370
  for hypertension, 414
Thiazolidinedione antidiabetic agents, 280
Third-degree heart block, 300, 757, 758
Thoracentesis in lung cancer, 179
Thoracic aneurysm, 106–110
Thoracic outlet syndrome, 623
Thoracotomy for lung cancer, 178
Thought processes, disturbed, in HIV/AIDS, 80–81
THP. See Tissue hydrostatic pressure.
THR. See Total hip replacement.
Threshold, pain, 3
Thrombectomy, 117
Thrombocytopenic purpura, autoimmune, 624–625
Thromboembolism, venous, 685
  following total hip replacement, 500
Thrombolic ischemic stroke, 610–611
Thrombolytic agents
  for coronary artery disease, 250
  for peripheral venous disease, 686
  for pulmonary embolism, 306–307
  for stroke, 613–614
Thrombophlebitis, 685
Thrombosis, deep venous, 685–688
  as complication of fractures, 323
Thrombus, 685
Thymectomy for myasthenia gravis, 486
Thyroid cancer, 201–202
Thyroid hormone
  excessive secretion of, 415–420
  low levels of, 437–441
Thyroid storm, 416
Thyroidectomy
  for hyperthyroidism, 418
  for thyroid cancer, 201
Thyroiditis, 625
Thyrotoxicosis, 416
TIA. See Transient ischemic attack.
Tibial fracture, 333–334
Tick bite, Lyme disease transmission from, 475

Tidal volume in mechanical ventilation, 761
Time cycle ventilators, 760
Timolol
  for glaucoma, 344
  for prevention of migraine headaches, 359
Tinea infection, 457
Tinel's sign, 212
Tinnitus in Ménière's disease, 479
Tissue hydrostatic pressure, 704
Tissue integrity, impaired, perioperative, 26–27
Tissue osmotic pressure, 704
Tissue perfusion
  assessment of following amputation, 94–95
  ineffective
    in cardiac dysrhythmias, 301
    in coronary artery disease, 250–251
    in diabetes mellitus, 287
    due to burns, 138–139
    in spinal cord trauma, 647–649
    in stroke, 613–615
TJA. See Total joint arthroplasty.
TKA. See Total knee arthroplasty.
Tolerance, drug, 4
Tonic seizure, 592
Tonic-clonic seizure, 592
Tonsillectomy, 626
Tonsillitis, 626
TOP. See Tissue osmotic pressure.
Topical anesthesia, 24
Topical medications
  for burn injury, 143
  for pain management, 7
Total ankle arthroplasty, 502
Total elbow arthroplasty, 502
Total hip replacement, 499–501
Total joint arthroplasty, 499
Total knee arthroplasty, 501–502
Total shoulder arthroplasty, 502
Toxic shock syndrome, 626–627
Toxins
  cataracts due to, 214
  cirrhosis due to, 230
  hepatitis due to, 379
Toxoplasmosis in AIDS, 76
Trabeculoplasty, laser, 344
Tracheobronchial trauma, 652–653
Tracheostomy
  in burn injury treatment, 139–140
  in oropharyngeal cancer, 182
Trachoma, 627–628
Traction for treatment of fractures, 328–329